Third Edition

GERIATRIC NUTRITION

Daphne A. Roe
Division of Nutritional Sciences
Cornell University

PRENTICE HALL, Englewood Cliffs, New Jersey 07632

Library of Congress Cataloging-in-Publication Data

Roe, Daphne A.,
    Geriatric nutrition / Daphne A. Roe. -- 3rd ed.
        p.   cm.
    Includes bibliographical references and index.
    ISBN 0-13-353046-9
    1. Aged--Nutrition. 2. Geriatrics.   I. Title.
    [DNLM: 1. Nurition--in old age.   WT 100 R698g]
TX361.A3R63 1991
613.2'084'6--dc20
DNLM/DLC
for Library of Congress

Editorial/production supervision and
   interior design: Shelly Kupperman
Cover design: Karen Salzbach
Prepress buyer: Kelly Behr
Manufacturing buyer: Mary Ann Gloriande
Acquisitions editor: Carol Wada

© 1992, 1987, 1983 by Prentice-Hall, Inc.
A Simon & Schuster Company
Englewood Cliffs, New Jersey 07632

Printed in the United States of America
10 9 8 7 6 5 4 3 2

ISBN   0-13-353046-9

PRENTICE-HALL INTERNATIONAL (UK) LIMITED, *London*
PRENTICE-HALL OF AUSTRALIA PTY. LIMITED, *Sydney*
PRENTICE-HALL CANADA INC., *Toronto*
PRENTICE-HALL HISPANOAMERICANA, S.A., *Mexico*
PRENTICE-HALL OF INDIA PRIVATE LIMITED, *New Delhi*
PRENTICE-HALL OF JAPAN, INC., *Tokyo*
SIMON & SCHUSTER ASIA PTE. LTD., *Singapore*
EDITORA PRENTICE-HALL DO BRASIL, LTDA., *Rio de Janeiro*

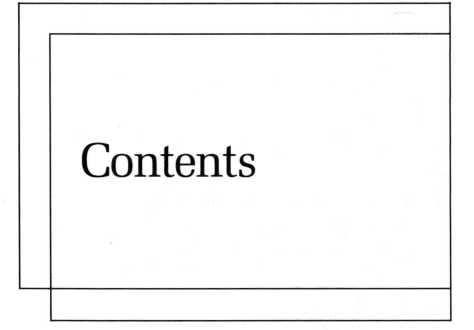

Contents

Preface

The decision to produce a third edition of *Geriatric Nutrition* is explained in part by the need to modify and expand the discussion of dietary influences on the aging process and on the development of chronic disease, but in greater part by the need to acquaint readers with recent knowledge of how best to identify and reduce nutritional risk in the elderly population. Yet another reason for this latest edition was the desire to answer the requests from teachers and students of the subject to bring the literature citations up to date.

In the section describing theories of the aging process, this third edition provides information on recent work pertaining to the glycosylation process and on how diet can modify this process which leads to premature aging of the tissues. The chapter on nutritional requirements has been revised to include a discussion of major changes in dietary recommendations for the aging population, which are derived both from the 1988 Surgeon General's Report and from the 1989 book *Diet and Health*, which expresses the consensus of the Committee on Diet and Health of the U.S. Food and Nutrition Board on diet and chronic disease risk. Information on the 1989 Recommended Dietary Allowances is also provided in the same chapter. In the chapter on nutritional deficiencies, there is new focus on the special risk of protein-energy malnutrition in the institutionalized elderly who need to be fed.

Major updating has been carried out in Chapter 9, "Drugs and Nutrition in the Elderly," which now includes a discussion of drugs in current usage and practical suggestions to dietitians about how to identify the risks of drug and nutrient interactions in their patients.

In a number of places, greater emphasis has been given to the inequalities of nutrition knowledge and health care access, which may explain the greater prevalence of diet-related diseases, such as non-insulin dependent diabetes, in socially disadvantaged populations.

As in previous editions of the book, the major aim is to provide a readable text for undergraduate and graduate students in nutrition as well as for medical students and health care professionals already working in the field. Since many more nutrition departments in universities are now providing courses in geriatric nutrition, this book provides a text that is readable in one-semester, around which a course may be built. Furthermore, in this edition there is an explicit description of the roles and tasks of geriatric dietitians which is intended for students and practitioners in the field.

Since no text of this size can claim to be comprehensive in its coverage of the subject, those using this book are provided with a list of further references with which to expand their knowledge.

As the author of this book, I hope I will continue to excite students not only to learn about the field of geriatric nutrition but also to become committed enough to serve the needs of the older population with nutritional advice, preventive medicine, and effective care.

Acknowledgments

First, I want to acknowledge the contributions of my current and recent graduate students, with whom I have learned about the nutrition of the elderly. Those students and former students whom I would particularly like to acknowledge are Gerita HoSang, Sharmeen Gettner, Elizabeth Andersen, Elvira Conde Pitzrick, and Laura Ellis, whose findings in the field of nutritional survey methodology have been incorporated into this third edition.

I would like to thank Donna Abrahams, Dr. Ellen Schiaffino-Purvis, and YanFang Wang for giving me new insights into the problem of protein-energy malnutrition in dependent eaters in nursing homes. I would like to express my deep appreciation for the work of Drs. Harold Faulkner and Dorothea Faulkner, who have given me inestimable help in our research on the nutritional requirements of the elderly and who have worked with me on studies in the human nutrition research unit at Cornell University.

I would like to express my deep appreciation for the opportunity I have been given over the last seven years to work with Thea Jackson and Robert O'Connell and their colleagues at the New York State Office for Aging. And I wish to thank Mary Cannata and the directors and staffs of the county and city nutrition programs in New York State for their help in my performing surveys of elderly living outside of institutions.

I am much indebted to Dr. Ray Vickers, Medical Director of the New York State Veterans' Home at Oxford, New York, who afforded me the opportunity to study patients and to develop methods of nutritional assessment of patients in the intermediate and skilled nursing facilities.

My secretary, Beverly Hastings, has given me inestimable help and encouragement by collating new material and by assisting me in checking references and in reading proofs.

I would also like to thank the Prentice Hall reviewers for their helpful suggestions: Catherine Justice, Professor Emerita, Purdue University, and Barbara B. North, North Dakota State University.

Finally I would like to thank my family, the students in my geriatric nutrition course, and colleagues who have helped me to prepare this third edition.

Daphne A. Roe

chapter 1

The Elderly in Our Society

In the United States, about 12 percent of the population is over 65 years of age. Ten years ago it was estimated that by the year 2030, 20 percent of the population will be over the age of 65 (Kane and Kane, 1980). In the past two decades, there has also been a very marked decline in mortality among the very old, those over the age of 85. Not only have the current numbers of this subgroup of the elderly surpassed the 1984 projections of the U.S. Census Bureau, but it now seems likely that those over 85 years of age will continue to be the fastest growing age group in the United States and in other industrialized countries (U.S. Bureau of the Census, 1984; Guralnik et al., 1988; Schneider and Guralnik, 1990). While the possibility exists that if the acquired immunodeficiency syndrome (AIDS) is not contained the numbers of men and women surviving will be less than predicted, this eventuality appears unlikely since progress is already being made in the containment of this fatal disease.

This change in the age structure of the population can be attributed to a recent decline in the fertility rate and a long-term decline in the mortality rate. The decline in the mortality rate is due to improved means of combating disease in middle-aged and older people.

The demographic changes pertaining to the increased size of the very old population have led to projections that health care costs will escalate in the United States because the very old have the greatest need for medical and nursing care (Guralnik et al., 1987). In The People's Republic of China another concern is that the one child per family policy will mean the

1

burden of care for two dependent, very old parents will fall on that one child (Goldstein and Goldstein, 1986).

Physiological as well as disease-related changes that occur with aging are highly variable and are potentially modifiable by limiting adverse environmental exposures and by instituting long-term dietary changes aimed at health promotion and disease prevention (Rowe, 1988).

"Getting old" is a derogatory term suggesting that a person can no longer function efficiently, that thought processes are slowed down, or that senility is imminent. The expressed or implied goals of programs for the elderly are to create unequal opportunities in the workplace, to segregate them in living situations, to offer them an inferior social position, to deny them decision-making roles in community policymaking, and to provide them with health and nutrition programs which deny them freedom to choose their own facility, physician, or food. The elderly in our society are you, me, and the next person grown older. Demographically, the elderly are heterogeneous. They vary in age, sex, marital status, education, job skills, work experience, social background, living situation, and health (Shanas, 1974). Variability in the health status of the elderly has been attributed to the presence or absence of health-seeking behavior earlier in life. We assume (without very good evidence) that the healthy elderly have had "healthy" eating patterns throughout life and have maintained the nutritional quality of their diets. Likewise, we assume that the unhealthy elderly have indulged in self-abusive behaviors such as smoking; abusing alcohol; overeating; consuming an excessive amount of sodium, cholesterol, fat, or sugar; and leading a sedentary life. We have not, however, identified many of the factors which contribute to good physical and mental health in later years. In the present state of knowledge, it appears that "biological intactness," the ability to function well to an advanced age, is the outcome of life advantages, including:

1. *Genetic potential for extended longevity.* Stated differently, this means that the individual has inherited characteristics which confer protection from, or lack of susceptibility to, degenerative diseases.
2. *Intelligence.* Highly intelligent people tend to retain their capacity for productive intellectual pursuits longer.
3. *Motivation.* Individuals who believe they can shape their own destiny and plan their own lives can resist societal pressures to play a passive role in later life.
4. *Curiosity.* The continued desire for new knowledge and new experience means that as a person grows older, he or she can find new and challenging occupations and activities.
5. *Socialization.* Older people who maintain an active role in local affairs find they are still indispensable. Senior citizens' groups foster this idea.
6. *Religious belief.* Religious conviction, with or without external observation, allows celebration of life and reduces fear of death.
7. *Responsibility.* Elderly people function well when they have responsibility for the care of others, including other elderly and young children.
8. *Family integrity.* Older people thrive in situations where family bonds are strong. The traditional responsibility of the family is to take care of their own

membership. Older people function best in a family atmosphere in which love, understanding, respect, and sharing of household duties are combined to give meaning to life.

9. *Intimacy.* Marriage or sustained intimate friendships based on love and mutual understanding bring joy. The partners also accept responsibility for each other's welfare. When two older people live together, keeping up personal appearance, organizing of the daily routine, cooking of nutritious meals, and sharing of experiences are common benefits which have positive impact on health and social functioning.

10. *Prudent diet.* Adherence to a prudent diet with avoidance of dietary excesses of food-energy, fat, cholesterol, and sodium diminishes the risk of killer diseases such as atherosclerotic vascular disease, essential hypertension, and maturity-onset diabetes. Complications of these diseases such as angina, late effects of stroke, and diabetic gangrene with amputation restrict the mobility of the elderly inside and outside the home. For the prudent diet to have a protective effect against these diseases and their complications, it is assumed that the elderly individual has followed such a dietary pattern throughout adult life or, better still, since childhood.

11. *Slimness.* In addition to increasing the agility of the elderly, slimness is associated with dietary moderation, which lowers the risk of hypertension, maturity-onset diabetes, and the disabling symptoms of osteoarthritis.

12. *Avoidance of substance abuse.* Nonsmokers who have never smoked heavily or who stopped smoking in early middle life have a substantially reduced risk of chronic disease, including bronchitis and emphysema, lung cancer, and heart attacks. Lifelong nonsmokers and ex-smokers tend to be more health conscious than smokers and follow general guidelines for health maintenance. Moderate drinkers and abstainers avoid alcohol-related disease.

Avoidance of over-the-counter self-medication and prescription drugs other than with specific indication reduces the risk of adverse drug reactions, including drug-induced nutritional deficiencies.

13. *Community health care.* Lack of access to health care in younger life explains why low-income elderly become disabled at younger ages than the more affluent, and why they frequently require home care with nutritional services at a younger age than do higher-income individuals (The Black Report, 1982).

Community health personnel necessary to the elderly include a family physician who knows and cares about his or her older patients; a health clinic which provides a broad range of medical, dental, and ancillary services without financial barriers to the elderly; an efficiently organized public health nursing service which can provide health care to the elderly in their own homes; a podiatrist to supply care for the feet of the elderly; a dentist who has special knowledge of the dental needs of the elderly, including servicing of dentures; a physical therapist who can instruct elderly persons in exercise to promote mobility and offer advice on the purchase and use of special cooking appliances for the elderly disabled; a pharmacist who can interpret prescriptions; and a community nutritionist who can give guidance on the selection and preparation of foods to meet nutritional needs and comply with special diets.

14. *Living arrangements.* Housing for the elderly in an urban setting is most successful in low-level apartment complexes providing units for one or two persons. Each apartment unit should be designed to allow tenants to prepare

their own food, and a ground floor congregate meal center should provide tenants with a main meal on weekdays. The facility should be within walking distance of food markets, or bus service could be provided for elderly people of limited mobility. Provision of low-income housing for the elderly is the responsibility of all urban communities. In rural areas, housing for the elderly may be arranged as grouped cottage homes. Housing units for the elderly in urban and rural areas should be served both by a public health nurse and by community nutritionists, who can define and address the health and nutritional needs of residents. It should be emphasized that better housing for the elderly is often with younger people, preferably family, and that the best housing for vigorous elderly people is in their own established homes, with or without a spouse or companion.

15. *Financial independence.* Elderly people are better able to live comfortably in their community if they have financial resources. These may include salary for part- or full-time work; business profits; money earned from the sale of handicrafts; earned income from services rendered, including provision of day care for others; pensions; savings; unearned income from investments; or money earned through the sale of personal property. Poverty restricts the choice of housing. Unless community, low-income housing for the elderly is provided, the elderly poor will often live in ill-lit, cold, or poorly ventilated single rooms having dangerous or inadequate facilities for cooking. Economic stability allows a greater choice of foods and an opportunity to purchase different foods of high nutrient value. Financial independence allows an elderly person to obtain domestic help to purchase food and prepare meals, thus freeing the elderly individual from those household chores—an advantage to those who find meal preparation a burden. Financial independence allows elderly people in the United States to obtain optimal health care.

The ability of the elderly to lead independent lives is reduced or lost in the following cases:

1. When severe chronic physical illness with permanent disability is present.
2. When the individual is an older, mentally retarded person.
3. When schizophrenia has begun in old age (paraphrenia) with development of a chronic delusional state and disorganized thought process.
4. When paranoid psychosis exists such that the patient is self-abusive or may inflict injury on others.
5. When Korsakoff's psychosis is present—an organic brain syndrome which occurs in chronic alcoholics who are thiamin deficient, leading to disorientation and confusion.
6. When depressive illness is present which does not lift in response to anti-depressant drugs. Depressive illness may be caused by manic-depressive psychosis or neurosis. The depressed elderly may stop eating.
7. When Alzheimer's disease or other presenile or senile dementia has impaired the ability to fulfill the activities of daily living.
8. When skid-row alcoholism has led to eviction or imprisonment.
9. When sight is lost and the individual has adjusted poorly to blindness.
10. When family support and care are not forthcoming.

Major determinants of life setting for the elderly are as follows:

1. Age
2. Motivation
3. Education
4. Job skills
5. Job availability
6. Family support
7. Presence or absence of disabling physical illness
8. Dementia
9. Antisocial tendencies
10. Ability to carry out activities of daily living (ADL)

These determinants are illustrated in Figure 1-1 on next page.

Comparative studies of old people have shown that in industrialized societies there is a wide range of physical capacity and functional ability which is independent of culture. In each of several countries studied, including the United States, Britain, Denmark, Israel, Poland, and Yugoslavia, from 2 to 4 percent of the elderly are bedridden. The number of elderly people who are housebound varies from 12 to 24 percent. Four to eight percent of old people living at home and not bedridden need help with simple physical tasks. About 75 percent of the elderly are ambulatory or report only minimal impairment of ability for performance of tasks related to daily living (Muir Gray, 1980). One quarter of the elderly are in need of medical care and other supportive services in their own homes (Kane and Kane, 1980).

The institutionalized elderly have less support available from community services (including nutritional services) and from family members and friends. They are more impaired in their access to mental health and social resources and are more likely to have had previous need of support or placement. Premature institutionalization of the rural elderly, i.e., institutionalization at a younger age and with less impairment, may be explained by lack of community services in some areas of the country (Greene, 1984). The implications are that expansion of home-care services would reduce the number of elderly in institutions, whereas mobility and the capacity to live independently are determined by physical, mental, and emotional health.

Although health, nutrition, and social services share the goal of helping elderly people remain in the community as long as possible, excessive control over the lives of elderly individuals is unacceptable.

However, it has been shown that for the highly disabled elderly person the selection of nursing-home care over community care by the family is based on cultural norms as well as on financial means, rather than on the personal preference of the disabled older family member (Shapiro and Roos, 1989).

Among the frail elderly, whether in urban or rural areas, determi-

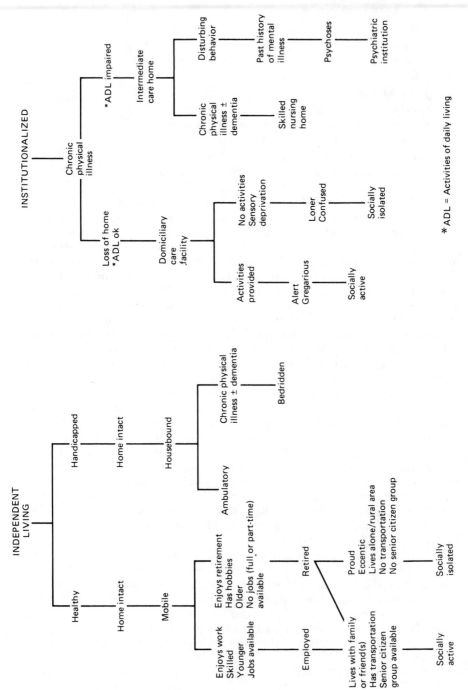

FIGURE 1-1 Determinants of Life Setting for the Elderly.

INDEPENDENT LIVING

Healthy — Home intact — Mobile

Enjoys work / Skilled / Younger / Jobs available — Employed

Lives with family or friend(s) / Has transportation / Senior citizen group available — Socially active

Enjoys retirement / Has hobbies / Older / No jobs (full or part-time) available — Retired

Proud / Eccentic / Lives alone/rural area / No transportation / No senior citizen group — Socially isolated

Handicapped — Home intact — Housebound

Ambulatory

Chronic physical illness ± dementia — Bedridden

INSTITUTIONALIZED

Chronic physical illness

Loss of home *ADL ok — Domiciliary care facility

Activities provided — Alert / Gregarious — Socially active

No activities / Sensory deprivation — Loner / Confused — Socially isolated

*ADL impaired — Intermediate care home

Chronic physical illness ± dementia — Skilled nursing home

Disturbing behavior — Past history of mental illness — Psychoses — Psychiatric institution

*ADL = Activities of daily living

6

nants of hunger, as measured by insufficient meals per week or going one or more days a week without food, include loss of mobility, poverty, and inadequate assistance in obtaining food. Dependency and the need for long-term geriatric care may be explained by inadequate community services, particularly lack of coverage by home-delivered meals programs (Figure 1-2) (Davies, 1984; Roe et al., 1985).

These problems cannot be solved by providing more nursing homes and clinics or by more efficient placement of the elderly. Health, nutritional, and social services should, as far as possible, allow the elderly to make

FIGURE 1-2   Overview of Sociodemographic and Health Characteristics of the Frail Elderly which Contribute to Nutritional Risk and Need for Services.

A. SOCIODEMOGRAPHIC FACTORS	PLUS	B. HEALTH FACTORS
Low income		Acute infections
Living alone		Fractured hip
Minority		Congestive heart failure
		Chronic lung disease
		Late effects of stroke
		Amputations resulting from diabetes
		Arthritis
		Cancer

lead to . . .

C. *Disabilities*
Loss of mobility resulting in . . .

D. *Failure of Food Access*
Can't do food shopping
Can't cook
Can't manage special diet
which explains . . .

E. *Nutritional Risk*
Less than 7 hot meals per week . . .
Days without food . . .
Causing dependency and need for geriatric care unless food needs are met by . . .

F. *Community Services*
Home-delivered meals
Food shopping assistance
Special diets
Nutrition counseling
Homemaker services

decisions for themselves as to health, nutrition, and housing. Even where independent living is no longer feasible and a move to a nursing home is a must, personnel in these geriatric institutions (including dietary service staff) should not make the elderly eat food, play games, or follow routines set up for the convenience of the staff.

Better nutrition for elderly people, whether they live in the community or reside in institutions, requires knowledge of their nutritional needs and wants, as well as provision of food and food services designed to meet their physical, emotional, social, and economic needs.

QUESTIONS

Circle all correct answers (there may be more than one correct answer to each question).

1. Constraints on independent living for the elderly include:
   a. lack of community health care
   b. chronic physical illness with disability
   c. paranoid psychosis
   d. dementia
   e. mental retardation
2. What percent of the elderly are ambulatory?
   a. 25
   b. 25–50
   c. 75
3. The percent of the elderly in industrial societies who are bedridden is:
   a. 2–4
   b. 5–10
   c. 10
   d. 20
4. The percentage of elderly in institutions would be decreased by:
   a. home visits by a doctor
   b. the expansion of home health care services
   c. the provision of more home-delivered meals
5. Which of the following factors are thought to explain why some elderly remain healthy till an advanced age? (Circle the letter beside the correct answers)
   a. Avoidance of substance abuse
   b. Genetic potential for extended longevity
   c. More exposure to the sun
   d. High intake of nutrients that protect against chronic disease
   e. High protein intake

6. Check which of the following statements are true.
   a. Men live longer than women.
   b. The fastest growing segment of the elderly population is made up of those over 85.
   c. Inequalities of health care access explain the earlier onset of disability in low-income groups.
   d. Those under 65 who are among the homebound include alcoholics and smokers.
   e. Once an older person is homebound, they need long-term home care.

REFERENCES

DAVIES, L., "Nutrition and the elderly: identifying those at risk," *Proc. Nutr. Soc.,* 43 (1984), 295.

GOLDSTEIN, A., and S. GOLDSTEIN, "The challenge of an aging population: The case of The People's Republic of China." *Research on Aging,* Vol. 8, No. 2. Sage Publications, Inc., 1986, pp. 179–199.

GREENE, V. L., "Premature institutionalization among the rural elderly in Arizona," *Public Health Rep.,* 99 (1984), 58–63.

GURALNIK, J. M., D. B. BROCK, and J. A. BRODY, "The changing demography of the elderly in the United States, in *Advanced Geriatric Medicine,* eds. F. I. Caird and J. Grimley Evans. Bristol: Wright, 1987, pp. 3–20.

GURALNIK, J. M., M. YANAGISHITA, and E. L. SCHNEIDER, "Projecting the older population of the United States: Lessons from the past and prospects for the future," *Millbank Quart.* 66 (1988), 283–308.

KANE, R. L., and R. A. KANE, "Long-term care: can our society meet the needs of its elderly?" *Ann. Rev. Public Health,* 1 (1980), 227–53.

KAPLAN, O. J., ed., *Psychopathology of Aging.* New York: Academic Press, Inc., 1979.

MUIR GRAY, J. A., "Do we care too much for our elders?" *Lancet,* 1 (1980), 1289.

ROE, D. A., D. F. WILLIAMS, and E. A. FRONGILLO, *1984–85 Survey of Elderly Recipients of SNAP Home-Delivered Meals in New York State.* Final Cornell Report, July, 1985 (Unpublished).

ROWE, J. W. "Aging reconsidered: Strategies to promote health and prevent disease in old age," *Quart. J. Med,* 66 (1988), 1–4.

SCHNEIDER, E. L., and J. M. GURALNIK, "The aging of America," *J. Amer. Med. Assoc.* 263 (1990); 2335–40.

SHAPIRO, E., and N. ROOS, "Predictors and patterns of nursing home and home care use," in *Health Care of the Elderly,* eds. M. D. Petersen and D. L. White. London: Sage Publications, 1989, pp. 127–66.

SHANAS, E., "Health status of older people. Cross-national implications," *Amer. J. Public Health,* 64 (1974), 261–64.

SMYER, M. A., "The differential usage of services by impaired elderly," *J. Gerontol.* 35 (1980), 249–55.

"The Black Report," In *Inequalities of Health,* eds. P. Townsend and N. Davidson. London: Penguin Books, 1988, pp. 124–25 (first published 1982).

U.S. BUREAU OF THE CENSUS. *Current Projections of the Population of the United States by Age, Sex and Race:* 1983–2080. Washington, DC: U.S. Govt. Printing Office, 1984.

chapter 2

The Physiology and Pathology of Aging

THE AGING PROCESS

It is presently believed that aging is a dual process of progressively impaired self-protection and increased self-destruction (Butler, 1979). Aging is inherent and genetically determined such that within species and between species there is a variability in the time frame of the process. Impaired self-protection is due both to immunodeficiency and loss of chemical protector mechanisms. The self-destruction of cells also occurs because the immune system is deranged and because the reparative functions of cells are lost. Changes in immune function, somatic mutation, hormonal insufficiency, irreversible changes in structural proteins, acquired metabolic error, and free radical lipid peroxidation reactions all contribute to aging. The senescence of tissues and organ systems is associated with the loss of cells and a decline in function (Mauderly, 1979).

The rate of the aging process is influenced by the physical and chemical environment. For example, exposure to sunlight ages the skin (Lavker, 1979). Aging within certain organs, such as the pancreas, is increased by chronic intake of food-energy beyond the body's needs (Gerritsen, 1976; Andres, 1972). Aging of the lungs is more rapid in smokers (Barnett, 1972). The rate of aging varies between individuals so that at specific ages different people show different degrees of aging as well as differences in aging between tissues and organ systems.

Pathological changes occur as a result of secondary disease of the elderly, and these may also affect the rate of aging. All components of the aging process are moderated by nutritional factors. Secondary diseases of the elderly can also be prevented or favorably influenced by diet.

Genetic Components of Aging

The expected duration of life is dependent on genetic and acquired factors. It is generally accepted that the life span of a warm-blooded animal, including the human, is predestined. Thus the expected life span of a man or woman is about 70 years, whereas the expected life span of a mouse is about 2 years. It is the predestined component of the prediction of survival which is genetically determined (Hayflick, 1979). Survival at the cellular level implies regenerative activity. The regeneration of cells requires that the genetic material of a cell retain the formula of how to make a cell of the same type as itself. The formula for cell replication is contained in DNA molecules, which must be faithfully duplicated for new cells to be produced having the characteristics of their predecessors. Accurate replication of DNA requires a constant surveillance because of the presence in the cell of repair enzymes (DNA polymerases).

Whereas a low level of DNA error is a condition of life and accounts for evolutionary change, failure to repair DNA is a condition of death. It means either that abnormal cells will be produced and retained, giving rise to cancer, or that the abnormality of the cell is "recognized" by the cellular immune system and deleted.

Aging may result from an accumulation of DNA damage caused by a progressive failure of DNA repair. Support for this hypothesis rests in part on the finding that in a rare genetic disease, progeria, which is characterized by premature aging, fibroblasts cannot repair DNA damage induced by ionizing radiation. It has been suggested that in this disease a repair enzyme is missing (Martin, Sprague, and Epstein, 1970). It seems that in normal aging the DNA repair mechanism may become progressively less efficient and that the rate of decline of DNA repair is genetically determined, leading to different periods of survival. Other genetic determinants of aging reside in the immune system and also in the mixed-function oxidase system, which is responsible for the metabolism of foreign compounds. The ability of cells to activate environmental chemicals to produce cell-damaging metabolites and the ability of cells to detoxify foreign compounds are related inversely to life span (O'Malley et al., 1971; Vestal, 1980).

Aging and Immune Function

The efficiency of immune function decreases with age. There are both decreases in immune response and inappropriate responses. Aging is not a passive wearing out of tissue but an active process which is mediated by the immune system. The number of cells responding to antigenic stimulation decreases, and there is also a decline in activity of antigen-stimulated cells. Cellular immune function, rather than humoral immunity, is affected by the aging changes (Makinodan and Adler, 1975; Matzner et al., 1979).

There is also a decreased ability for the body to distinguish self (normal cells) from nonself (foreign or abnormal cells), which is expressed in a destructive process directed or aimed toward cells which are normal components of tissues. Signs of cellular self-destruction, called autoimmune manifestations, are analogous to chronic graft-verus-host reactions which occur when foreign tissues are introduced into the body. In the adult, prior to aging, potentially autoreactive cell lines (lymphocytic clones) are maintained in a quiescent state by homeostatic mechanisms. With aging, these homeostatic mechanisms are lost (Weksler, Innes, and Goldstein, 1979).

Change in Hormone Responsiveness

Hormone function requires prior attachment of hormones to specific receptor sites located within cells or on the plasma membrane. Receptors are functionally linked to enzyme systems which mediate hormonal activity. Hormones become reversibly bound to specific receptors, forming hormone-receptor complexes ($H + R \rightleftharpoons HR$, where H is the concentration of free hormone, R the concentration of the receptors, and HR the concentration of the hormone-receptor complex). The binding affinity of the receptor may vary with the occupancy of receptor sites by the hormone. Receptor concentration (R) and affinity are influenced by genetic factors, by growth, age and aging, as well as by disease states, including "insulin-resistant" diabetes.

Altered hormonal responsiveness which occurs with advancing age is related mainly to a change in the concentration of hormone receptors (R). Receptor concentrations decline in many organs and tissues as age advances. Age-related changes in the concentration of hormone receptors (R), and hence hormone-receptor complexes (HR), vary with hormone, organ, and, ultimately, physiological need for survival.

Decreased receptor concentration is associated with hormone resistance and lack of adaptability to hormone concentration (Gregerman and Bierman, 1974).

Decreased secretion of growth hormone is partially responsible for the decrease in lean body mass, the increase in fat mass, and the thinning of skin that occur with aging. Injections of growth hormone can induce increases in lean body mass, decreases in the fat mass, and an increase in the thickness of the skin in older men (Rudman et al., 1990).

Free Radical Lipid Peroxidation Reactions

Oxidative damage can be induced by oxygen, ozone, hydrogen peroxide, or other environmental oxidants. Cells of the body are normally protected against oxidative damage (Slater, 1972).

In the process of cellular and membrane aging, lipid peroxidation plays a significant role. Lipid peroxidation involves the formation of semistable peroxides from free radical intermediates by reaction of oxygen and unsaturated lipid. Further reactions occur with the formation of peroxy-, alkoxy-, and hydroxy-free radicals, which cause cell damage even in low concentration. Lipid peroxidation damage occurs mainly in the membranes of subcellular organelles, including microsomal, mitochondrial membranes which contain large amounts of polyunsaturated fatty acids. These membranes are key sites for lipid peroxidation because they contain, or are in proximity to, powerful catalysts of the reaction. Fluorescent products of lipid peroxidation which occur in aging cells are ceroid and lipofucsin. Sources of oxidants which trigger lipid peroxidation are contained in the atmosphere and in foreign compounds within the chemical environment.

Free radicals which are generated in lipid peroxidation are important in the development of degenerative diseases associated with aging.

Biological protector systems which prevent oxidant damage to cells include peroxidases and antioxidants. In the membrane portions of cells the antioxidant function of vitamin E is to protect against lipid peroxidation. Within the cytosol and the mitochondria, the selenium-glutathione peroxidase complex can prevent or minimize oxidative damage.

Tissues most vulnerable to damage through free radical lipid peroxidation are the lungs, heart, and brain (Slater, 1972).

AGING AND THE GLYCOSYLATION PROCESS

Diabetes has long been known to accelerate the aging processes. Recently, the underlying mechanisms that explain this association have been unraveled. It is now known that all proteins with amino groups involved in their stabilization or in a critical site for activity can be functionally impaired when exposed to reducing sugars such as glucose (Monnier, 1990). Irreversible linkages are known to be formed in the body between lens protein and glucose and also between glucose and other blood and tissue proteins, including lipoproteins and collagen. This process, known as glycation or glycosylation, is known to inhibit tissue integrity and system functions. Examples of age-related problems that are linked to glycosylation include cataract formation and nephropathy. Furthermore, it is this process of glycosylation that is accelerated in diabetes.

Aging of Connective Tissue

Fibrous elements of connective tissue, including collagen and elastin, undergo qualitative and quantitative changes in the process of biological aging. The relative amounts of different types of collagen in connective tissue are altered. There are also changes in collagen turnover (Chvapil and Hvuza, 1959).

Although in adults most body collagen is stable, a fraction of the body collagen is continually degraded and replaced. With aging, less of this collagen is degraded and less is synthesized. Changes in cross-linking of collagen occur with aging, but it is not clear that these changes are an integral part of the aging process.

Elastin is a connective tissue component which consists of microfibrils surrounding a nonfibrillar core. In elastogenesis, the microfibrils are formed before the aggregation about the core takes place. With aging, at least in the connective tissue of the skin, there is an increased microfibril formation, which may either represent an attempt to replace old elastin with new material or signify that in older connective tissue there is a loss in functional capacity to produce mature elastin.

There is a progressive loss of elastic recovery of skin after compression stress. Evidence points to changes in the ground substance of the skin as being responsible for the observed change in the mechanical properties of the skin rather than change in the fibrillar components (Daly and Odland, 1979; Prockop et al., 1979).

Relative Effect of Genetic and Acquired Factors in the Aging Process

The term "aging" is used to denote irreversible changes in the tissues which develop with time. Implications of the time element are not only that tissues show a progressive loss of repair mechanisms, which is in part genetically determined, but also that tissue changes result from chronic environmental exposure to physical or chemical agents which are damaging. Whether diet can affect molecular changes of aging is not clear. The thermal contractility of tail collagen from rats, maintained on calorie-restricted diets, has been reported to show the characteristics of tail collagen from younger animals on an unrestricted diet (Porta, 1980).

FIGURE 2-1   Genetic and Environmental Determinants of Geriatric Diseases.

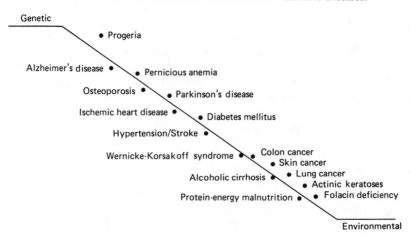

Aging of the skin is highly influenced by ultraviolet light exposure. Persons who develop premature changes of aging in the skin may have genetically determined disorders of DNA repair (Montagna and Carlisle, 1979).

Similarly, aging of other tissues is highly influenced by exposure to environmental toxicants. Aging of the lungs is promoted by air pollutants which cause oxidative damage (Barnett, 1972). Aging of bone leading to osteoporosis is influenced by the toxic effects of chronic alcohol abuse (Albanese et al., 1975). Aging of different tissues occurs at different rates, the time frame of aging in any one tissue being dependent on exposure of that tissue to an environmental damage.

Relationships of aging in different tissues to genetic influences and to the chemical environment are shown in Figure 2-1.

EFFECTS OF NUTRITIONAL VARIABLES ON THE AGING PROCESS

Investigations carried out over the last 50 years indicate that functional deficits in physiological systems, which many believe occur as an inevitable outcome of aging, can in fact be modified by diet. Long-term moderate caloric restriction is known to retard aging processes in rodents (McCay and Crowell, 1934). Further, caloric restriction in rats delays age-dependent losses in androgen function (Chatterjee et al., 1989). Studies in mice indicate that the so-called age-dependent defects in glucose homeostasis may depend on genetic variables that define whether or not the pancreatic islets functionally adapt to glucose load. Obesity and pancreatic fibrosis, rather than aging, may explain impaired glucose handling that occurs in certain strains of rodents as they age (Leiter et al., 1988). These findings are relevant to people as they age since it is known that progressive impairment in the ability to handle a glucose load in humans is associated with insulin resistance and also with obesity (Chen et al., 1985). Prevention of obesity is a major factor in reducing the risk of non-insulin dependent diabetes. Furthermore, the glycosylation process, which is integral to the process of tissue aging, is reduced by caloric restriction at least in laboratory animals (Masoro et al., 1989).

Processes linked to aging, including DNA damage and cancer initiation by ultraviolet light exposure, may be reduced by carotenoids (Suter and Russell, 1989).

Exercise, which certainly influences body composition and nutritional status, delays functional decrements in the cardiovascular system, as well as maintaining muscle function (Fiatarone et al., 1990).

Cellular Aging

Cellular aging can be studied in human cells which have a short life span and are easily accessible, such as red blood cells (Ganzoni, Oakes, and Hillman, 1971). They are produced and undergo maturation in the bone marrow. The process of maturation actually is a process of aging in that the cell loses its capability for reproduction by expulsion of the nucleus from the precursor cell, which is called a normoblast. The cell which is the intermediate between the normoblast and the mature red cell (erythrocyte) is the reticulocyte. When the change takes place in which the reticulocyte turns into a mature red cell, intracellular organelles are lost. Reticulocytes retain capability for protein synthesis because they contain the necessary machinery, including polyribosomes, messenger RNA, transfer RNA, and the required enzymes, for protein synthesis. Protein synthetic activity is important in the reticulocyte, but this activity is lost in the red blood cell. Similarly, the reticulocyte contains mitochondria which allow a high rate of oxygen consumption by the reticulocyte. Mitochondria are lost when the reticulocyte becomes a red blood cell.

The mature red blood cell is a biconcave disc with a cell membrane containing enzymes which catalzye processes necessary to physiological function of the cell. New enzyme proteins cannot be produced because the apparatus for protein synthesis no longer exists.

When red blood cells complete their normal life span, they are re-moved by the reticuloendothelial system. Macrophages, or scavenger cells, in the reticuloendothelial system recognize the aging red cell as being no longer needed (aging self) because of biophysical and immunological changes which have taken place in the cell with time. The ability of the cell to undergo reversible changes in shape to get through narrow blood vessels is lost.

The density of membrane antigens increases in old red blood cells. There is also a decrease in the surface charge on the aging red blood cell. It is presently believed that the aging red blood cell may be "identified" by the macrophage as having completed its normal life and being ready for destruction by engulfment or phagocytosis both by the change in surface antigens and by the change in surface.

There is evidence that events occurring in the aging of other cells may be analogous to those occurring in red blood cells.

PHYSIOLOGY OF AGING IN TISSUES AND ORGANS

The Skin and Its Appendages

The changes in the skin with aging include dryness; wrinkling; mottled pigmentation; loss of elasticity; dilatation of capillaries, particularly on the face; senile purpura (bleeding into the skin in response to minor trauma); and growth of seborrhoeic warts, skin tags, and cherry angiomata, which are red vascular lesions having a similar appearance to "blood blisters" but appearing and remaining usually on the abdomen and back.

The skin is divided into the epidermis, or cellular surface layers, and the underlying dermis. The epidermis is anchored to the dermis at the epidermodermal junction, characterized by a ridged structure. Aging of the epidermis is associated with flattening of the epidermodermal junction and loss of the ridged structure. The epidermis in aged skin is less well anchored to the dermis and more liable to be torn off or rubbed off by shearing stress. Similarly, it is because of the looser attachment of the epidermis to the dermis in aged skin that blister formation can occur with less trauma than in young skin (Verbov, 1974).

The epidermis retains some of its important functions despite changes in aging. A normal horny surface layer is formed. Barrier function, whereby the epidermis can limit water loss from the body, is also retained. However, increased losses of water from the surface layers of the epidermis occur because of decreased water-holding capacity, and this accounts in large part for the dryness of the aged skin.

The skin also becomes drier because of a decrease in sebaceous (oil) gland activity. However, sebaceous glands enlarge with age in men and in women, and the enlarged glands may be prominent on the nose or on the cheeks, forehead, and temples.

In the dermis the cells which produce elastic and collagen fibers, the fibroblasts, become less active, and those that become inactive contain lipofucsin granules. Elastic fibers of the dermis become denser with age, and with time, the elastic fibers shrink and lose their attachment to the epidermis. It is because of these changes in elastic tissue, as well as the degenerative changes in the interfibrillar "ground substance" of the dermis, that wrinkling occurs.

Skin capillaries become more fragile, which accounts for bleeding into the skin with very mild trauma in the elderly (purpura). Senile purpura is more common on light-exposed areas such as the forearms. The capillaries also become sparser and functionally less responsive to cold. Coldness is experienced as soon as the ambient temperature begins to fall.

Decline in cellular immune function, which is a general phenomenon of aging, explains in part the greater prevalence of fungal infections in older persons and their increased susceptibility to malignant tumors.

Hair changes include greying of the hair and hair loss. Hair loss in men initially has the distribution of male patterns of baldness, with thinning and loss of hair being most prominent over the frontal areas of the scalp. In older men, extensive loss of scalp hair may be accompanied by growth of coarse hair in the nostrils and ears. In women the scalp hair tends to become sparser over the entire scalp, though thinning of the hair is most noticeable over the vertex. Secondary sex hair on the body decreases in both sexes in the process of aging, and in the female loss of body hair may begin soon after the menopause.

Changes in the nails include slowed rate of growth, thickening, and deformity (onychogryposis).

Prematurely aging skin occurs with chronic exposure to sunlight. Aging of the skin occurs earlier and most prominently on light-exposed areas. Changes seen in the skin with actinic skin damage include wrinkling, pigmentary changes, and loss of elasticity. Actinic keratoses are rough, red areas of the light-exposed skin which, on histological examination, may show precancerous changes. If untreated, they have a strong tendency to develop skin cancer (Montagna and Carlisle, 1979).

Aging of the skin is influenced by genetic factors. Early aging of the skin occurs in light-skinned Caucasians. Premature aging of the skin occurs in general diseases of premature aging, such as progeria. In the very serious skin disorder xeroderma pigmentosum, DNA of the epidermal cells fails to undergo repair after ultraviolet-induced injury. Persons with this disease develop skin cancer very early in life, as well as skin changes resembling, in some respects, those seen with aging.

Chronic exposure to sunlight accelerates aging both in the epidermis and in the dermis. In the epidermis the life span of the keratinocytes (hair-forming cells) is decreased, and in the dermis collagen fiber synthesis and degradation are slowed.

Pathophysiology of the Oral Cavity

The flow of saliva is decreased with aging. Dehydration and thinning of the gum tissue and shrinking of the connective tissue of the mouth occur. Sensory changes which may occur include impaired taste and glossodynia (pain in the tongue) (Schiffman, 1977).

Masticatory efficiency may be impaired by loss of mobility of the mandibular joint caused by osteoarthrosis, periodontal disease, inflammation under a denture, or the edentulous or partially dentulous state. Periodontal disease is common and is associated with inflammation of the gums, loosening of the teeth, and dental abscesses. The bone surrounding the teeth shows rarification. It has been suggested that periodontal disease is a calcium deficiency state, but this has not been proven.

Age-related changes in the teeth that are not associated with periodontal disease include abrasion or wearing down of the crowns, formation of secondary dentine, and resorption of the dental tip roots.

Angular cheilitis and stomatitis are common. They may or may not be associated with riboflavin deficiency. Frequently both angular cheilitis and stomatitis, i.e., cracks at the corners of the lips or mouth, are associated with deep skin creases and local secondary yeast infection.

Common diseases of the oral mucosa include candidiasis (thrush/yeast infection); leukoplakia (premalignant mucosal changes); cancer of the mouth or oral cavity, including the tongue; and xerostomia, associated with Sjögren's syndrome (an autoimmune disease).

Dental caries is uncommon in the elderly; with age, resistance to caries increases. This has generally been explained as being caused by maturation of enamel and dentine (Soremark and Nilsson, 1972).

The Gastrointestinal System

Secretory activity into and within the gastrointestinal tract is reduced with aging. The most marked change in secretory activity is in the stomach, where gastric hydrochloric acid production is diminished. Pepsin and gastric mucus secretion also decline.

In pernicious anemia, a disease which is not uncommon in elderly people, the production of gastric intrinsic factor ceases, and there is also achlorhydria (complete lack of gastric acid production) (Steinberg and Toskes, 1978). Pernicious anemia is an autoimmune disease in which megaloblastic and neurological signs are caused by vitamin B_{12} deficiency. Vitamin B_{12} from the diet cannot be absorbed in the absence of gastric intrinsic factor. The aging process increases the risk of autoimmune disease within the gut.

Physiological decreases in absorptive capacity within the small intestine are moderate. Tolerance of fat is slightly reduced such that with high fat intake, the fat content of the feces is raised. The screening test for malabsorption of sugars using D-xylose may be used to indicate impairment of intestinal absorption, but caution must be used in interpreting the test, which is dependent on retention of normal renal function, a condition which may not be present in the elderly (Steinheber, 1976).

Calcium absorption in the elderly is frequently decreased, and there is also a reduced ability for adaptation to low calcium intake, which may be caused by change in vitamin D status.

Constipation is common in the elderly. General causes of constipation in the elderly, as in persons of younger age groups, are (1) delayed transit of feces throughout the colon and (2) prolonged retention of feces within the rectum. Slowed colonic transmit may be caused by a low-residue diet, semistarvation, drugs (narcotic analgesics), hypothyroidism, laxative abuse, late radiation damage to the gut wall, or chronic intestinal obstruction caused by colonic or rectal cancer or inflammatory bowel disease. Slow passage of the colonic contents is associated with dehydration and hardening of the fecal mass. The dehydration of feces occurs when the feces remain longer than normal in the large intestine and more water is extracted because of continued exposure of the feces to the water-absorbing surface of the colon.

In the elderly constipation is also characterized by fecal hoarding in the rectum resulting from habitual postponement of defecation or inability to defecate easily.

Habitual postponement of defecation is termed dyschezia. Dyschezia may be caused by (1) fear of pain, (2) anxiety and depression, (3) situational factors (inadequate privacy of toilet arrangements), (4) fecal impaction, (5) debility as a result of chronic disease states or malnutrition of dietary or disease origin, and (6) "loss" of the gastrocolic reflex which initiates propulsive movement of feces from the colon and rectum, producing the desire to defecate. The gastrocolic reflex is normally triggered by intake of warm food or beverages (Berman and Kirschner, 1972).

The Cardiovascular System

Anatomical changes which take place in the heart with aging include an overall decrease in size, decrease in the size of the cavity of the left ventricle, and increase in the size of the left atrium. The heart valves become more rigid and thickened, and collagen increases in the valves. Calcification occurs in the aortic valve. The heart muscle (myocardium) becomes brownish because of increased lipochrome (lipofucsin) deposition. There is enlargement or hypertrophy of individual muscle fibers of the myocardium, which apparently occurs to compensate for other muscle fibers which are lost. Fat deposition occurs beneath the surface membrane of the heart (pericardium), and thickened whitish plaques appear in the membrane lining the heart (endocardium).

Dilatation of the aorta occurs because of loss of elasticity.

Physiological changes of the heart with aging include decreased myocardial contractility and decreased cardiac output. There is a decreased ability of the heart to utilize oxygen. The aging heart does not tolerate physical stress, such as increase in blood pressure, fever, and strenuous exercise, as well as the younger heart, because these stresses can precipitate cardiac failure. Although large arteries dilate with aging, there is generally a loss of arterial distensibility with age.

Systolic blood pressure usually increases with age, but changes in diastolic blood pressure are slight (Hurst et al., 1974; Harris, 1975).

The Respiratory System

Anatomical changes in the lungs with aging include enlargement of the alveoli (air sacs) with weakening of septal membranes and a reduction in the alveolar surface area. Changes in alveolar surface are accompanied by deterioration of elastic properties of the tissue. Decreases in the alveolar surface area are almost linear between the ages of 20 and 80 years, such that by age 80 the surface is approximately 30 percent of the maximal young adult valve.

Changes in the lung elastic tissue are both quantitative and qualitative. The lungs become stiffer and the alveolar tissue less distensible.

Vital capacity decreases with age, and the ability to adapt to exercise is reduced. Maximal breathing capacity and maximal voluntary ventilation of the lungs also decrease with age. The lungs are, of course, the organs of gaseous exchange whereby oxygen enters and carbon dioxide leaves the body. Gas exchange capacity is lowered with aging because of the combined effects of reduced alveolar surface area, increased thickness of alveolar membrane, decreased permeability of the alveoli to respiratory gases, and reduced capillary blood volume (Hook, 1972).

The Renal System

A morphological change in the kidney associated with aging is a loss of nephrons (renal excretory units). Renal functional changes which occur with aging include a reduction in total renal blood flow, glomerular filtration rate, daily urinary creatinine excretion, sodium conservation, and renal concentrating ability. The renal capacity for reabsorption of glucose declines, and the secretory function of the renal tubule is diminished. The physiological adaptation to sodium load, as well as to dietary sodium restriction, is also progressively less efficient with aging. Because of decreased efficiency of sodium handling, the elderly risk developing both hyponatremia and hypernatremia. These abnormalities of sodium homeostases may be life-threatening conditions when elderly people are subjected to physical stress such as injury or infection (Epstein, 1979).

The Endocrine System

Aging produces marked physiological changes in the endocrine system, but failure of endocrine function is not a generalized phenomenon. Indeed, endocrine dysfunction in the elderly, as in other age groups, is disease related.

The pituitary-hypothalamic system. Hypothalamic aging influences endocrine function in the peripheral endocrine system, including the pituitary, thyroid, parathyroid, and reproductive glands. Events associated with aging include diminished production of hypothalamic-releasing hormones and a lessened sensitivity of the pituitary to the action of hypothalamic-releasing hormones. Decreased growth hormone release occurs in the elderly following the stimulus of hypoglycemia, and this may be explained by loss of growth hormone–releasing hormone. On the other hand, aging induces impairment in direct renal response to the posterior pituitary antidiuretic hormone (ADH), with less effect of ADH on water conservation or urine concentrating ability. In elderly people there is also a reduced pituitary response to thyrotropin-releasing hormone.

Thyroid glands. Aging of the thyroid is associated with anatomical alterations in the gland, including fibrosis, follicular change, and nodularity. There is no change in plasma levels of thyroxine (T) in healthy elderly people, but circulating levels of the other thyroid hormone, triiodothyronine (T_3), are reduced. Aging does not produce hypofunction of the gland.

Parathyroid gland. Aging is associated with slightly decreased blood parathyroid hormone (PTH) levels. The normal PTH drop with age is not seen in osteoporotic individuals. Neither hypoparathyroidism nor hyperparathyroidism is an outcome of aging, although hyperparathyroidism does increase in incidence in older people.

Reproductive glands. Ovarian aging is associated with loss of oocytes (ova/egg–producing cells), but this process of oocyte reduction actually begins in infancy and continues throughout life. The cause of human reproductive failure with age is not loss of oocytes. Ova produced by older ovaries are less viable and do not undergo the maturation which occurs in the ova of younger individuals. Estrogen production is reduced in women over about 40 years, and there is a further decrease in estrogen production which occurs after menopause.

Reduction in plasma total testosterone levels does not occur uniformly with increasing age, and, indeed, variability in testosterone production among elderly men is noteworthy. However, physiologically active testosterone is reduced in the elderly male. The loss of libido with age and the impairment of sexual performance is multifactorial. Sterility in the elderly male is commonly disease related. Disease-related causes of sterility in the elderly male include alcoholism (Gregerman and Bierman, 1974).

Endocrine pancreas. Glucose tolerance decreases with age, and production of insulin is reduced in response to physiological stimulation. Reduced end-organ sensitivity to the effects of insulin occurs with obesity, which is common in older people, but end-organ sensitivity to insulin is normal in elderly, nonobese individuals (Andres, 1972).

Adrenal glands. Decreased secretion of the sodium-conserving hormone aldosterone occurs with age. With sodium restriction, older persons, like younger persons, do increase aldosterone production, but the increase is smaller in people over 60. The secretion of renin shows an age-related decrease, which is correlated with the decrease in aldosterone secretion.

Decreased glucocorticoid secretion in response to adrenocorticotropic hormone (ACTH) may occur in the elderly but is not a uniform finding.

Physiological Changes in Hemopoiesis

Decreased efficiency of hemopoiesis occurs with aging. In the healthy aged, hemoglobin concentrations are similar to those in younger people. Absorption of available iron sources is also similar in elderly and younger groups. However, the percentage of absorbed iron that is utilized for hemopoiesis is less in the elderly than in the young. In the healthy elderly, iron stores are increased, and it has therefore been assumed that ineffective erythropoiesis is increased. The red cell incorporation of iron decreases with age, and it has been suggested, although it is at present unproven, that in the aged some absorbed iron may be retained in the liver or in other storage tissues. Both the aged and the young respond to iron deficiency by increased iron absorption. Iron deficiency anemia in the aged is not explained by the change of efficiency of hemopoiesis (Marx, 1979; Matzner et al., 1979).

Limited studies of folacin absorption in the aged suggest that there is a decrease in utilization of ingested polyglutamate forms of folacin derived from foods but that synthetic sources of folic acid are as well absorbed by the elderly as by the young. Whether or not absorbed folacin is as well utilized for hemopoiesis in the elderly as in the young is currently unknown (Rodriguez, 1978). Present evidence does not suggest that absorption of other B vitamins, including vitamin B_6, vitamin B_{12}, and riboflavin (which are required in hemopoiesis), is decreased with aging. Information is lacking as to whether utilization of any one of these B vitamins for hemopoiesis is decreased in older persons.

The Central and Peripheral Nervous Systems

Changes in the central nervous system with aging are structural and functional. Aging, independent of disease processes, is associated with a progressive loss of brain cells, particularly in the cortical areas (Brody and Vijayashankar, 1977).

Memory declines, but memory losses vary greatly among individuals.

Although the loss of memory always affects the ability to learn and retain information, those people who are intellectually gifted and continue to be intellectually active and socially stimulated are less likely to show severe impairment. Past skills are retained or may be relearned, provided that the necessary motivation is provided. New skills are acquired with increasing difficulty as aging progresses.

Sensory perceptivity decreases in the elderly. The blunting of sensory perception is related to the special senses; hearing, smell, and taste are less acute. The anguish of pain is lessened (Schiffman, 1977).

Sleep is usually unchanged in duration, but sleeping patterns may be reversed so that elderly tend to sleep more during the day and less at night.

Muscle response to nerve stimulation declines, both because nerve impulses to muscles are conducted more slowly and because of loss of muscle mass.

The Eye

Aging affects multiple components of the eye concerned with vision. These include the reduction in visual acuity and a decline in accommodation, or the loss of ability to focus on near objects, which usually begins in middle life. This is due to an inability of the aging lens to change in curvature in response to the needs of near vision. The loss of the power of accommodation is designated *presbyopia*. Senile cataract, causing opacity of the lens, is due to condensation or an increased density of fibers within the lens. Cataract in the aging eye is classified as cortical and nuclear according to the distribution of the opacity (Weale, 1973). The opacity of the lens limits the usefulness of the lens as a light filter. The development of cataract, even in the early stages, reduces night vision. Approaching lighted objects, such as the headlights of cars, appear fuzzy, and the glare of lights impedes visual judgment. Later cataracts impose a progressive loss of vision, which can be relieved by extraction of the lens. The rate of development of cataract usually differs between the two eyes.

With aging, the lens not only becomes rigid and loses translucency, but it also increases in size. This increase in size may lead to impaired drainage of the fluid (the aqueous humor) which is present in the anterior chamber of the eye (in front of the lens). Narrowing the angle between the iris and the cornea occludes drainage of this fluid into the canal of Schlemm. Intraocular pressure builds up with resultant glaucoma, which also imposes a threat to vision because of excessive pressure on the retina or visual membrane. The central area of the retina, called the macula, which is the most sensitive site of visual perception, tends to degenerate in the elderly.

The changes of aging within the eye are subject to wide interperson variability. Important factors which contribute to the early development of these eye changes are familial predisposition (genetic factors), exposure to ionizing radiation (leading to cataract), and diabetes (Passmore and Robson, 1974).

The Effect of Age on Hearing

Hearing defects of the elderly account for the greatest number of sensorineural hearing loss disorders. Sensorineural hearing loss disorders comprise hearing loss arising from impaired function of the inner ear (cochlea) and/or connections of the auditory nerve close to or within the brain.

The hearing disorders of the elderly may result from several factors operating during an individual's life. These factors include genetic determinants of deafness, occupational noise exposure, and chronic middle ear disease. In addition, common health problems associated with hearing loss include Meniere's disease, which increases in incidence with age. Hearing loss in the elderly has been correlated with the extent or severity of atherosclerosis.

Most elderly people have poorer high-frequency hearing levels. However, chronological age does not determine the rate of decline in hearing (Goldstein and Reichel, 1978).

PATHOLOGY OF AGING IN TISSUES AND ORGANS

Skin Diseases

Skin diseases of the elderly should be familiar to the nutritionist for one or more of the following reasons:

1. They may be manifestations of specific forms of malnutrition, e.g., avitaminoses.
2. They require nutritional intervention to heal, e.g., decubitus ulcers.
3. They are indicators of metabolic disease, e.g., diabetes.
4. They cause malnutrition, e.g., systemic sclerosis.
5. They suggest gross personal neglect, e.g., scabies.
6. They are self-induced because of organic brain syndromes or senile psychoses.
7. They require therapy which may compromise nutrition.
8. They are associated with alcoholism.
9. They are caused by misuse or abuse of medications.
10. They interfere with food intake.

Cutaneous signs of malnutrition. In the presence of a *riboflavin deficiency*, seborrhoic dermatitis is present with redness and scaling of the nasolabial folds (skinfold between the nose and the corners of the mouth), and similar scaly lesions of the wrinkles around the eyes may be present. Patients exhibit a dermatitis of the scrotum or vulva. Angular stomatitis (fissures at the corners of the mouth) is also present. The tongue is smooth, purplish, and sore.

These changes of the skin and mucous membranes disappear when therapeutic doses of riboflavin are given.

Riboflavin deficiency may be secondary to malabsorption or alcoholic liver disease (Sebrell and Butler, 1938).

Skin changes in the elderly which clinically resemble riboflavin deficiency but which do not respond to riboflavin administration are due to causes other than riboflavin deficiency, e.g., intertrigo (Verbov, 1974).

A niacin deficiency, or *pellagra*, is characterized by dermatitis and brownish pigmentation of light-exposed areas of skin. Soreness of the mouth and diarrhea also occur. The patient exhibits signs of an organic brain syndrome characterized by fearfulness, depression, and suicidal thoughts. Cutaneous, gastrointestinal signs of pellagra, as well as the characteristic psychoses, disappear following niacin administration (Fouts et al., 1937).

Vitamin B_6 deficiency (pyridoxine) is signaled by dermatitis of the face, ears, trunk, and limbs associated with redness and bran-like scales; neuritis with complaint of burning feet; depression; confusion or disorientation; and hypochromic anemia. Cutaneous and noncutaneous signs of vitamin B_6 deficiency usually clear when therapeutic doses of vitamin B_6 are given, but it should be noted that since vitamin B_6 deficiency is usually due to chronic intake of drugs such as L-dopa, which are vitamin B_6 antagonists, change in the dose of the drug or discontinuation of the drug may be necessary to promote resolution of the deficiency.

Scurvy is associated with prominence of hair follicles on the limbs and perifollicular hemorrhage into the skin. More widespread purpura may be present. Scorbutic gums which are swollen and bleeding do not occur in elderly people who are edentulous. Signs of scurvy disappear when vitamin C is given in therapeutic doses (Irwin, 1976).

In the presence of a *vitamin A deficiency* the skin is dry and permanent goose pimples are visible on the limbs. Night blindness is a common complaint. Vitamin A deficiency is very rare in the United States, except in alcoholics or in patients with severe malabsorption syndromes (Steinberg and Toskes, 1978).

Purpura occurs in association with *vitamin K deficiency* (hypoprothrombinemia). The cause is intake of either anticoagulant drugs or other drugs which interfere with vitamin K absorption, e.g., cholestyramine (Roe, 1976).

With an *essential fatty acid deficiency*, the skin shows widespread or generalized scaling and redness. Skinfolds are particularly involved. Other signs include hair loss and poor wound healing. Patients are likely to be receiving semisynthetic enteral or parenteral formulas (Wene, Connor, and Denbensten, 1975).

Cutaneous signs of *zinc deficiency* include dermatitis of the backs of the hands, forearms, and lower legs, which in severe cases becomes generalized. The dermatitis does not respond to any topical medications. Wound healing is impaired. Patients complain of loss of taste. Patients are often alcoholics. Cutaneous and noncutaneous signs of zinc deficiency disappear when zinc supplements are administered (Ecker and Schroeter, 1978).

Lesions of the skin requiring nutritional intervention for optimal healing. Wound healing is dependent on adequate nutrition with respect to protein, B vitamins (niacin, folacin, and riboflavin), ascorbic acid, zinc, and essential fatty acids. The retarded healing of surgical wounds, decubitus ulcers (bed sores), and stasis ulcers (leg ulcers) is associated with deficiency of one or more of these nutrients. Scar formation with deposition of collagen requires vitamin C. Epithelialization (surface closure) of wounds and ulcers requires optimal B vitamins and zinc nutrition. Wound edema, associated with protein deficiency, retards healing (Steffee, 1980).

Cutaneous signs of metabolic disease. *Gout* is a disorder of purine metabolism associated with hyperuricemia. Cutaneous signs of gout include chalky deposits of urate around finger and toe joints and also on the ears. In acute gouty attacks, local redness, swelling, and tenderness of the tophi occur (Verbov, 1974).

Cutaneous signs of *diabetes* are fat atrophy at the sites of insulin injections; widespread fungus and yeast infections of the skin involving primarily the feet and legs; ulcers and abscesses of the feet with diabetic neuropathy, recurrent boils, and carbuncles; other recurrent pyodermas (bacterial infections of the skin); gangrene (usually of the toes or feet); and necrobiosis lipoidica diabeticorum (NLD). NLD consists of oval areas of thinned skin over the shins in which small underlying blood vessels are clearly visible. Dermatitis of skinfolds *(intertrigo)* is common in obese patients with maturity-onset diabetes (Passmore and Robson, 1974; Verbov, 1974).

Signs of *atherosclerosis* include xanthomata, which are yellow skin nodules around the elbows and knees, on the hands, and along the Achilles tendon consisting of deposits of cholesterol, and cholesterol esters in the skin. They are present in patients with genetically determined hyperlipoproteinemias. Many patients with these lesions (Type IIA, IIB, III, and IV) do not survive to be senior citizens because of predisposition to atherosclerotic heart disease in early or middle life. Xanthelasma, which is a variant of xanthomatous lesions, consists of unilateral or bilateral small, yellow, plaque-like lesions in or below the lower eyelids. They are more common in the elderly. Half of the patients with xanthelasmas have elevated serum cholesterol values (Verbov, 1974).

Hemochromatosis is an iron-storage disorder, sometimes primary, caused by genetically determined hyperabsorption of iron or secondary to alcoholism or certain hematological diseases such as thalassemia. Signs appear in middle life or later. The skin is greyish in color because of deposition of iron. Loss of secondary sex hair is usual. Patients with this disease have cirrhosis and diabetes mellitus (Braverman, 1970).

Cutaneous diseases causing malnutrition. *Systemic sclerosis* is a progressive connective tissue disease leading to hardening of the skin and progressive impairment of upper and lower GI function. Decreased pulmonary and renal function are also common. Signs related to the skin are

Raynaud's phenomenon (blanching of the fingers in response to cold) and ulceration of the fingers and toes.

Dysphagia and regurgitation of food occur with upper GI tract involvement. Intestinal malabsorption is found in a high percentage of cases. The combination of poor food retention and malabsorption leads to malnutrition.

Bullous pemphigoid and *pemphigus* are both generalized blistering eruptions of the skin. Bullous pemphigoid is mainly seen in people over 60 years of age, whereas pemphigus is more common in younger age groups. Loss of serum proteins from the skin because of blistering can cause protein malnutrition in both of these diseases.

In *exfoliative dermatitis* the whole skin surface (or most of it) is red, dry, and peeling. Exudation of serum may be present, and edema is common. Nails and hair are often lost. In many cases, itching is intense. Common causes are adverse drug reaction, psoriasis, Norwegian scabies, neurodermatitis, and lymphomas. A severe loss of protein from the skin occurs as epidermal keratin and serum. Malnutrition is a result of low food energy intake associated with anorexia and protein loss. Folacin deficiency may occur because of an increased rate of turnover of epidermal cells.

Cutaneous indicators of neglect. Gross personal neglect in the elderly is strongly suggested by the presence of infestation. Common parasitic skin diseases in the elderly are (1) pediculosis corporis caused by infestation with body lice and (2) scabies caused by infestation with the scabies mite. Generalized scabies with exfoliation is called Norwegian scabies. Malnutrition caused by a faulty diet and infestation associated with lack of personal hygiene occur together in socially isolated elderly people.

Self-induced skin lesions. *Delusions of parasitosis* occur when elderly people become convinced that they are infested (Verbov, 1974). They scratch themselves obsessionally and will bring to the doctor's office containers of skin fragments and/or small bits of thread which they insist are insects which are infecting them. Patients with this obsession are usually paranoid. Obsessions may not be limited to skin parasites but frequently extend to food. Ideas that certain foods are poisonous or poisoned may also be present.

With *factitial dermatitis*, self-inflicted skin lesions, including self-inflicted thermal or chemical burns, may occur. Patients are psychotic, and associated psychoses include organic brain syndromes. Patients who burn or mutilate their own skin may also rub feces into the wound and develop severe infections which can compromise nutritional status.

Chemotherapy and radiation therapy of cutaneous disease. Cancer and lymphomas of the skin may require either radiation therapy or chemotherapy for curative or palliative treatment. Basal and squamous cell cancers of the skin are treated by radiation therapy and by surgery. Cutaneous diseases which require chemotherapy include Kaposi's sarcoma and mycosis fungoides.

Both radiation therapy and chemotherapy are likely to cause nausea and anorexia, which diminish food intake and can be responsible for protein-energy malnutrition, which in turn diminishes tolerance for treatment (Bergevin, 1976).

Dermatoses associated with alcoholism. Elderly people are unlikely to give an accurate account of their drinking habits to a dietitian or clinical nutritionist, especially if they are alcoholics.

Skin diseases and disorders which are commonly associated with alcohol abuse and may offer presumptive evidence of alcoholism in the elderly are rosacea (a red and bulbous nose); raindrop-like pigmentation of the shoulders and upper back; dilated capillaries ("spiders") over the face, back, and chest; and light sensitivity appearing in later life caused by porphyria (porphyria cutanea tarda). See also the discussion of grey skin pigmentation in hemochrometosis (Braverman, 1970).

Eruptions caused by medications. The elderly are common drug users. Laxative abusers are found particularly among older people, and secrecy about the habit may be maintained. Malnutrition with potassium depletion and fat malabsorption can result from laxative abuse or a particularly high intake of phenolphthalein-containing preparations. Phenolphthalein may cause a fixed drug eruption which consists of reddish, hyperpigmented circular skin lesions, which become very red when the drug is ingested. The finding of a fixed drug eruption in elderly people can lead to discovery of laxative abuse, although fixed drug eruptions are also associated with intake of drugs other than phenolphthalein (Verbov, 1974).

Dermatoses interfering with food intake. Dermatoses which interfere with food intake include those which cause intractable itching (such as exfoliative dermatitis) or pain (such as herpes zoster, or shingles), those which are skin manifestations of internal cancer, those which require radiation or chemotherapy, those which may also involve the mucous membrane of the mouth and throat (such as pemphigus and avitaminoses), and those which are associated with disease of the esophagus (such as systemic sclerosis) (Wormsley, 1964).

COMMON DISEASES OF THE ORAL CAVITY

Ulceromembranous Stomatitis (Vincent's Angina)

Multiple painful greyish ulcers occur with ulceromembranous stomatitis *(Vincent's angina)*, involving the mouth and, most commonly, the pharynx. The mouth has a foul odor, and swallowing is difficult. The lymph glands in the neck are enlarged, and there may be a fever. Patients are frequently malnourished, and resistance to infection is often impaired. Vincent's organisms, which normally live within the mouth without causing infection, become pathogenic.

Candidiasis

Yeast infections of the mouth are frequently seen in the elderly. Whitish patches are present on the mucous membranes of the mouth. Localization may be to the tongue, gums, or lips, but it is not unusual to see generalized candidiasis infections of the mouth. Malnutrition and poor oral hygiene accompany this disease.

Black Hairy Tongue

In black hairy tongue the upper surface of the tongue appears blackish in color, the pigmentary development on the tongue being caused by proliferation of pigment-producing microorganisms. Factors which promote development include prolonged intake of antibiotics and poor oral hygiene.

Glossitis

Glossitis may be nutritional or non-nutritional in origin. Common nutritional causes are iron deficiency, riboflavin deficiency, and folacin deficiency (Baker, Jaslow, and Frank, 1978). Pellagra is now a very uncommon cause of glossitis in the United States. All nutritional disorders which cause glossitis are associated with loss of the projections on papillae normally occurring on the surface of the tongue.

Geographic tongue is a benign condition of the tongue in which irregular areas on the upper surface of the tongue become denuded of papillae. The disorder may be accompanied by soreness when hot food is eaten or hot beverages drunk.

Leukoplakia

Leukoplakia causes whitish, persistent thickened patches or streaks on the lips and on the mucous membrane within the mouth. The lesions, if untreated, are sites of cancer development.

Plummer-Vinson Syndrome (Sideropenic Dysphagia)

Plummer-Vinson syndrome is characterized by dysphagia, angular stomatitis, atrophic tongue (denuded of papillae), brittle and/or spoon-shaped nails, and pharyngeal or esophageal web. The patients are mostly women and are all chronically iron deficient. A high percentage of patients with this condition develop cancer of the pharynx or esophagus.

Cancer (Squamous Cell Carcinoma)

Cancer of the lips, tongue, and the mucous membrane lining the buccal cavity is most likely to develop in areas of leukoplakia. Cancers may appear as a lump or ulcer. With early lesions pain is often absent. Spread to a regional (neck) gland occurs. More advanced lesions are extremely painful and cause dysphagia, such that food intake by mouth becomes difficult or virtually impossible (Shaw and Sweeney, 1980).

DISEASES OF THE GASTROINTESTINAL TRACT

Diseases of the GI tract encountered in the elderly fall into one of two categories:

1. Diseases that are age related
2. Diseases that are not age related

In the first category there are three subgroups:

1. Diseases which occur as complications of aging in the gut, e.g., diverticulitis
2. Diseases caused by systemic degenerative disease which is progressive with age, e.g., mesenteric infarction (a block of the mesenteric artery causing gangrene of the gut, which is secondary to generalized atherosclerosis)
3. Diseases caused by previous chemical or physical insult characterized by slow development, e.g., colon cancer, radiation enteritis

In the second category are diseases which can occur at any age. Subgroups are:

1. Diseases of long duration, e.g., gluten-sensitive enteropathy
2. Diseases of short duration, e.g., peptic ulcer

Diseases of the GI tract found in the elderly are commonly classified (as in Table 2-1) by location. Common symptoms of serious disease of the GI tract in the elderly are dysphagia, or difficulty in swallowing; gastrointestinal bleeding; change in frequency of defecation (diarrhea or constipation); abdominal pain; and jaundice. In the elderly it is often difficult to differentiate symptoms of minor disorders of the GI tract from symptoms of serious disease (Berman and Kirschner, 1972).

Dysphagia

Pharyngeal and esophageal diseases are recognized by dysphagia. Progressive dysphagia in the elderly is most frequently due to cancer. Dysphagia with or without nasal regurgitation of food is common in cerebrovascular disease involving the medulla, such as bulbar palsy. A list of diseases which most often cause dysphagia is given in Table 2-2 on page 32.

Gastrointestinal Bleeding

Severe or chronic GI bleeding is associated with iron deficiency anemia (an otherwise unusual condition in the elderly) and the lowering of blood pressure, most dramatic in people with previous hypertension. Upper GI bleeding, which if massive may be associated with hematemesis, or

TABLE 2-1 Diseases of the Gastrointestinal Tract Classified by Site of Involvement

SITE	DISEASE
Mouth (including tongue)	Nutritional stomatitis (niacin, riboflavin, folacin, ascorbic acid deficiencies) Candidiasis (thrush-yeast infection) Leukoplakia (precancerosis) Pemphigoid Cancer Sjogren's syndrome Mixed salivary tumors
Salivary glands	Mixed salivary tumors Cancer
Pharynx	Pharyngitis Pharyngeal paralysis Cancer
Esophagus	Zenker's diverticulum Esophageal varices Esophageal stricture Peptic esophagitis Plummer-Vinson syndrome Progressive systemic sclerosis Achalasia of the esophagus Cancer
Stomach	Hiatus hernia Gastric ulcer Acute gastritis Chronic gastritis Giant hypertrophic gastritis Post-gastrectomy syndrome Pyloric stenosis Zollinger-Ellison syndrome Cancer
Duodenum	Duodenal ulcer
Exocrine pancreas	Acute pancreatitis Chronic pancreatitis Cancer
Small intestine	Tropical sprue Acute enteritis Gluten-sensitive enteropathy Progressive systemic sclerosis Whipple's disease Intestinal lymphagiectasia Crohn's disease (Regional enteritis) Malignant lymphomas Carcinoid tumors Radiation enteritis Amyloidosis Mesenteric arterial insufficiency and infarction

TABLE 2-1   (Continued)

SITE	DISEASE
Large intestine	Crohn's disease
	Ulcerative colitis
	Diverticulosis
	Diverticulitis
	Appendicitis
	Ischemic colitis
	Colonic polyposis
	Cancer of the colon or rectum

Adapted from I. A. D. Bouchier, *Gastroenterology*, 2nd Ed. (London: Bailliere Tindall, 1977).

vomiting of blood, is most often silent except for a gradual onset of anemia. Upper GI bleeding is characteristic of disease of the esophagus and particularly the stomach. Common causes in the elderly are listed in Table 2-3.

Rectal bleeding with blood in the stool may be caused by colon or rectal cancer. Other common causes are diverticulosis and ischemic (atherosclerotic) colonic diseases.

Diarrhea

Causes of diarrhea can be divided into causes of acute and of chronic diarrhea. Acute (or short duration) diarrhea occurs in the presence of bacterial gastroenteritis, pseudomembranous colitis (due to drugs), and

TABLE 2-2   Diseases of the Elderly Associated with Dysphagia

Acute	Pharyngitis } due to infection, drugs, radiation
	Stomatitis }
	Pharyngeal abscess
	Foreign body
	Trauma, including surgery
	Esophagitis
Chronic	Neurological disorders*
	Oropharyngeal tumors
	Xerostomia
	Plummer Vinson syndrome
	Esophageal strictures
	Reflux esophagitis
	Systemic sclerosis
	Esophageal ulcer
	Esophageal cancer
	Zenker's diverticulum

*Commonly late effects of cerebrovascular accidents, amyotrophic lateral sclerosis of Alzheimer's disease.

Adapted from J. Loren Pitcher, "Dysphagia in the elderly: causes and diagnosis," *Geriatrics*, 28 (1973), 64–69.

TABLE 2-3   Causes of Upper GI Bleeding in the Elderly

Gastritis due to aspirin
Esophageal varices associated with alcoholic cirrhosis
Gastric or duodenal ulcer
Esophageal tear
Esophagitis
Cancer of the esophagus or stomach

Adapted from E. L. Rogers, "Emergency management of gastrointestinal bleeding," *Geriatrics*, 35 (1980), 35–40.

laxative abuse. Chronic diarrhea is characteristic of inflammatory bowel disease, including regional enteritis and diseases of the small intestine which lead to maldigestion and malabsorption. Maldigestion occurs in diseases shown in Table 2-4. Malabsorption occurs in diseases shown in Table 2-5 on page 34.

In the elderly, when diarrhea is associated with abdominal pain, acute ischemic colitis is a common cause. Frequent, very small stools occur with fecal impaction.

Constipation

Constipation is related to low dietary fiber ingestion and debility. Misuse of laxatives as well as diverticular disease causes intermittent constipation. Constipation of short duration is usually due to colon pathology, including colon cancer. Chronic constipation occurs in hypothyroidism and early ischemic colitis and with drugs, including narcotic analgesics.

TABLE 2-4   Causes of Maldigestion of Fat in the Elderly

Due to decreased production, activity, release or contact with:
  Pancreatic lipase
  Chronic pancreatitis
  Cancer of the pancreas
  Gastric surgery (partial or total gastrectomy)
  Zollinger–Ellison syndrome
  Neomycin therapy
Due to decreased quantity of bile acids:
  Obstructive jaundice
  Hepatocellular disease
  Ileal resection
  Cholestyramine therapy
  Crohn's disease
  Bacterial overgrowth in the small intestine due to blind loops, diverticula, progressive systemic sclerosis, diabetes, partial obstruction, fistulae or amyloidosis

Adapted from W. M. Steinberg and P. P. Toskes, "A practical approach to evaluating maldigestion and malabsorption," *Geriatrics*, 33 (1978), 73–85.

TABLE 2-5   Causes of Malabsorption in the Elderly

Decreased number of absorptive cells due to intestinal resection.

Mucosal and submucosal disease or damage including tropical sprue, gluten-sensitive enteropathy, progressive systemic sclerosis, blind loop syndrome (bacterial overgrowth in small intestine), amyloidosis, ischemic bowel disease, drugs including neomycin, colchicine and methotrexate.

Decrease in lymphatic drainage due to:
Intestinal lymphangiectasia
Lymphoma
Congestive heart failure
Constrictive pericarditis
Abdominal tuberculosis
Whipple's disease
Crohn's disease

Transfer defect
Pernicious anemia
Alcohol abuse

Causes of malabsorption unknown
Drug-associated, laxatives and cathartics
Hormonally mediated—carcinoid, hypoparathyroidism, and hyperthyroidism
Addison's disease, mast cell disease
Parasitic diseases, e.g. giardiasis

Adapted from I. A. D. Bouchier, *Gastroenterology*, 2nd Ed. (London: Bailliere Tindall, 1977), p. 84.

Abdominal Pain

Common causes of acute abdominal pain are the following:

1. Intestinal obstruction (caused by cancer, volvulus, or appendicitis)
2. Acute myocardial infarction
3. Cardiac failure
4. Lung disease plus pleural involvement
5. Disease of the urinary tract
6. Acute cholecystitis
7. Acute pancreatitis
8. Acute mesenteric infarction
9. Dissecting aneurysm

A common cause of chronic or recurrent abdominal pain is cancer of the pancreas.

It should be remembered that causes of abdominal pain in the elderly may be local or referred and may be from disease of the GI tract or disease of other organs.

DISEASES OF THE CARDIOVASCULAR SYSTEM

Atherosclerosis is a progressive degenerative condition of the arteries, characterized by appearance of fatty streaks (cholesterol deposits), fibrous plaques, and raised lesions as deep as and involving the inner arterial lining. Complications involving the raised lesions are ulceration, calcification, and thrombosis. Thrombosis of an arteriosclerotic artery leads to occlusion, which results in partial or complete loss of arterial blood supply to tissues normally receiving blood from this vessel (Hurst et al., 1974).

Atherosclerotic changes in the arteries begin in childhood, but clinical signs of atherosclerosis do not usually appear until later in life. An exception is when a kindred or individuals within families with a genetic trait have antecedent hypercholesterolemia resulting from inborn errors of lipoprotein metabolism.

Risk factors for the development of atherosclerotic vascular disease are genetic factors, male sex, high intake of cholesterol and saturated fat, hypercholesterolemia, cigarette smoking, diabetes, hypertension, possibly oral hypoglycemic agents, and stress-related and/or type A behavior pattern. (Type A behavior indicates excessive competitiveness, aggressiveness, restlessness, haste, and impatience [Friedman and Roseman, 1959].) Softness of the drinking water has also been associated with death caused by atherosclerotic heart disease (Vavrik, 1974).

Factors conditioning the distribution of atherosclerotic lesions within the cardiovascular system include the internal diameter of the artery and multiple factors related to local blood flow and blood pressure.

Manifestations of atherosclerotic vascular disease are myocardial infarction (heart attack), angina pectoris, cerebral thrombosis and cerebral hemorrhage (both commonly designated as strokes), cerebrovascular ischemic episodes (minor strokes), atherosclerotic leg ulcers, and gangrene and uremia caused by atherosclerosis of the renal vessels.

Morbidity and mortality from specific atherosclerotic vascular diseases are influenced by factors which directly or indirectly affect atherosclerotic development in particular organs. For example, strokes are the end results in hypertensives of atherosclerosis of the arteries of the brain and particularly of the middle cerebral artery.

Proximate causes of death in people with atherosclerotic vascular diseases are:

1. Heart attack
2. Cardiac failure
3. Respiratory failure
4. Stroke
5. Hemorrhage or shock from auto accidents sustained during heart attacks
6. Carbon monoxide poisoning

COMMON RESPIRATORY DISEASES

Chronic bronchitis has been so defined on the basis of symptoms including chronic cough and sputum production. Etiological factors include smoking, air pollution, and recurrent respiratory infection. The disorder consists of obstructive inflammation of the smaller air passages. Patients with chronic bronchitis are at particular risk of developing pneumonia.

Pulmonary emphysema occurs with aging but is far more extensive in elderly people who are or have been smokers. Both chronic bronchitis and emphysema cause progressive reduction in pulmonary function. Associated breathlessness may cause the patient to reduce food intake (Barnett, 1972).

The *pneumonias* are acute or chronic diseases of the lungs, characterized by "consolidation" of the alveoli or a filling up of these air sacs with inflammatory cells and fluid. Pneumonia may be caused by bacterial, viral, fungus, or mold infection or by inhalation of vomited food or inert substances, such as mineral oil. Despite the availability of antibiotics, pneumonias are life threatening to the elderly, especially to those whose immune function is compromised by malnutrition or cancer chemotherapeutic drugs.

Influenza pneumonia is particularly serious in the aged, particularly in elderly people with pre-existing cardiac and respiratory disease, in whom it is likely to lead to respiratory failure. High fever, cough, malaise, and chest pain caused by accompanying pleurisy reduce food intake. Low intake of food and the catabolic effects of the disease can rapidly lead to protein-energy malnutrition (Hook, 1972).

The development of *carcinoma,* or *cancer, of the lung* has been clearly associated with cigarette smoking. Cancer is more likely to develop in emphysematous lungs than in nonemphysematous lungs. Occupational exposure to carcinogens (such as occurs in men working for a long time around coke ovens) can also cause lung cancer. Peak incidence is in the sixth decade of life, but occurrence in the elderly is also common. Early stages of lung cancer are asymptomatic. Symptoms include cough, chest pain, hemoptysis (coughing up of blood), and symptoms of pneumonia. Systemic manifestations include fever, phlebitis, and most important for the nutritionist, anorexia and rapid weight loss. With metastatic lung cancer, particularly when liver metastases are present, the sense of smell is often perverted so that meat tastes rotten. Tolerance of cancer chemotherapy or radiation therapy is related to nutritional support (Pool, 1972; Bergevin, 1976).

RENAL DISEASE

The physiological decline in functional capacity of the kidney is symptom free and does not per se cause renal failure, because of its normal functional reserve (Epstein, 1979).

Renal disease of the elderly is commonly chronic. Chronic diseases of the kidney in the elderly include conditions arising in later life as well as end stages of pre-existing disease. Common to many diseases of the kidney are the signs of chronic renal failure (uremia), including polyuria (passage of large volumes of dilute urine); neurological signs such as headache, convulsions, tremor, and coma; and bleeding episodes. Secondary bone disease may occur both because of impaired metabolic synthesis of the active form of vitamin D in the kidney and because of secondary hyperparathyroidism. Anemia may be caused by the bleeding episodes, but a more common cause is failure of the diseased kidney to produce erythropoietin, a hormone-like substance which normally stimulates red cell production and output from the bone marrow into the blood stream. General signs of uremia include nausea, anorexia, and vomiting. Low output of urine (oliguria) and failure of urinary output (anuria) may occur terminally. Renovascular hypertension is a major complication of chronic renal disease.

Laboratory data indicative of renal disease in the elderly include elevation of the blood urea and blood urea nitrogen. Increased serum creatinine is present, but levels are less indicative of renal failure than in the younger patients because of diminished production of creatinine by the elderly.

Diseases of the elderly which commonly lead to chronic renal failure are chronic nephritis, chronic pyelonephritis, and renovascular disease, which may be associated with diabetes. Other causes of renal failure in the elderly are lupus nephritis and renal complications of systemic sclerosis. Pyelonephritis (inflammatory disease of the kidney) may be secondary to obstructive renal disease (kidney stones). Acute renal failure in the elderly is most often caused by an adverse drug reaction.

Causes of oliguria in the elderly male include prostatic enlargement caused by simple hypertrophy or by cancer that obstructs urine outflow. Urinary retention can be caused by prostatic disease or disease of the bladder (Rosen, 1976).

DIABETES

Diabetes in the elderly may be insulin dependent or insulin insensitive. When diabetes develops in later life, it is commonly of non-insulin dependent (NIDDM) type. Glucose tolerance decreases with age, and there is a decreased response of the beta cells of the Islets of Langerhans of the pancreas to a rise in blood sugar. However, the glucose uptake of the tissues in response to insulin does not appear to be age related. When a glucose load is given to older people, their blood sugar (glucose) levels increase more than in younger persons, and the return of the blood glucose to preload levels is slower.

Risk factors for the development of NIDDM include genetic predisposition, prolonged excessive food-energy intake, obesity, and genetically determined hyperlipoproteinemias. The assumption that diabetes of this type is related to high carbohydrate intakes now seems untenable, unless the high carbohydrate intake is also associated with high total food-energy intake. It has been shown that approximately 75 percent of patients with maturity-onset diabetes are obese at the time that diabetes is diagnosed (Gerritsen, 1976). Reduction in energy expenditure and increase in food intake may account for the increased prevalence of diabetes in developing societies within and outside the United States (e.g., Pima Indians and Polynesians). Plasma insulin levels are high in maturity-onset diabetes, but the level decreases when weight reduction is achieved. In the elderly, reduction in body weight alone may be sufficient to control the diabetes.

Whereas diabetes in the elderly is usually of the insulin-insensitive type, insulin-dependent or insulin-requiring diabetes may also be found among older people. Older people with insulin-dependent diabetes are (1) those who have had this form of diabetes since early or middle life and (2) those who have developed insulin insensitivity (maturity-onset diabetes) and in whom the diabetic state has changed over time. It has been postulated that in the obese with maturity-onset diabetes overfunctioning of the pancreas with hyperproduction of insulin can lead to a state of exhaustion of the beta cells of the pancreas. Although this theory is not generally accepted, it is true that with time some patients who have not previously required insulin may alter their diabetic state such that they require insulin for glucose homeostasis and control of the diabetic state.

Older diabetics without complications of the disease show few, if any, physical signs of a specific nature. Complaints and physical findings which should alert the physician to investigate for the presence of the disease are:

1. *Generalized or local itching.* The itching is frequently localized to the scalp, although it may involve the hands, feet, or legs.
2. *Dermatitis.* The diabetic may develop dermatitis in areas which are persistently scratched because of intractable itching. Dermatitis in skinfolds (intertrigo) is common, and infections in these areas are usually caused by yeasts or fungi. Severe mycotic infection of the feet and legs is common (athlete's foot). The athlete's foot may show moist macerated lesions between the toes and blisters on the feet, as in the classic form, but more often lesions are dry and scaly and may extend both over the feet and up the legs. Involvement of the toenails with the fungus infection is also very common. This leads to a distortion and thickening of nail growth.
3. *Boils and abscesses.* Recurrent boils that are slow to heal, as well as carbuncles (infection of multiple hair follicles with cellulitis), are common in diabetics. "Silent infections" of the feet, with large collar stud abscesses, occur in diabetics who have sensory loss in the feet. They are unable to feel the pain from stepping on small objects, resulting in injury to the sole of the foot which, if untreated, may infect and produce a large abscess in the deep tissues of the sole.
4. *Neuropathies.* Elderly people may complain of pain in the legs, particularly the lower legs, which is often burning in character and may only occur at night. The pain is usually associated with unpleasant sensations in the feet and lower legs, including prickling; excessive or abnormal perception of heat, cold, pain or touch; and/or a feeling that he or she is walking on cotton.

5. *Failing vision.* Failing vision is a common complaint of elderly diabetics. The condition may be caused by cataract or diabetic retinopathy. Diabetic retinopathy is associated with obliterative changes occurring in the retinal arterioles. Retinal ischemia occurs as well as microaneurysms, hemorrhage, and exudates. This ischemic retinal disorder can lead to blindness, which may be unilateral or bilateral.

Frequently in the elderly the classical symptoms of diabetes, including excessive thirst and excessive urination, do not occur. Excessive thirst is uncommon in elderly diabetics; excessive urination (polyuria) may occur but is frequently confused by the elderly patient with frequency of urination associated with increasing age.

Common complications of diabetes in the elderly include cardiovascular accidents. High-risk factors in the development of atherosclerotic cardiovascular disease are diabetes, hypertension, and hypercholesterolemia. Arterial disease is the most common cause of death in diabetics over the age of 50, and the mortality rate for these diseases is much higher than in nondiabetic persons. Ischemic heart disease and peripheral arterial disease are particularly common. Peripheral arterial disease is the precursor of gangrene. Because elderly diabetics often have poor eyesight and impaired sensation in the feet (because of neuropathy) as well as an increased susceptibility to cutaneous infection (because of the presence of glucose in sweat), trivial injuries to the feet are common, and these are very likely to become infected. The infection is often neglected and may progress to tissue necrosis, and this, together with the impaired circulation to the foot, leads to a gangrenous state which may progress to a "wet" gangrene, requiring amputation.

Diabetic retinopathy, as described above, may lead to blindness and is indeed the most important ocular complication of diabetes which can result in loss of eyesight.

Although vascular complications are particularly common in elderly diabetics having the insulin-insensitive form of the disease, in insulin-requiring diabetics, diabetic ketoacidosis may develop. Prognosis is poor in severe diabetic ketoacidosis in the elderly unless treatment is prompt. Insulin reactions may also occur because of hypoglycemia. Diabetic nephropathy leading to end-stage renal failure is more likely to occur in diabetics of the insulin-requiring type (Passmore and Robson, 1974).

ANEMIAS

Anemias in the elderly, as in other age groups, may be nutritional or nonnutritional in origin. Common types of anemia and etiological factors are summarized in Table 2-6 on next page.

Iron deficiency anemia may be caused by low iron intake, which is particularly likely when the daily diet is low in food energy and consists of foods which are of low total iron content. Inadequate intake of heme iron may also contribute to iron deficiency, since heme iron is better utilized

TABLE 2-6   Classification of Anemias of the Elderly and Common Etiological Factors

TYPE OF ANEMIA	ETIOLOGY
Microcytic hypochromic anemia Iron deficiency	a. Low iron intake b. Intake of foods/beverages which decrease iron absorption c. Blood loss due to disease or drugs
Vitamin B₆ deficiency	a. Drugs, alcohol
Macrocytic hyperchromic anemia Folacin deficiency	a. Low folacin intake b. Malabsorption due to disease or drugs c. Intake of folate antagonists d. Intake of drugs which increase catabolism of folacin
Vitamin B₁₂ deficiency	a. Pernicious anemia b. Vegan diet c. Ileal resection or disease d. Postgastrectomy anemia
Hemolytic anemia	a. Drugs ± glucose-6-phosphate dehydrogenase deficiency (G6PD deficiency)
Aplastic anemia	a. Drugs, radiation to bone marrow, cancer, leukemia
Hypoplastic anemia	a. Erythropoietin deficiency in end-stage renal disease

Adapted from B. A. Brown, *Hematology: Principles and Procedures* (Philadelphia: Lea & Febiger, 1973), p. 191.

than non-heme iron. Other factors of dietary origin which increase the risk of iron deficiency anemia are low intake of ascorbic acid and high intakes of foods or beverages which contain non-nutrient substances. Iron absorption is decreased by high intake of tea (because of formation of iron tannates), oatmeal (because of formation of iron phytates), and bran (because of absorption of iron on fiber particles). In the elderly, chronic blood loss is a frequent cause of anemia. The major route of chronic blood loss is the GI tract. Causes of blood loss via the GI tract are (1) high and prolonged intake of aspirin or indomethacin, (2) hemorrhage from colonic or diverticular polyps, and (3) hemorrhage from colon or rectal cancer. Blood loss from leaking esophageal varices may cause iron deficiency anemia in alcoholics with cirrhosis.

Nutritional macrocytic anemia in the elderly is most commonly caused by inadequate intake of dietary folacin. Low intake of foods rich in folacin, such as raw and cooked green, leafy vegetables and liver, is particularly likely with advanced age. Also, the aged, because of lack of familiarity with or dislike of fortified cold breakfast cereals, may not obtain synthetic folic acid from this source. Folacin malabsorption occurs in elderly people who are alcoholics, and also in those with GI disease, including systemic sclerosis, mesenteric vascular insufficiency, tropical sprue, gluten-sensitive enteropathy, chronic radiation enteritis, and intestinal resection. Drugs contributing to the production of folacin deficiency in the elderly include phenytoin, barbiturates, glutethimide, and folate antagonists, including methotrexate and triamterene. In the elderly, folacin deficiency also has been associated with congestive heart failure and with chronic liver disease, whether or not this is alcoholic cirrhosis.

Vitamin B_{12} deficiency in the elderly is most commonly caused by pernicious anemia. Pernicious anemia results from an autoimmune process, whereby gastric intrinsic factor is no longer produced or is produced in inadequate amounts, causing insufficient vitamin B_{12} absorption. Pernicious anemia is particularly liable to occur in Caucasians of Northern European origin. Patients may show signs of dyspnea caused by severe anemia, weakness, loss of balance, and sensory changes, including parasthesias in the lower limbs. Vitamin B_{12} deficiency occurs less commonly in the elderly as a late complication after partial or total gastrectomy or after ilial resection. A rare cause of vitamin B_{12} deficiency is prolonged adherence to a totally vegetarian (vegan) diet.

Sideroblastic anemia caused by vitamin B_6 deficiency may occur in elderly alcoholics or may be caused by intake of drugs which are vitamin B_6 antagonists, including isonicotinic acid hydrazide or hydralazine.

Hemolytic anemias may occur in older people, usually because of ingestion of drugs which carry a risk of immunologically determined hemolysis. The drug methyldopa is a cause of a hemolytic anemia of this type. In the elderly, as in younger people, susceptibility to drug-induced hemolytic anemia is markedly increased if they carry the genotype of glucose-6-phosphate dehydrogenase deficiency.

Aplastic anemia in the elderly may be drug induced or may follow chronic radiation to long bones for the treatment of cancer. Metastatic involvement of bone marrow by cancer can also lead to aplastic anemia, and chronic leukemia can lead to aplasia of normal cells of the hemopoietic system.

Anemia is commonly present in elderly people with end-stage renal disease because of inadequate synthesis and release of the renal hormone erythropoietin.

Studies of elderly anemic patients have indicated that anemia was secondary to underlying disease in about 50 percent of the cases. Patients with anemia caused by underlying disease rather than an inadequate intake of nutrients required in hemopoiesis may fail to respond to hematinics, including iron and folic acid (Baker, Jaslow, and Frank, 1978). In elderly hospitalized patients, severe anemias with very low hemoglobin values have been most commonly found in patients with GI bleeding, chronic renal disease, pernicious and hemolytic anemia, and hypothyroidism. Elderly patients with metastatic cancer as well as those with chronic infections, i.e., tuberculosis or recurrent infections, including those of the urinary tract, may exhibit anemia. Causes of anemia in cancer and in infection include inadequate intake of iron and folacin, increased or decreased life span of red blood cells, block in the release of iron from storage sites, or a combination of these factors. Blood loss is a common cause of anemia in cancer patients (Kalchthaler and Tan, 1980)

ORGANIC BRAIN SYNDROMES

The term "organic brain syndrome" is used to denote a group of disorders associated with loss of mental function caused by a known pathology in the absence of manic-depressive psychosis and other psychiatric illnesses. Organic brain syndromes now include Alzheimer's disease and other diseases of the brain which disturb cerebration and other brain functions. Table 2-7 gives a classification of organic brain syndromes grouped according to type and cause.

Alzheimer's Disease

Alzheimer's disease is a progressive, degenerative condition of the brain which always causes dementia. The disease can be considered to

TABLE 2-7 Classification of Organic Brain Syndromes in the Elderly

CLASSIFICATION	SYNDROMES	CAUSE
Nutritional	Korsakoff's syndrome	Thiamin deficiency in alcoholics
	Pellagrous psychosis	Niacin deficiency
	Pernicious anemia (mental changes in)	Vitamin B_{12} deficiency
	Nutritional dementia	Folacin deficiency
Metabolic	Myxedema	Hypothyroidism
	Uremia	End stage renal disease (e.g. chronic nephritis)
Toxic	Drug-induced encephalopathies	Alcohol
		Morphine
		Barbiturates
		Phenothiazines
Vascular	"Stroke" [atherosclerotic brain atrophy]	Cerebrovascular atherosclerosis + hypertension
Neoplastic	"Brain cancer"	Primary or secondary malignant brain tumor
Infective	General paralysis of the insane	Syphilis
Degenerative	Alzheimer's disease	Unknown
	Senile dementia	Unknown

Adapted from A. McGee Harvey, R. J. Johns, V. A. McKusick, A. H. Owens, and R. S. Ross, *The Principles and Practice of Medicine*, 20th Ed. (Englewood Cliffs, NJ: Prentice-Hall, Inc., 1980), p. 1193.

represent a cerebral form of premature aging, although in syndromes of premature aging such as Werner's syndrome, signs of Alzheimer's disease are absent. A familial form of Alzheimer's disease is recognized in which the disease is transmitted as an autosomal dominant trait. In families in which this form of the disease occurs, clinical signs appear earlier, sometimes by the age of 40-45 years. The disease is otherwise similar both in evolution and neuropathology to that of the non-familial form which usually does not become clinically apparent until the individual is over the age of 65 years. The gene defect in familial Alzheimer's disease (FAD) has been localized to chromosome 21. This is of particular interest in that this is also the aberrant gene in Down's syndrome, in which, if survival to adult life occurs, an Alzheimer's type dementia may supervene. The so-called non-FAD form of Alzheimer's disease, which makes its appearance later, may also have a genetic etiology (Gusella, 1989).

Three stages are defined. In the first stage, which may last from 2 to 4 years, there is loss of memory, spatial disorientation, and a lack of spontaneous emotional response. The second stage is characterized by progressive dementia with peculiar focal signs, including inability to identify or interpret familiar sounds (including the spoken word), sights, or smell. In the third stage, seizures develop and speech is lost. The patient is indifferent to his or her environment. Compulsive eating may occur, with consumption of inedible objects. More commonly all interest in food is lost, and when the patient is fed, food is pushed out of his or her mouth by tongue movement.

Autopsy examination reveals atrophy of the brain, a reduction in brain weight, loss of cortical neurons, and widespread neurofibrillary tangles. The cause of Alzheimer's disease is unknown (Sowrander and Sjögren, 1970).

HUNTINGTON'S DISEASE

Huntington's disease, formerly known as Huntington's chorea, is a degenerative neurological disease that is transmitted by an autosomal dominant gene. The disease usually begins between the ages of 35 and 50 years. After onset, the average length of life is about 16 years. The disease is characterized in its early stages by sinuous (choreiform) movements of the arms, cognitive loss, and marked personality changes. Later the movements involve the lower limbs and the trunk, and, unless the patient is sedated, the movements continue night and day. Because of the large energy expenditure associated with these movements, those with the late form of the disease become extremely wasted (Henderson and Gillespie, 1943). Severe weight loss can be minimized by providing sufficient food-energy to balance the energy expenditure. It is not unusual for these patients to require 4000 calories a day. However, whether or not the food is actually consumed depends both on appropriate drug therapy to lessen head movements and on skilled nursing care.

CEREBROVASCULAR DISEASE

Cerebrovascular disease occurs as a complication of hypertension that, in the elderly, is usually associated with cerebral atherosclerosis. In the common multi-infarct syndrome, patients have frequent transient ischemic episodes in which areas of the brain are deprived of their normal blood supply. Long-term effects include loss of recent memory, periodic confusion, and the loss of cognitive skills. The ability to prepare food may be limited or lost. It is particularly difficult for the person to prepare a special diet that may have been prescribed. In addition, choking attacks may occur or the patient may complain of difficulty in swallowing.

Late effects of stroke also include hemiplegia, which causes partial paralysis of one side of the body and which also impairs the individual's ability to purchase and prepare food (Wilcock and Middleton, 1984).

KORSAKOFF'S PSYCHOSIS

Korsakoff's psychosis, which is a late effect of thiamin deficiency in alcoholics, is characterized by memory loss and a degree of cognitive loss that usually prohibits independent living. Special nutritional risks of elderly individuals with this disease include protein-energy malnutrition which is secondary to inadequate intake or secondary to co-existent alcoholic liver disease. Dietary assessment requires direct observation of the patient since confabulation is usual, and the ability to remember what was actually eaten is lost (Dreyfus, 1974).

SUBACUTE COMBINED SYSTEM DISEASE

Subacute combined system disease is the neurological disorder which occurs from vitamin B_{12} (cobalamin) deficiency. Until recently, it was assumed that this condition always occurred in association with megaloblastic anemia, However, cases have been described of vitamin B_{12} deficiency with this neuropsychiatric illness in which the megaloblastic anemia has been absent (Lindenbaum et al., 1988). Signs include ataxia, sensory loss, and mental confusion. Marked improvement occurs following injections of vitamin B_{12}.

ORGANIC BRAIN SYNDROMES AND NUTRITION

Organic brain syndromes may be nutritional in origin, caused by thiamin, niacin, folacin, or vitamin B_{12} deficiencies. Reversibility of these syndromes may be possible, but nutritional therapy is not always successful because of irreversible brain changes. Organic brain syndromes always result early in diminished ability to obtain and prepare food. In the later stages, intake of food is severely reduced. Patients have to be fed, and even then food is frequently not swallowed and may be pushed out of the mouth (Roth, 1978).

CHRONIC NEUROLOGICAL DISEASE

Parkinson's disease is a degenerative condition of the basal ganglia of the brain in which production of the neurotransmitter dopamine is greatly reduced. The disease is characterized by slowness of movement *(bradykinesia)*, rigidity, tremor, and loss of facial expression. Treatment is with levo-dopa given in combination with a peripheral decarboxylase inhibitor (Yahr, 1975; McGee-Harvey et al., 1980).

DEPRESSION

Depression in the elderly may be due to a long-term manic depressive psychosis or, quite commonly, to antihypertensive therapy with β-Adrenergic drugs such as propranolol. Other less common causes include hypothyroidism and pellagra. Elderly individuals with depression do not show cognitive impairment but their decision making may be extremely poor. The loss of decision-making skills often makes food selection very difficult. Depressed elderly are also very preoccupied with bodily functions, particularly bowel function. This preoccupation may lead to laxative abuse with the subsequent risk of hypokalemia and malabsorption. Depressive episodes are best treated with small doses of tricyclic antidepressants, which can completely relieve the symptoms. However, recurrence of the depression is likely to occur when treatment is discontinued. β-Adrenergic blocking agents should be avoided (Blazer, 1989).

GERIATRIC DISEASES OF THE MUSCULOSKELETAL SYSTEM

Diseases of the musculoskeletal system which are commonly seen in older people may begin in later life or may develop in youth or middle age and be progressive or more disabling with age. The relationship of joint and bone diseases of the elderly to the aging process is popularly accepted, but except in the case of osteoporosis this theory remains largely unproven (Garn, 1975). Genetic and acquired factors determine the occurrence, localization of the disease process, severity, complications, and disability of musculoskeletal diseases in the elderly.

Common musculoskeletal diseases which begin in middle or later life include osteoarthrosis, pseudogout, osteoporosis, Paget's disease, infectious arthritis, and rheumatic polymyalgia (Smith, 1976). Characteristics of these diseases are summarized in Table 2-8 on pages 46 and 47. Whereas these diseases all occur in both sexes, osteoporosis and osteomalacia are more common in women.

Diseases of muscle, connective tissue, joints, and bone which usually start in early life but are seen as major causes of disability in older people include polymyositis, progressive systemic sclerosis, rheumatoid arthritis,

TABLE 2-8 Characteristics of Common Musculoskeletal Diseases in the Elderly

DISEASE	USUAL AGE OF ONSET	PATHOLOGY	SYMPTOMS	COMPLICATIONS AND DISABILITY	ETIOLOGY/RISK FACTORS
Osteoarthrosis	50 or above	Cartilage degeneration Bony outgrowths	Pain on motion Stiffness after rest	Limp Deformity Muscle wasting	Preexisting disease of the joints Trauma Obesity Acromegaly Gram toxin Intracellular corticosteroids Aging(?)
Pseudogout (Chondrocalcinosis)	60 or above	Calcium pyrophosphate in joint fluid Acute recurrent or chronic arthritis	Pain Joint swelling	Intermittent or progressive lameness	Diabetes Parathyroid disease Hypothyroidism Aging(?)
Osteoporosis	40 or above	Progressive reduction in skeletal mass	None except with fractures	Fracture of femoral neck Compressed fracture vertebra	Aging Menopause Disuse Alcoholism Low calcium intake

Disease	Age	Pathology	Symptoms	Signs	Causes
Osteomalacia	70	Decalcification of bone Incomplete fractures	Bone pain Bone tenderness Muscle weakness	Deformities of spine, chest, pelvis, and legs	Vitamin D deficiency Lack of sunlight Low intake vitamin D Drug intake (barbiturates, diphenylhydantoin)
Paget's disease	40 or above	Disorganized bone structure Sarcoma as complication	Bone pain Girdle pain	Deformity of long bones Enlargement of head	Unknown
Infectious arthritis	60 or above	Joint infection	Pain Fever	Joint destruction	Diabetes Cancer Alcoholism Uremia Pneumonia Subacute bacterial endocarditis
Rheumatic polymyalgia	50 or above	Tuberculosis Fungi Giant cells Arteritis	Shoulder or pelvic stiffness and pain Morning stiffness Fatigue	Intermittent claudication Raynaud's phenomena Headache Loss of vision	Unknown

Adapted from A. McGee Harvey et al., 1980, p. 1165.

ankylosing spondylitis, psoriatic arthropathy, and alveolar bone loss with periodontal disease (Brenenstock and Fernanto, 1976).

CANCER

The increased incidence of cancer and other malignant diseases in the elderly has three main causes:

1. Long-term exposure to environmental carcinogens, including diet-related carcinogens, smoking, ultraviolet light, and industrial chemicals
2. Failure of cellular immune defense mechanisms against cancer, usually age related
3. Inadequate treatment of precancerous conditions, e.g., Plummer-Vinson syndrome associated with chronic iron deficiency or other precancerous conditions, including actinic keratoses and leukoplakia. (Diagnosis of cancer in the elderly may be missed because symptoms are confused with those of other diseases common in the elderly.)

Common forms of cancer in the elderly are (1) cancer of the breast, (2) cancer of the colon and rectum, (3) cancer of the lung, (4) cancer of the pancreas, (5) cancer of the uterus, (6) cancer of the prostate, (7) cancer of the bladder, and (8) cancer of the skin (Pool, 1975; Bergevin, 1976). Common symptoms and/or signs which point to cancer of one or the other of these organs are summarized in Table 2-9, which also indicates the nutritional significance of particular clinical indicators of these cancers.

Paraneoplastic syndromes may develop in patients with cancer and are either caused by secretion of hormones or other biologically active compounds by the tumor cells or represent autoimmune phenomena. Some of these syndromes have adverse nutritional effects (see Table 2-10). These syndromes are usually resolved with effective or temporarily suppressive therapy of the underlying cancer.

Leukemia

Recent mortality statistics indicate a rise in details from leukemia in the elderly. Whether this represents a true increase in the incidence of leukemia has been questioned. An alternate and plausible explanation of the increased reported deaths from leukemia in older age groups is improved diagnosis, whereby more cases of leukemia are identified.

Acute leukemia occurs most frequently in two groups: children under 5 years old and adults over 60. Chronic myeloid leukemia is most common in people over 50. Chronic lymphatic leukemia is essentially a disease of the elderly, with the incidence increasing with age.

Signs of leukemia may include (1) profound and progressive weakness, (2) weight loss, (3) breathlessness (caused by anemia), (4) hemorrhage, (5) enlargement of the abdomen (caused by progressive increase in the size of the spleen and/or lymphatic masses), and (6) susceptibility to infection.

TABLE 2-9 Symptoms and Signs of Common Forms of Cancer in the Elderly with Their Nutritional Significance

SITE OF CANCER	PRESENTING SIGNS	NUTRITIONAL EFFECT (early)
Breast	Mass Nipple discharge	
Colon and Rectum	Change in bowel habit Rectal bleeding Reduction in blood pressure	Iron deficiency anemia
Lung	Cough, wheeze, sputum Fever, chest pain	Loss of weight
Pancreas	Jaundice	
Uterus	Vaginal bleeding	Iron deficiency anemia
Prostate	Difficulty in urination Urinary retention	
Bladder	Blood in the urine Painful urination	Iron deficiency anemia
Skin	"Spot," "mole," nodule or ulcer that does not heal	

Adapted from M. E. Shils, "Nutritional problems induced by cancer," *Med. Clin. N. Amer.*, 63 (1979), 1011.

Chronic lymphatic leukemia is frequently asymptomatic in the elderly. Symptoms which may be present in this disease include breathlessness associated with anemia, cardiorespiratory embarrassment, jaundice caused by hemolysis, bleeding into the skin or from mucous membranes caused by thrombocytopenia, and pain caused by intestinal obstruction or glandular masses pressing on nerves. Weight loss and profound weakness also occur.

TABLE 2-10 Paraneoplastic (Ectopic Hormone) Syndromes, and Their Adverse Nutritional Effects

ENDOCRINE DISORDER	TUMOR ASSOCIATION	ADVERSE NUTRITIONAL AND METABOLIC EFFECTS
ACTH syndrome	Ca. lung Ca. pancreas	Weakness Hypokalemia
Inappropriate antidiuretic hormone secretion	Ca. lung	Urinary sodium wastage Hyponatremia
Ectopic parahormone secretion	Ca. kidney Ca. lung	Hypercalcemia
Ectopic insulin production	Ca. liver Ca. adrenal	Hypoglycemia
Serotonin hyperproduction	Carcinoid	Pellagra

Adapted from A. McGee Harvey et al., 1980, p. 592.

Treatment of leukemia is by chemotherapy and/or radiation therapy. Decision to treat chronic lymphatic leukemia in the elderly is based on the presence or absence of symptoms such as anemia, hemorrhage, glandular masses, or weight loss (Gibson, 1974).

INTERRELATIONSHIPS OF DISEASE PROCESSES

Disease processes which are found in life or at autopsy of the elderly may be of recent origin (acute), or they may be of long standing (chronic). Acute diseases such as pneumonia may be superimposed on chronic disease and may be the immediate cause of death (Hook, 1972). Origin, course, and outcome of disease processes of the elderly are illustrated in Figure 2-2. The process of aging predisposes elderly persons to certain diseases, including cancer, maturity-onset diabetes, osteoporosis, and autoimmune diseases such as pernicious anemia. On the other hand, chronic disease in the elderly may be the end result of disease which has developed over many years but which was originally independent of the aging process. Examples of such disease are congestive heart failure caused by rheumatic heart disease and chronic nephritis following long-term use of the drug phenacetin (Vavrik, 1974; Rosen, 1976). Widespread atherosclerosis in the elderly is the end result of a disease which developed slowly over many years. Malnutrition may develop in the elderly as a result of inadequate diet, disease, drugs, or a combination of these factors. Further, the elderly who are conspicuous users of medications and have a diminished drug tolerance are prone to develop adverse drug reactions which contribute to

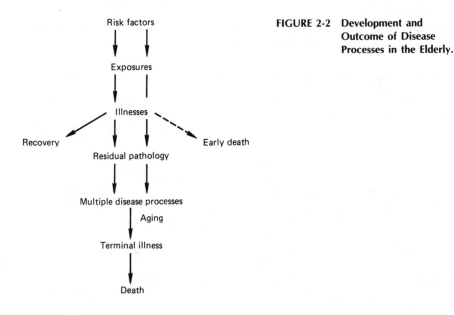

FIGURE 2-2 Development and Outcome of Disease Processes in the Elderly.

organ pathology and may be the proximal cause of death (Caranases, Stewart, and Cluff, 1974).

In the elderly, disease processes are often of complex origins, as for example strokes (cerebral hemorrhage or cerebral thrombosis), which are the end result of hypertension and atherosclerosis of the arteries of the brain. Diseases are also commonly multiple, and it is not unusual to find several related or unrelated diseases in any one elderly person (Baker and Baker, 1975).

QUESTIONS

Circle all correct answers (there may be more than one correct answer to each question).

1. What are the consequences of failure of DNA repair?
   a. production of abnormal cells
   b. regeneration of cells
   c. death of cells
   d. evolutional changes
   e. premature aging
2. Which of the following contribute to the process of aging?
   a. autoimmune cell destruction
   b. atherosclerosis
   c. free radical lipid peroxidation reactions
   d. chronic exposure to sunlight
   e. not using a skin moisturizer
3. Which of the following statements are correct?
   a. The aging heart tolerates physical stress badly.
   b. Vital capacity decreases with age.
   c. Aging causes night blindness.
   d. Glucose tolerance decreases with age.
   e. Calcium absorption is increased in the elderly.
4. In the elderly, chronic constipation is commonly caused by:
   a. not taking a laxative
   b. depression
   c. debility
   d. low residue diet
   e. obesity
5. Which of the following geriatric diseases are influenced by diet?
   a. Alzheimer's disease
   b. osteoporosis
   c. diabetes mellitus

    d. colon cancer
    e. lung cancer
6. Which of the following are not risk factors for the development of atherosclerotic heart disease?
    a. hypercholesterolemia
    b. high intake of cholesterol
    c. diabetes mellitus
    d. daily intake of alcoholic beverages
    e. tuberculosis

REFERENCES

ALBANESE, A. A., A. H. EDELSON, E. J. LORENZE, M. L. WOODHULL, and E. H. WEIN, "Problems of bone health in elderly: ten-year study," N.Y. State J. Med., 75 (1975), 326–36.

ANDRES, R., "Aging and carbohydrate metabolism," in Nutrition in Old Age, Symp. Swedish Nutrition Foundation, ed. L. A. Carlson. Uppsala: Almqvist and Wiksell, 1972, pp. 24–31.

BAKER, A. B., and L. H. BAKER, eds., Clinical Neurology. New York: Harper & Row Publishers, Inc., 1975.

BAKER, H., S. P. JASLOW, and O. FRANK, "Severe impairment of dietary folate utilization in the elderly," J. Amer. Geriat. Soc., 26 (1978), 218–29.

BARNETT, T. B., "Chronic bronchitis and pulmonary emphysema," Vol. 2, in Bronchopulmonary Diseases and Related Disorders, eds. C. W. Holman and C. Muschenheim. New York: Harper & Row Publishers, Inc., 1972, pp. 632–64.

BERGEVIN, P. R., "The increasing problem of malignancy in the elderly: new concepts in diagnosis and management," Med. Clin. N. Amer., 60, No. 6 (1976), 1241–51.

BERMAN, P. M., and J. B. KIRSCHNER, "The aging gut. II. Diseases of the colon, pancreas, liver and gall bladder: functional bowel disease and iatrogenic disease," Geriatrics, 27 (1972), 117–24.

BLAZER, D., "Depression in the Elderly," New Eng. J. Med., 320 (1989), 164–66.

BOUCHIER, I. A. D., Gastroenterology, 2nd Ed. London: Balliere Tindall, 1977.

BRAVERMAN, I. M., Skin Signs of Systemic Disease, Philadelphia: W. B. Saunders Co., 1970, p. 344.

BRENENSTOCK, H., and K. R. FERNANTO, "Arthritis in the elderly," Med. Clin. N. Amer., 60 (1976), 459–1211.

BRODY, H., and N. VIJAYASHANKAR, "Anatomical changes in the nervous system," in Handbook of the Biology of Aging, eds. C. E. Finch and L. Hayflick. New York: Van Nostrand, 1977, pp. 241–61.

BROWN, B. A., Hematology: Principles and Procedures. Lea & Febiger, 1973, p. 191.

BUTLER, R. N., "Overview of the biology of aging," Fed. Proc., 38 (1979), 1955–71.

CARANASES, C. J., R. B. STEWART, and L. E. CLUFF, "Drug-induced illness leading to hospitalization," J. Amer. Med. Assoc., 228 (1974), 713–17.

CHATTERJEE, B., G. FERNANDES, C. YU SONG, et al., "Caloric restriction delays age-dependent loss in androgen responsiveness of the rat liver," FASEB J., 3 (1989), 169–73.

CHEN, M., R. N. BERGMAN, G. PACINI, and D. PORTE, JR., "Pathogenesis of age-related glucose intolerance in man: Insulin resistance and decreased beta cell function," *J. Clin. Endocrinol. Metab.*, 60(1985), 13–20.

CHVAPIL, M., and Z. HVUZA, "The influence of aging and undernutrition on chemical contractility and relaxation of collagen fibers in rats," *Gerontologia* 3 (1959), 241–52.

DALY, C. H., and G. F. ODLAND, "Age-related changes in the mechanical properties of human skin," *J. Invest. Dermat.* 73 (1979), 84–7.

DREYFUS, P. M., "Diseases of the nervous system in chronic alcoholics," in *The Biology of Alcoholism*, Vol. 3, eds. B. Kissin, and H. Begleiter. New York: Plenum Press, 1974, pp. 267–72.

ECKER, R. I., and A. L. SCHROETER, "Acrodermatitis and acquired zinc deficiency," *Arch. Dermatol.*, 114 (9178), 937–39.

EPSTEIN, M., "Effects of aging on the kidney," *Fed. Proc.*, 38 (1979), 168–71.

FIATARONE, M. A., E. C. MARKS, N. D. RYAN, et al., "High-intensity strength training in nonagenarians," *J. Amer. Med. Assoc.* 263 (1990), 3029–34.

FOUTS, P. J., O. M. HELMER, S. LEPKOVSKY, and T. H. JUKES, "Treatment of human pellagra with nicotinic acid," *Proc. Soc. Exp. Biol. Med.*, 37, 405–7.

FRIEDMAN, M., and R. H. ROSEMAN, "Association of specific overt behavior pattern with blood and cardiovascular findings: blood cholesterol level, blood clotting time, incidence of arcus senilis, and clinical coronary artery disease," *J. Amer. Med. Assoc.*, 169 (1959), 1286–96.

GARN, S. M., "Bone loss and aging," in *The Physiology and Pathology of Human Aging*, eds. R. Goldman, M. Rockstein, and M. L. Sussman. New York: Academic Press, Inc., 1975, pp. 39–57.

GANZONI, A. M., R. OAKES, and R. S. HILLMAN, "Red cell aging in vivo," *J. Clin. Invest.*, 50 (1971), 1373–78.

GERRITSEN, G. C., "The role of nutrition to diabetes in relation to age," in *Nutrition, Longevity, and Aging*, eds. M. Rockstein and M. L. Sussman. New York: Academic Press, Inc., 1976, pp. 229–52.

GIBSON, I. I. J. M., "Advances in the treatment of leukemia," in *Geriatric Medicine*, eds. W. Ferguson-Anderson and T. G. Judge. New York: Academic Press, Inc., 1974, pp. 184–90.

GOLDSTEIN, S., and W. REICHEL, in *Clinical Aspects of Aging*, ed. W. Reichel. Baltimore: Williams & Wilkins Co., 1978, pp. 429–33.

GREGERMAN, R. I., and E. L. BIERMAN, "Aging and hormones," in *Textbook of Endocrinology* 5th ed., ed. R. H. Williams. Philadelphia: W. B. Saunders Co., 1974, pp. 1056–69.

GUSELLA, J. F., "Location cloning strategy for characterizing genetic defects in Huntington's disease and Alzheimer's disease," *FASEB. J.*, 3(1989) 2036–41.

HARRIS, R., "Cardiac changes with age," in *The Physiology and Pathology of Human Aging*, eds. R. Goldman and M. Rockstein, New York: Academic Press, Inc., 1975, pp. 109–22.

HAYFLICK, L., "Cell biology of aging," *Fed. Proc.*, 38 (1979), 1847–50.

HENDERSON, D. K., and R. D. GILLESPIE, *A Textbook of Psychiatry*. London: Oxford University Press, 1943, pp. 398–400.

HOOK, E. W., "The pneumonias and viral respiratory infections," Vol. 1, in *Bronchopulmonary Diseases and Related Disorders*, eds. C. W. Holman and C. Muschenheim. New York: Harper & Row Publishers, Inc., 1972, pp. 279–340.

HURST, J. W., R. B. LOGUE, R. C. SCHLANT, and N. K. WENGER, eds., *The Heart, Arteries, and Veins*, 3rd Ed. New York: McGraw-Hill Book Co., 1974.

54 The Physiology and Pathology of Aging

IRWIN, M. I., "A conspectus of research on vitamin C requirements of man," *J. Nutr.*, 106 (1976), 821–97.
KALCHTHALER, T., and M. E. RIGOR TAN, "Anemia in institutionalized elderly patients," *J. Amer. Geriat. Soc.*, 28 (1980), 108–13.
LAVKER, R. M., "Structural alterations in exposed and unexposed aged skin," *J. Invest. Dermat.*, 73 (1979), 59–66.
LEITER, E. H., F. PREMDAS, D. E. HARRISON, et al., "Aging and glucose homeostasis in C57BL/6J male mice, *FASEB J.*, 2 (1988), 2807–11.
LINDENBAUM, J., E. B. HEALTON, D. G. SAVAGE, et al., "Neuropsychiatric disorders caused by cobalamin deficiency in the absence of anemia or macrocytosis." *New Eng. J. Med.*, 318 (1988), 1720–28.
MAKINODAN, T., and W. H. ADLER, "The effects of aging on the differentiation and proliferation of cells of the immune system," *Fed Proc.*, 34 (1975), 153–58.
MARTIN, G. M., C. A. SPRAGUE, and C. J. EPSTEIN, "Replicative life-span of cultivated human cells: effects of donor's age, tissue, and genotype," *Lab. Invest.*, 23 (1970), 86.
MARX, J. J. M., "Normal iron absorption and decreased red cell iron uptake in the aged," *Blood*, 53 (1979), 204–11.
MASORO, E. J., M. S. KATZ, and C. A. McMAHON, "Evidence for the glycation hypothesis of aging from the food-restricted rodent model," *J. Gerontol.* 44 (1989), B20–22.
MATZNER, Y., S. LEEVY, N. GROSSOWICZ, G. IZAK, C. HERSHKO, "Prevalence and causes of anemia in elderly hospitalized patients," *Gerontology*, 25 (1979), 113–19.
MAUDERLY, J. L., "Effect of age on preliminary structure and function of immature and adult animals and man," *Fed. Proc.*, 38 (1979), 173–77.
McCAY, C. M., and M. F. CROWELL, "Prolonging the life span," *Sci. Monthly*, 39 (1934), 405–14.
McGEE-HARVEY, A., et al., *The Principles and Practice of Medicine*, 20th Ed. Englewood Cliffs, NJ: Prentice-Hall, Inc., 1980, p. 1193.
MONNIER, V. M. Nonenzymatic glycosylation, the Maillard reaction and the aging process," *J. Gerontol.*, 45 (1990), B105–B111.
MONTAGNA, W., and K. CARLISLE, "Structural changes in aging human skin," *J. Invest. Dermat.*, 73 (1979), 47–53.
O'MALLEY, K., J. CROOKS, E. DUKE, and I. H. STEVENSON, "Effect of age and sex on human drug metabolism," *Brit. Med. J.*, 3 (1971), 607–9.
PASSMORE, R., and J. S. ROBSON, eds., *A Companion to Medical Studies*, Vol. 3, Part I. Oxford: Blackwell Scientific Publications, Ltd., 1974, pp. 23.74–23.101.
PITCHER, J. L., "Dysphagia in the elderly: causes and diagnosis," *Geriatrics*, 28 (1973), 64–69.
POOL, J. L., *Carcinoma of the Lung and Trachea in Bronchopulmonary Diseases and Related Disorders*, eds. C. W. Holman and C. Muschenheim. Hagerstown, MD: Harper & Row, Publishers, Inc., 1972.
PORTA, E. A., "Nutritional factors and aging," in *Advances in Modern Human Nutrition*, eds. R. B. Tobin and M. A. Mehlman. Park Forest South, IL: Pathotox Publishing Co., 1980, pp. 65–119.
PROCKOP, J. D., et al., "The biosynthesis of collagen and its disorders. II.," *New Eng. J. Med.*, 301 (1979), 77–85.
RODRIGUEZ, M. S., "Conspectus of research on folacin requirements of man," *J. Nutr.*, 108 (1978), 1983–2103.
ROE, D. A., *Drug-Induced Nutritional Deficiencies*. Westport, CT: AVI Publishing Co., 1976, pp. 36–38.

ROGERS, E. L., "Emergency management of gastrointestinal bleeding," *Geriatrics,* 35 (1980), 35–40.

ROSEN, H., "Renal disease in the elderly," *Med. Clin. N. Amer.,* 60 (1976), 1105–19.

ROTH, M., "Diagnosis of senile and related forms of dementia," in *Alzheimer's Disease: Senile Dementia and Related Disorders* (Aging, Vol. 7), eds. R. Katzman, R. D. Terry, and K. L. Bich. New York: Raven Press, 1978, pp. 71–85.

RUDMAN, D., A. G. FELLER, H. S. NAGRAJ, et al., "Effects of human growth hormone in men over 60 years old," *New Eng. J. Med.,* 323 (1990), 1–5.

SCHIFFMAN, S. S., "Food recognition by the elderly," *J. Gerontol.,* 32 (1977), 586–92.

SEBRELL, W. H., and R. E. BUTLER, "Riboflavin deficiency in man," *Public Health Rep.,* 53 (1938), 2282.

SHAW, J. H., and E. A. SWEENEY, "Nutrition in relation to dental medicine," in *Modern Nutrition in Health and Disease,* 6th Ed., eds. R. S. Goodhart and M. E. Shils. Philadelphia: Lea & Febiger, 1980, pp. 886–90.

SHILS, M. E., "Nutritional problems induced by cancer," *Med. Clin N. Amer.,* 63 (1979), 1011.

SLATER, T. F., *Free Radical Mechanisms in Tissue Injury.* London: Pion, Ltd., 1972.

SMITH, R., "Bone disease in the elderly," *Proc. Roy. Soc. Med.,* 69 (1976), 925–26.

SOREMARK, R., and B. NILSSON, "Dental status and nutrition in old age," in *Nutrition in Old Age,* Symp. Swedish Nutrition Foundation, ed. L. A. Carlson. Uppsala: Almqvist and Wiksell, 1972, pp. 147–66.

SOWRANDER, P., and H. SJÖGREN, "The concept of Alzheimer's disease and its clinical implications," in *Alzheimer's Disease and Related Conditions.* London: J. & A. Churchill, 1970. pp. 11–32.

STEFFEE, W. P., "Nutrition intervention in hospitalized geriatric patients," *Bull. N.Y. Acad. Med.,* 56 (1980), 564–74.

STEINBERG, W. M., and P. P. TOSKES, "A practical approach to evaluating maldigestion and malabsorption," *Geriatrics,* 33 (1978), 73–85.

STEINHEBER, F. U., "Interpretation of gastrointestinal symptoms in the elderly," *Med. Clin. N. Amer.,* 60 (1976), 1141–57.

SUTER, P. M., and R. M. RUSSELL, "Vitamin nutriture and requirements of the elderly," in *Nutrition, Aging and the Elderly,* eds. H. N. Munro, and D. E. Danford. New York: Plenum Press, 1989, pp. 245–91.

VAVRIK, M., " 'High risk' factors and atherosclerotic cardiovascular diseases in the aged," *J. Amer. Geriat. Soc.,* 22 (1974), 203–7.

VERBOV, N. J., *Skin Diseases in the Elderly.* London: Wm. Heinemann Medical Books, Ltd., 1974, p. 187.

VESTAL, R. E., "Methodological problems associated with studies of drug metabolism in the elderly," in *Clinical Pharmacology and Therapeutics,* Proc. First World Conf. Clin. Pharmacol. Therap., London, Aug. 3–9, 1980. London: Macmillan Publishing Co., 1980.

WEALE, R. A., "The effects of the ageing lens on vision," in *The Human Lens in Relation to Cataract,* Ciba Foundation Series 19. Amsterdam: Elsevier North-Holland, Inc., 1973, pp. 5–20.

WEKSLER, M. E., J. E. INNES, and G. GOLDSTEIN, "The role of the thymus in the senescence of the immune response," in *Aging and Immunity,* eds. S. K. Singal, N. R. Sinclair, and C. R. Stiller. New York: Elsevier North-Holland, Inc., 1979, pp. 165–72.

WENE, J. D., W. E. CONNOR, and L. DENBENSTEN, "The development of essential fatty acid deficiency in men fed fat-free diets intravenously and orally," *J. Clin. Invest.,* 56 (1975), 127–34.

WILCOCK, G. K., and A. M. MIDDLETON,   *Geriatrics*. London: Blackwell Scientific
    Publications, 1984, pp. 23, 58–63.
WORMSLEY, K. G.,   *The Skin and Gut in Disease*. London: Pitman Medical Publish-
    ing Co., Ltd., 1964.
YAHR, M. D.,   "Levodopa," *Ann. Intern Med.*, 83 (1975), 677–82.

chapter 3

The Nutritional Status of the Elderly

Epidemiological studies have been conducted in a number of countries, including the United States, to determine the association between diet, nutritional status, and health variables in aging populations. Study goals and survey methods, however, have varied with the research question being asked and the survey population being studied. The goals of cross-sectional surveys of well elderly have mainly been to determine the food-energy and nutrient intakes of elderly that are associated with the acceptable anthropometric and biochemical indicators of adequate nutritional status as well as with good health and the maintenance of cognitive function (Garry et al., 1982; Goodwin et al., 1983). Other study goals of current cross-sectional surveys of healthy elderly have been to define diet and lifestyle variables that are associated with extended longevity (Kouris, 1989).

Longitudinal studies of healthy populations have been carried out with the aim of defining changes in diet and in nutritional status that occur with normal aging (O'Hanlon and Kohrs, 1978). Other goals of longitudinal surveys have examined those lifestyle or dietary variables that are predictive of chronic disease, disability, or premature mortality. Interesting new findings of the Baltimore Longitudinal Study (Hallfrisch et al., 1990) are that men may make beneficial changes in intake of nutrients that affect health.

Surveys of frail elderly living in their own homes have been conducted to define those subgroups of this population that are at highest risk of hunger and malnutrition. These surveys have concurrently attempted to define the nutritional support services that such elderly need to continue to live in their own homes.

Major questions asked in the surveys have been whether the elderly have too little to eat, whether they exhibit clinical signs of nutritional disease, and whether they show hematological or biochemical evidence of subclinical nutritional deficiencies. Another survey goal has been to determine, by repeated surveys of the same population, whether nutritional status deteriorates with advancing age. Longitudinal studies have also looked at changes in anthropometric measurements and body composition with age. Findings have been that the nutrition of the elderly varies according to chronological age, sex, health status, and living situations (O'Hanlon and Kohrs, 1978).

Difficulties have been encountered in obtaining reliable estimates of food-energy and nutrient intakes. Most surveys have found a low prevalence of clinical signs which could be proven to be caused by nutritional deficiency. Severely malnourished persons among the independently living sample populations have been eccentric, socially isolated, and lacking in interest in their own well-being (Clark, Mankikar, and Gray, 1975). Severely malnourished institutionalized patients have chronic severe physical and mental disorders, including dementias. Biochemical evidence of the presence of one or more vitamin deficiencies has been common, especially among persons over 75 years of age (Exton-Smith, 1972; Kalchthaler and Rigor Tan, 1980; Steffee, 1980). Change in body composition with age has been found with increase in body fat in certain age groups.

SURVEYS OF INDEPENDENTLY LIVING ELDERLY POPULATIONS

Longitudinal nutritional surveys of the elderly have been conducted in the United Kingdom by Exton-Smith and his co-workers. The first extensive survey by this group was conducted from 1967 to 1968. The study population consisted of independently living people over the age of 65 living in four areas of England and two areas in Scotland (Nutrition and Health, 1979). The survey, published in 1972, showed differences in nutrient intakes between men and women, between people of different age groups, and also between the different study areas. For the most part, differences in nutrient intake reflected variations in total food-energy consumption. Malnutrition was diagnosed in 3 percent of the total study population of 879 persons. For the most part, malnutrition was associated with disease, but in about 2 percent of those who were malnourished, no obvious medical cause was found, nor could malnutrition be attributed to dietary inadequacy on the basis of poverty. The incidence of subclinical malnutrition was difficult to assess because normal ranges of biochemical indices of nutritional status for the older-age groups are unknown.

A subsample of the same study population agreed to participate in another nutritional survey in 1972 to 1973. The subsample participants were still living in their own homes. The 1979 report by Exton-Smith's group describes findings in 365 subjects who participated fully in both surveys (Nutrition Survey, 1979). It was found that in the total group, men and women aged 80 years or over had lower mean daily intakes of food-energy than younger persons. However, the healthy persons who were 80 years or over had mean daily food-energy intakes that were not significantly different from those of persons less than 80 years of age. It was therefore assumed that lower intakes of food-energy were in those who were not in good health. Housebound men and women had lower food-energy intakes than those who were mobile. Men had higher food-energy intakes than women. Food-energy intakes were not statistically greater in obese subjects but were greater in taller men and women and in men with larger arm muscle measurements, which may reflect total muscle mass. Tentative explanation of this finding was that physical activity, which would be reflected in large muscle mass, is an important determinant of food-energy intake.

The nutrient density of the diet was similar for both men and women. Of the 365 participants, 26 (7.1 percent) were considered to be clinically malnourished. Malnutrition was more than twice as common in subjects of 80 years or more than in subjects under that age. Malnutrition included scurvy, osteomalacia, and nutritional anemias. Several people had multiple nutritional deficiencies. Diets of the malnourished were of poor nutritional quality. Medical factors related to malnutrition were history of partial gastrectomy, chronic bronchitis and emphysema, depression, dementia, difficulty in swallowing, and non-use or nonavailability of dentures. Housebound individuals were more likely to be malnourished. The housebound had lower nutrient intakes. There was an association between lower nutrient intakes of the housebound elderly and the presence of chronic disease. It was inferred that lower nutrient intakes of the housebound elderly could also be related to decreased physical activity and poorer choice of food. The housebound had less satisfactory vitamin D status, which was probably caused by lack of sunlight exposure.

A gerontological survey was carried out in the city of Göteborg, Sweden, in which food-energy and nutrient intakes, meal habits, body composition, and laboratory tests of the nutritional status of 70-year-old men and women were observed (Göteborg Study, 1977). In Sweden the life expectancy for males is 73 years and for females 77 years. The study was started in 1971 and 1972, with an investigation of a representative sample of about three tenths of the 70 year olds in the city population. Only about 3 percent of these 70 year olds had handicaps or diseases for which institutionalization was required. The physical and mental condition of the subjects was generally good.

The dietary habits of a subsample of 191 males and 199 females were studied and among these, 182 males and 188 females took part in the complete dietary interview. In this population the dietary history method gave a better estimate of food intake than 24-hour recalls. On an average, 1.8 hot meals and 0.9 light meals of a beverage and a sandwich were consumed daily. Intakes of energy and nutrients were variable but generally satisfactory. Significant associations were found between sources of intake of energy and nutrients. Subjects with an education beyond elementary school showed a higher proportion of energy intake from protein than other subjects. Males who lived alone had lower iron intakes than other males.

In comparison between this study and a study of middle-aged women in Göteborg, it was shown that energy intakes and body composition were similar in the two groups.

Body composition studies were carried out on a subsample of 49 males and 56 females. Average values for body weight were 76.2 kg for males and 66.3 kg for females. Males at the age of 70 years had a higher relative body cell mass than females and slightly more extracellular water, but their body fat mass, as calculated, was little over half that of the females (Table 3-1).

Biochemical indicators of nutritional status showed intersubject variability but no consistent differences between men and women. Hemoglobin levels were lower in females than in males.

Anthropometric data and information on body composition were also obtained for women living in Göteborg (Noppa et al., 1980). The women were studied in 1968 and 1969 and again from 1971 to 1975. Body height was found to decrease with age. The reduction in body height was greater at higher ages. Body weight increased with age, but the change was partly a cohort effect and partly a time effect of age. Arm muscle mass decreased with age. The increase in subcutaneous fat with age was both in the arm and in the trunk. However, between the initial study and the follow-up, body fat did not change significantly.

A study of the nutritional status of apparently healthy, independently living elderly people in Corvallis, Oregon, included dietary and biochem-

TABLE 3-1   Body Composition of Elderly Men and Women
in the Göteborg Study

	MALES		FEMALES	
	MEAN	SD	MEAN	SD
Height (cm)	173	5.9	160	6.0
Body weight (kg)	76.2	11.1	66.3	12.4
Absolute values (kg)				
BCM	28.1	3.5	20.3	2.7
ECW	26.5	5.0	20.0	4.3
BF	12.5	6.5	18.1	7.2
Relative values (percent of BW)				
BCM	37.1	4.0	30.9	4.0
ECW	34.9	5.6	30.2	4.9
BF	16.1	7.0	26.6	6.7

Adapted from B. Steen et al., "Body composition in 70-year-old males and females in Göteborg, Sweden, a population study," *Acta Med. Scand.*, *Suppl. 611 (1977)*, p. 97.

ical assessment (Yearick, Wang, and Pisias, 1980). The total sample consisted of 100 persons (75 women and 25 men). Calcium, vitamin A, and thiamin were the dietary nutrients most likely to be low, particularly in women. Nutrient supplements taken were frequently inappropriate and often excessive. The mean biochemical indices of nutritional status were within acceptable limits.

In a randomly selected subsample of 20 persons, 11 subjects had serum folacin below an acceptable level of 6 ng/ml, and of these, three had values in the deficiency range. Mean calculated intake of folacin for this group was very low, but the author would caution interpretation because of missing and inaccurate values in food comparison tables.

CROSS-CULTURAL SURVEYS OF HEALTHY ELDERLY

Cross-cultural studies of elderly are now being carried out in a number of countries to determine the long-term dietary characteristics and lifestyle patterns that are predictive of men and women living to a healthy old age (Kouris et al., 1989). In each country where these studies are being carried out (in Australia, the United States, the United Kingdom, Greece, New Zealand, China, Japan, and Kenya), representative samples of men and women are being interviewed and stratified according to the broad categories of healthy and unhealthy. Information is being obtained, using a common survey instrument, on their long-term dietary patterns, social activities, social networks, and on their nutritional and health status. Initial analysis of the data has not indicated any association between food variety and good health, as had previously been suggested.

NATIONAL NUTRITION SURVEYS IN THE UNITED STATES

The Ten-State Nutrition Survey 1968–1970 was limited to Washington, California, Texas, Louisiana, South Carolina, Kentucky, West Virginia, Missouri, Massachusetts, and New York, including a separate survey of New York City (DHEW Publ. 72-8131; 72-8133; 72-8134). The primary interest in each of these states was the evaluation of malnutrition among the poor. Sampling procedures used are believed to have produced a representative sample of low-income families, but higher income families, also included in the sample, are not thought to have been representative of middle- and high-income families.

The evaluation of nutritional status involved 40,000 individuals. High-risk subgroup populations included in the sample were persons over 60 years of age.

The total survey included more than 86,000 individuals (23,846 families), of which 10.9 percent were 60 years of age or more. According to the survey report, these people consumed less food than was needed to meet nutrient standards for their age, sex, and weight. However, the reliability of the data is in some doubt, because of dependence on 24-hour recalls in all states surveyed except Missouri, where a dietary history was obtained. Limiting nutrients were protein, iron, vitamin A, and calcium in older men. There was no strong relationship between dietary intake and income. Dietary intakes were positively related to biochemical findings. Although there was a high incidence of obesity in the total adult population sample studied, the mean triceps skinfold thickness was lower in females and (more strikingly) in males over 60 years.

The First Health and Nutrition Examination Survey (NHANES I) was conducted between 1971 and 1974 (O'Hanlon and Kohrs, 1978). The population sample for NHANES I was meant to be a representative sample of the U.S. population. In fact, it was a stratified probability sample of the noninstitutionalized population between the ages of 1 and 74 years. Dietary information was obtained from a 24-hour recall and a food frequency interview. In the preliminary report of NHANES I, low intakes of iron were prevalent in the low-income older group.

O'Hanlon and Kohrs (1978) point out that it is difficult to compare nutritional surveys which include or focus on the elderly because of differences in dietary methodology and standards.

The NHANES III survey which will be completed in 1994, is oversampling the elderly and is expected therefore to provide better reference data on their nutritional status (*Diet and Health*, 1989).

SURVEYS OF HUNGER PREVALENCE IN THE ELDERLY AND EFFECTS OF INTERVENTION

Surveys have been carried out in several parts of the United States to determine the extent to which hunger is reported by the frail elderly. The focus of these surveys has been on those who are homebound. Follow-up surveys have then been performed to assess the impact of the home-delivered meals program in reducing hunger. Findings have been that in the homebound population hunger is associated with impaired mobility and extreme poverty. Those receiving home-delivered meals are less likely to report hunger, but there is still a problem because the geographically isolated elderly may not get these meals (Roe, 1990).

COMPARISON OF INDEPENDENTLY LIVING AND INSTITUTIONALIZED ELDERLY

The nutritional status of institutionalized and independently living elderly has been studied in Belfast, Northern Ireland (Vir and Love, 1979). There were 196 subjects over 65 years of age who were either in hospital geriatric units, in sheltered living facilities, or in residential accommodation. All subjects were grouped according to whether they did or did not take multivitamin supplements.

Three-day weighed diet records were obtained, clinical examination was undertaken, and there was biochemical assessment of nutritional status. Energy intake of females in the geriatric units and in sheltered dwellings was considered to be "comparatively low." The energy intakes of these institutionalized groups were lower than those of the noninstitutionalized group.

Dietary nutrients which were least often adequate in amount were potassium, magnesium, vitamin D, and vitamin B_6. Clinical signs of malnutrition were rare. According to the definition of anemia used (<13 g/dl hemoglobin for males and <12 g/dl for females), 18.6 percent of the sample were anemic. Of the subjects not on multivitamin preparations, 91.3 percent had some biochemical evidence of nutritional deficiency; among subjects who were receiving multivitamin preparations, 64.3 percent had biochemical evidence of a vitamin or mineral deficiency.

The authors conclude that although intake of multivitamin preparations may help to alleviate subclinical deficiencies, vitamin A requirements were not met by these preparations. The question to be asked is whether patients took the nutrient supplements regularly.

The prevalence and causes of anemia in the elderly have been studied. A study was carried out by Matzner et al. (1979) in Jerusalem of 104 patients over 60 admitted to a general ward. In males and females, mean hemoglobin levels were approximately 1 g/dl less than in healthy younger persons. Of the patients who had hemoglobin values of less than 11 g/dl, none could be identified as having a primary nutritional anemia. Most common causes of anemia were chronic renal failure, metastatic carcinoma, GI bleeding, and infection.

Major areas needing further research include:

1. Food-energy needs of sedentary and bedridden nursing home patients
2. Nutrient needs of these same patients
3. The means to best carry out nutritional screening and assessment of geriatric patients in these facilities
4. The interpretation of clinical, anthropometric, hematological, and biochemical indices of nutritional status in chronically sick elderly patients with or without skin disease, with or without disease-related muscle wasting, with or without anemia (which may be multifactorial), and with or without renal failure (which will influence blood levels and urinary levels of nutrients)
5. The responsiveness of patients showing one or more indices of malnutrition to nutrient supplementation
6. Acceptable values for nutritional status indicators in nursing-home patients

It is necessary to develop and carry out a national survey of geriatric patients in institutions in the United States, as well as homebound individuals.

Constraints on performance of major nutritional surveys of institutionalized geriatric patients are:

1. Lack of planning
2. Inadequate methodology

3. Need for informed consent of participants
4. Lack of funds
5. Lack of commitment

RECOMMENDATIONS FOR NUTRITIONAL SURVEY DATA REQUIREMENTS FOR ELDERLY POPULATIONS

Recommendations for the preliminary data collection necessary for the conduct of new nutritional survey of elderly populations have been made relative to dietary, anthropometric, and biochemical assessments. There is a particular need to overcome the problem of nonrespondent bias, and measures are actually being taken to do this in NHANES III. These measures include checking demographic and health characteristics during an in-home visit to determine whether or not the potential elderly survey subject will actually participate in the survey. This allows comparison between the respondents and nonrespondents within survey areas (Harris et al., 1989). Another priority is the development of a standard diet history questionnaire, which is tested for reliability and validity (Hankin, 1989; Block and Hartman, 1989). Another pressing need is for reference data on the anthropometric, biochemical, and functional parameters of nutritional status (Chumlea and Baumgartner, 1989; Garry et al., 1989; Shephard, 1989).

QUESTIONS

Circle all correct answers (there may be more than one correct answer to each question).

1. Which of the following statements are true?
    a. Nutrition of the elderly varies with chronological age.
    b. Differences in nutrient intake frequency reflect change in food-energy consumption.
    c. Malnutrition in the elderly is usually associated with disease.
    d. Normal ranges for biochemical indices of nutritional status for the elderly are not known.
2. Indicate which of the following statements are true:
    a. A representative sample of elderly in the United States was included in the NHANES I survey.
    b. Cross-cultural studies of healthy elderly are currently being conducted with the aim of defining common diet and lifestyle variables associated with early mortality.
    c. In longitudinal surveys, preanalytical and analytical sources of variability in blood nutrient levels are due to age differences of the sample population.

   d. Cross-cultural studies of healthy elderly are being conducted with the aim of defining common dietary and lifestyle factors associated with a healthy old age.

   e. There is definite evidence from surveys that loss of teeth is associated with low nutrient intake.

3. Common causes of anemia in elderly hospitalized patients are:
   a. low intake of liver
   b. chronic renal failure
   c. GI bleeding
   d. low iron absorption
   e. anticoagulant therapy

4. Malnutrition in the elderly may be related to one or more causes. Separate the causes into two groups, specifying which causes are more likely to occur in (1) independently living and (2) institutionalized (or hospitalized) patients.
   a. social isolation
   b. dementias
   c. psychoses
   d. lack of self-interest
   e. chronic renal failure

5. Which of the following statements are true?
   a. The nutritional status of patients in nursing homes in the United States is known from a recent national survey.
   b. Most patients in nursing homes in the United States are malnourished.
   c. In several independent studies of nursing home patients, there has been a high prevalence of anemia.

REFERENCES

BLOCK, G., and A. M. HARTMAN, "Issues in reproducibility and validity of dietary studies," *Amer. J. Clin. Nutr.*, 50 (1989), 1138–38.

CHUMLEA, W. C., and R. N. BAUMGARTNER, "Status of anthropometry and body composition data in elderly subjects," *Amer. J. Clin. Nutr.*, 50 (1989), 1158–66.

CLARK, A. N. G., G. D. MANKIKAR, and I. GRAY, "Diogenes syndrome, a clinical study of gross neglect in old age," *Lancet*, 1 (1975), 366–68.

Diet and Health: Implications for Reducing Chronic Disease Risk. NRC. Washington D.C.: National Academy Press, 1989, p. 49.

EXTON-SMITH, A. N., "Physiological aspects of aging: relationship to nutrition," *Amer. J. Clin. Nutr.*, 25 (1972), 853–59.

GARRY, P. J., J. S. GOODWIN, W. C. HUNT, et al., "Nutritional status in a healthy elderly population: dietary and supplemental intakes," *Amer. J. Clin. Nutr.*, 36 (1982), 319–31.

GARRY, P. J., W. C. HUNT, D. J. VANDERJAGT, and R. L. RHYNE, "Clinical chemistry reference intervals for healthy elderly subjects," *Amer. J. Clin. Nutr.*, 50 (1989), 1219–30.

"The gerontological and geriatric population study in Göteborg, Sweden," *Acta Med. Scand.*, Suppl. 611 (1977), 3–112.

GOODWIN, J. S., J. M. GOODWIN, and P. J. GARRY, "Association between nutritional status and cognitive functioning in a healthy elderly population," *J. Amer. Med. Assoc.*, 249 (1983), 2917–21.

HALLFRISCH, J., D. MULLER, D. DRINKWATER, J. TOBIN, and R. ANDRES, "Continuing diet trends of men," The Baltimore Longitudinal Study of Aging (1961–1987), *J. Gerontol.* 45. M 186-M191 (1990).

HANKIN, J. H., "Development of a diet history questionnaire for studies of older persons," *Amer. J. Clin. Nutr.*, 50 (1989), 1121–27.

HARRIS, T., C. WOTEKI, R. R. BRIEFEL, and J. C. KLEINMAN, "NHANES III for older persons: nutrition content and methodological considerations," *Amer. J. Clin. Nutr.*, 50 (1989) 1145–49.

KALCHTHALER, T., and M. E. RIGOR TAN, "Anemia in institutionalized elderly patients," *J. Amer. Geriat. Soc.*, 28 (1980), 108–13.

KERGOAT, M. J., "Determinants of total serum carotene concentrations in institutionalized elderly," *J. Amer. Geriatr. Soc.* 36, (1988), 430–36.

KOURIS, A., M. WAHLQVIST, A. TRICHOPOULOS, and E. POLYCHRONOPOULOS, "Food habits and health of elderly in Spata, Greece: Application of survey instrument." Presented at XIVth Int. Congr. Nutr., Seoul, Korea, August 1989.

MATZNER, Y., S. LEVY, N. GROSSOWICZ, G. IZAK, and C. HERSHKO, "Prevalence and causes of anemia in elderly hospitalized patients," *Gerontology*, 25 (1979), 113–19.

NOPPA, H., M. ANDERSSON, G. BERGTSSON, et al., "Longitudinal studies of anthropometric data and body composition: the population study of women in Göteborg, Sweden," *Amer. J. Clin. Nutr.*, 33 (1980), 155–62.

Nutrition and Health in Old Age: The Cross-sectional Analysis of the Findings of a Survey Made in 1972/3 of Elderly People Who Had Been Studied in 1967/8, Report by the Committee on Medical Aspects of Food Policy, Department of Health and Social Security Report on Health and Social Subjects #16. London: Her Majesty's Stationery Office, 1979.

A Nutrition Survey of the Elderly, Department of Health and Social Security, Report on Health and Social Subjects #3, London: Her Majesty's Stationery Office, 1972.

O'HANLON, P., and M. B. KOHRS, "Dietary studies of older Americans," *Amer. J. Clin. Nutr.*, 31 (1978), 1257–69.

ROE, D. A. "Development and current status of home-delivered meals programs in the United States: Who is served?" *Nutr. Rev.*, 48 (1990), 181–85.

SCHIAFFINO-PURVIS, E., "Nutritional status of nursing home residents in relation to their ability to eat independently." Presented at SAGE meeting, 1988.

SHEPHARD, R. J., "Assessment of physical activity and energy needs," *Amer. J. Clin. Nutr.*, 50 (1989) 1195–1200.

STEEN, B., et al., "Body composition in 70-year-old males and females in Göteborg, Sweden, a population study," *Acta Med. Scand.*, Suppl. 611 (1977), 97.

STEFFEE, W. P., "Nutritional intervention in hospitalized geriatric patients," *Bull. N.Y. Acad. Med.*, 56 (1980), 564–74.

SULLIVAN, D. H., G. A. PATCH, R. C. WALLS, and D. A. LIPSCHITZ, "Impact of nutrition status on morbidity and mortality in a select population of geriatric rehabilitation patients," *Amer. J. Clin. Nutr.*, 51 (1990), 749–58.

Ten-State Nutritional Survey 1968–70. III. Clinical; Anthropometry; Dental. DHEW Publ. No. (HSM) 72-8131.

Ten-State Nutritional Survey 1968–70. V. Dietary.   DHEW Publ. No. (HSM) 72-8133.
Ten-State Nutritional Survey 1968–70. Highlights.   DHEW Publ. No. (HSM) 72-8134.
VIR, S. C., and A. H. G. LOVE,   "Nutritional status of institutionalized and non-institutionalized aged in Belfast, Northern Ireland," *Amer. J. Clin. Nutr.*, 32 (1979), 1934–47.
WANG, Y-F.   "Biochemical and Anthropometric Characteristics of Elderly Independent and Dependent Eaters in a Nursing Home." M.S. Thesis, Cornell University, Ithaca, New York, 1990.
YEARICK, E. S., M-S. L. WANG, and S. J. PISIAS,   "Nutritional status of the elderly: dietary and biochemical findings," *J. Gerontol.*, 35 (1980), 663–71.

chapter 4

Nutritional Requirements and Tolerances

FOOD-ENERGY AND NUTRIENT NEEDS

The determinants of the food-energy and nutrient requirements of people as they get older are both genetic and acquired. Genetic factors that influence these requirements include inborn metabolic errors, disease susceptibility, and nutrient tolerance. Acquired factors that influence requirements include the extent of the aging process, the physical and chemical environments, the activity level, health problems present, medications being taken, and whether or not alcohol is consumed.

Previously there were two somewhat contradictory beliefs about the effects of aging on energy and nutrient requirements. The first of these beliefs was that all elderly have lowered food-energy requirements, because with aging there is always lessened physical activity as well as a reduction in metabolic rate (Durnin, 1964). The second belief was that aging increases nutrient requirements, because the ability to digest and absorb nutrients is less efficient (Munro, 1980). Although these ideas have not been proven conclusively incorrect, it is now known that if older people maintain their physical activity, either by engaging in physical work or by regular exercise, their food-energy requirements, just as those of younger people, are related to their energy expenditure. Whether nutrient requirements are decreased with aging depends on environmental variables, as well as on the presence or absence of disease, more than on the effects of aging on the digestive and absorptive functions of the gastrointestinal tract. Furthermore, new interpretations have arisen with respect to the nutrient requirements of the elderly because it is now recognized that the requirements are the acceptable range of values for caloric and nutrient intake that maintain the body in optimal function. In the past it was assumed that the requirements were necessary to prevent deficiency. In the aging body, the risks of caloric and nutrient excess are as dangerous as inadequate caloric and nutrient intake, and, in the United States, may impose a greater risk for the elderly than that of deficiency.

On the other hand, a requirement of infancy re-emerges with aging; namely, it is that the regularity of eating is critical to the preservation of functional normality.

More recent information about the nutritional needs of the elderly is summarized in the 1989 Surgeon General's Report. This report emphasizes that the variety of physiological, psychological, economic, and social changes that may occur with aging can, in turn, affect nutrient requirements. It is also brought out in this report that many of the changes, which in the past were thought to be inevitably associated with aging, may not, in fact, occur. It is also pointed out in the report that there are still major "unknowns" with respect to the nutrient requirements of the elderly. Some of these unknowns include the following:

1. Whether or not the nutrient requirements of elderly can be accurately extrapolated from those of younger age groups
2. What effects dietary restriction and overconsumption have on longevity
3. The role of nutrition in determining age-related impairments of the body
4. The effect of marginal nutrient and energy deficiencies on the mental and physical health of older people
5. How drugs affect the nutritional needs of the elderly

The total energy production per square meter of body surface falls progressively with advancing age. The average reduction in energy production is about 12 calories/m^2/hour between the ages of 20 and 90 years. These decrements may be caused by a loss of metabolizing tissue. The reduction in the energy metabolism of older people is related both to a decrease in physical activity, which becomes most pronounced after the age of 75, and to tissue loss (Exton-Smith, 1972).

Decreased nutrient absorption and increased nutrient losses will increase nutrient requirements. Nutrient absorption may decrease with aging. In catabolic states associated with injury or surgery or with acute or certain chronic diseases of the elderly, negative nitrogen balance occurs, implying that nitrogen losses exceed usual dietary nitrogen intake. In these conditions, protein deficiency can be averted if proteins of high biological value are fed at a level to meet the increased nitrogen requirements. However, there is no sound scientific evidence that, in the absence of catabolic states or states of malabsorption (when fecal nitrogen losses are high), the protein requirements would decrease. Since muscle mass decreases with age, it might be anticipated that nitrogen requirements of the elderly are greater than those of younger persons. Healthy elderly subjects have not been found to require more protein per unit of body weight than younger subjects studied under similar conditions.

In defining the individual protein or nitrogen requirements of the elderly, several factors need to be considered. Physiological changes that occur with aging which could alter protein requirement include reduced daily synthesis of body protein and reduction in lean body mass (Forbes and Reina, 1970; Winterer et al., 1976). However, there is no good evidence that these factors reduce protein requirements, perhaps because aging is also associated with a reduced efficiency of protein utilization (Zanni, Callaway, and Zezulka, 1979). There is a decline in renal function related to aging, and further chronic renal disease is common in the elderly. The work of the kidney is increased by the need to excrete nitrogenous end products of dietary protein when intake is high. Further reduction in renal function and retention of toxic nitrogenous waste are a result. When elderly patients have impaired renal function, total protein in the diet should be restricted, but proteins supplied should be of high biological value (Exton-Smith and Overstall, 1979).

On the other hand, in considering the protein needs of the elderly, it has to be remembered that animal protein foods are rich sources of heme iron, calcium, vitamins A and D, riboflavin, niacin, and vitamin B_{12} (Smith, 1965). Further prevention of protein deficiency with attendant hypoalbuminemia is most important in the elderly when protein-bound drugs are being taken. In the presence of hypoalbuminemia, less of the drug is bound to albumin and therefore more of the drug will reach receptor sites, which can result in drug toxicity. Dietary protein deficiency also increases the risk of certain hepatoxic drugs (Vestal, 1980).

Nutrient requirements are dependent on many environmental factors, including drug intake and exposure to sunlight. Drugs can increase nutrient requirements because of drug-induced malabsorption or malutilization of nutrients. Dietary requirements for vitamin D increase if the level of ultraviolet light exposure is reduced so that less of the vitamin is synthesized in the skin. Vitamin D requirements are also increased by intake of certain drugs, e.g., phenobarbital and phenytoin (Dilantin). Development of osteomalacia in elderly, housebound people is related to lack of adjustment upwards of the dietary intake of vitamin D when the patient is no longer exposed to sunlight and when the patient is taking drugs that affect vitamin D needs (Roe, 1976).

There is a lack of agreement as to whether the elderly have a high requirement for selected nutrients (Munro, 1980). The assumption is that if the nutritional requirements of elderly persons are in the same range as those of younger people, then, at similar levels of intake, nutritional status measurements would be similar. The logic of this approach would be satisfactory if we could be assured that our present means of determining nutritional adequacy are rational in that they determine functional adequacy. Currently we are concerned that it may be necessary to compute nutritional adequacy differently in the elderly than in younger persons. Correlations have been found in the elderly between dietary intake of specific nutrients and biochemical measurements of nutritional status.

These relationships can be assessed in elderly persons of above-average health. However, the relationship between dietary intake of nutrients and functional nutritional normalcy may be altered by disease or by drugs. Needs for specific nutrients may be increased by progressive loss of tissue function attendant on aging. In a British nutritional survey of the elderly and of younger people, none of the hematological indices of nutritional status showed significant differences between age groups (Nutrition and Health, 1979). On the other hand, mean values for serum iron, folacin, vitamin B_{12}, and pyridoxine concentration were lower for subjects in the survey who were above 65 years of age (Exton-Smith and Overstall, 1979). Considerations at present are the following:

1. Can we attempt dietary recommendations that mitigate against development of aging changes in body composition?
2. Since aging results in the accumulation of disease such as osteoporosis, atherosclerosis, and cancer, which are at least in part age related, can we offer guidelines for the diets of younger people to be continued throughout life which will protect them from the development of these diseases?
3. What are the criteria which we should be employing in order to understand the nutrient needs of the old?

Age-related changes in body composition, reduction in cardiac, respiratory, hepatic, and renal function as well as the decline in capacity for sustained exercise may influence nutritional needs. Further, in the elderly a slowed rate of homeostatic regulation and enzyme induction may affect nutrient requirements. Whereas we do have good evidence that the energy needs of the elderly are reduced, we do not as yet have any good basis for recommending that nutrient requirements of healthy elderly are different from those of the young, unless disease is present or drugs are being taken which increase specific nutrient needs (Harper, 1978). To reduce energy intakes in the elderly and to maintain nutrient intakes at levels which are optimal for health in young persons, the elderly will need to consume diets of higher nutrient-to-energy ratios.

It has been suggested that one way to determine needs of the elderly for particular nutrients could be by incremental addition of that nutrient to the basal diet while sequential tests of nutritional status are performed. This approach presupposes that it is possible to demonstrate a change in functional efficiency with nutrient intake. Our capabilities in this area are limited and, further, it is very possible that optimal nutrition for one physiological function, e.g. erythropoiesis (formation of red blood cells), is not the same as optimal nutrition for another function, e.g., metabolism of foreign compounds such as therapeutic drugs.

As we move toward a better definition of the nutritional needs of the elderly, two concepts must be born in mind. First, our goal is to provide guidelines for nutrient intakes by the elderly which will allow the best health protection of the most people in different age ranges 65 years and over; second, we must obtain more precise information about the long-term diets of very old people who have remained healthy until an advanced age. It is well documented that patterns of eating laid down in early life are generally maintained through the life span. Therefore, if particular patterns of food and nutrient consumption are correlated with extended longevity, a sensible recommendation might be to use such a diet as a guideline for nutrient needs of the elderly. Limitations of this approach are twofold; first, the diet of the long-lived healthy person may, for its desired effect, have to be maintained over a period of years and not suddenly imposed in later life; second, it must be remembered that all persons are not alike and that nutrient requirements for health maintenance are influenced by both genetic and environmental factors (Munro and Everett, 1981).

PROTEIN REQUIREMENTS

Age-related changes in protein nutriture and protein requirements include:

1. Lean body mass, particularly muscle mass, is lost (Steen et al., 1979; Cohn et al., 1980; Munro, 1981).
2. Capacity of the liver to synthesize albumin decreases, with associated decreases in plasma albumin levels (Gersovitz et al., 1975).
3. Protein tolerance decreases. A decline in renal function occurs with aging, and this is associated with a decrease in the glomerular filtration rate and a loss of functioning nephrons. These changes are related to the long-term high level of protein in the diet, and it has been demonstrated in experimental animals that the renal pathology can be reduced and renal function preserved longer when the protein in the diet is restricted (Hostetter, 1984).
4. The protein intake of elderly men and women, which is required to achieve zero nitrogen balance, may be increased over that of younger individuals. However, interpretation of the nitrogen balance studies that have provided this information is complex because of (1) differing food-energy intakes of the subjects, (2) chronic diseases in some of the studies' subjects, and (3) the differing activity levels of the subjects (Cheng et al., 1978; Uauy et al., 1978; Gersovitz et al., 1982).

Until further information is available, it is not possible to make a strong new recommendation about the safe and adequate protein requirement for elderly people. The recommended protein level at present is 0.8/ mg/kg body weight (Munro, 1980). However, further evaluation is required to determine whether this level of intake is best for conservation of renal function.

VITAMIN REQUIREMENTS

Fat-Soluble Vitamins

Vitamin A. Vitamin A is required both to maintain normal vision and to optimize normal differentiation of epithelial tissues (Linder, 1985).

The vitamin has been identified as a cancer-protective agent that functions in opposition to chemical promoters of tumorigenesis (Yuspa, 1983).

A significant body of epidemiological evidence indicates that individuals and populations whose intake of carotenoid sources of vitamin A is high and who have higher plasma carotenoid values may be at lower cancer risk (Mettlin, 1983).

The carotenoids are vitamin A precursors that are abundant in yellow and dark-green vegetables. Beta-carotene, which has the highest provitamin activity, is also used as a food colorant (Olson, 1985). Conversion of carotenoids to retinol occurs by a process of molecular cleavage in the gut mucosa.

It has been shown that several carotenoids enhance cellular immune responses. They also inhibit mutagenesis, reduce the extent of DNA damage, and have provided protection against light-induced skin cancer development in experimental animal models (Bendich and Olson, 1989). The protective role of carotenoids is further discussed in the section on antioxidant vitamins.

Pre-formed vitamin A is present in dairy products, including milk, cheese, butter, and ice cream. Rich food sources of the vitamin include liver, eggs, and fish such as herring, sardines, and tuna (Watt and Merrill, 1963).

Presently, 12 μg of mixed carotenoids in a typical food, or 6 μg of beta-carotene, is considered equivalent to 1 μg of retinol or pre-formed vitamin A (Olson, 1985).

Exposure to sunlight can degrade carotenoids and retinol in foods and in human plasma (Bauernfeind and Court, 1974; White and Roe, 1986). Loss of vitamin A because of oxidation occurs in foods that are exposed to a hot, humid environment in the absence of reducing agents and stabilizers (Olson, 1985).

Biochemical assessment of vitamin A status is by measurement of plasma vitamin A (retinol). Acceptable levels of plasma retinol are 20 to 50 μg/dl. Low plasma retinol values are from 10 to 20 μg/dl, and deficient values are less than 10 μg/dl. There is no general agreement as to whether aging affects plasma retinol values (Kirk and Chieffi, 1984; Rafsky, Newman, and Jolliffe, 1984; Gillum, Morgan, and Sailer, 1955).

Chronic disease that may occur in later life can influence plasma retinol levels. Abnormally elevated values occur with end-stage renal disease, and low levels are found in individuals with chronic lipid malabsorption syndromes, including alcoholic pancreatitis (Chytil, 1983; Olson, 1985). Night blindness, which is a specific sign of vitamin A deficiency in younger people, is not diagnostic of vitamin A deficiency in the elderly, in whom night blindness may occur because of cataracts.

The rise in plasma retinyl ester levels after administration of retinol with a high fat meal is greater in older people than in younger men and women. This is currently believed to be due to a delay in the plasma clearance of retinyl esters in triglyceride-rich lipoproteins of intestinal origin (Krasinski et al., 1990). These findings, however, do not in themselves presently suggest that the elderly have a lower need for vitamin A than younger people.

These allowances are considered to provide for individual variability in requirements. However, in view of the increasing evidence of a need for carotenoids to lessen cancer risk, it is recommended that the intake of vegetable sources of these forms of vitamin A be maintained at an adequate level.

Prolonged high intake of carotenoids results in yellowing of the skin, which is termed aurantiasis, or carotenemia. The condition is not associated with toxic manifestations. Excessive intake of pre-formed vitamin A causes vitamin overload (hypervitaminosis A), which is associated with severe headache, bone pain, dry skin, fissuring of the lips, alopecia, impaired liver function, and hypercalcemia. The risk for liver toxicity of vitamin A is increased by pre-existing hepatitis. For individuals with viral hepatitis, a daily dose of 25,000 IU of vitamin A may precipitate liver failure. However, elderly people with normal liver and kidney function may be able to tolerate 50,000 IU of vitamin A per day for periods up to 6 months without overt evidence of chronic toxicity (Bauernfeind, 1980; Hatoff et al., 1982; Farris and Erdman, 1982). However, such doses cannot be recommended, since there is no therapeutic justification for these megadoses of the vitamin in later life.

Vitamin D. A metabolically active form of vitamin D is required to optimize calcium absorption and to release calcium from bones so that plasma calcium levels are maintained within normal limits. Further, vitamin D is required for phosphate homeostasis. These major biological effects of vitamin D are mediated by calcitriol, or 1,25-dihydroxy-D_3, which is formed from vitamin D_3, or cholecalciferol (Fraser, 1980). Vitamin D_3 is synthesized from 7-dehydrocholesterol in the epidermis when the skin is exposed to natural or artificial forms of ultraviolet light. The ultraviolet light actually converts the parent sterol to previtamin D, which is then converted to vitamin D through thermal isomerization (MacLaughlin and Holick, 1983). The vitamin D so formed is transported in the plasma to the liver, where it is hydroxylated to form 25-hydroxycholecalciferol, or calcidiol. The level of 25-hydroxycholecalciferol in the plasma is increased by sunlight exposure. Calcitriol is formed from 25-cholecalciferol in the kidney, and it forms the physiological stimulus to the intestinal transport of calcium. When calcitriol acts to release calcium from the skeleton, its effect is dependent on a concurrent release of parathyroid hormone (PTH) (Miller and Norman, 1984).

Vitamin D is also obtained from milk and margarine, which in the United States are enriched with this vitamin. Fish oils and liver are also rich sources of the vitamin (Neer et al., 1977).

Elderly individuals are at risk for vitamin D deficiency if they are in institutions, are homebound, or are excessively clothed, particularly if they also refrain from drinking milk or consuming other food sources of the vitamin. For those elderly whose outdoor exposure is in cloudy or air-polluted environments, the duration of light exposure to effect adequate skin synthesis of vitamin D is longer than for those who live in sunnier climates. Ultraviolet light absorption is also reduced by melanin, the normal skin pigment, and is therefore less in blacks than in whites for a given duration of light exposure. Also, ultraviolet light of the appropriate short wavelength for vitamin D synthesis is screened out with topical sunscreens, particularly those containing para-aminobenzoic acid or its esters (Devgun et al., 1981).

However, Newton et al. (1985) showed that in the elderly, plasma 25-hydroxycholecalciferol values can be maintained at the lower level of the acceptable range (20 nmol/l) when the daily intake of vitamin D is 4 μg and there is no exposure to sunlight.

Evidence is accumulating that elderly individuals may have an increased requirement for vitamin D to reduce the degree of bone loss which occurs with age. For example, Nordin et al. (1985) reported that normal elderly women in the north of England who have low plasma 25-hydroxycholecalciferol levels, indicative of vitamin D depletion, respond to vitamin D supplementation by gaining bone, whereas those not receiving such supplementation lose bone. However, while an increased need for vitamin D to prevent the bone loss of aging is advocated by certain investigators, McKenna et al. (1985) emphasize that the need for higher intake of vitamin D to prevent bone loss may occur only in populations who live in a sun-deprived climate.

Vitamin K. Vitamin K is required for the synthesis of the blood clotting factors II (prothrombin), VII, IX, and X, and it is therefore the vitamin which is required for the normal maintenance of blood coagulation (Suttie and Olsen, 1984). There are several forms of vitamin K. Vitamin K_1 is found in foods of vegetable and animal origin. Foods rich in vitamin K include such leafy green vegetables as spinach, broccoli, and brussels sprouts (Suttie, 1984). However, liver is also an excellent source of vitamin K_1. Diets of the elderly are adequate in their vitamin K_1 contents unless the individual is subsisting on bread, oatmeal, or formula foods that do not have added vitamin K. Vitamin K_2 is synthesized by the intestinal bacteria. Bacterial synthesis of vitamin K_2 is inhibited by administration of broad-spectrum antibiotics. Absorption of vitamin K_1, and probably of vitamin K_2, is impaired by concurrent intake of mineral oil. The human requirement for vitamin K is 1 μg/day. However, this requirement may be increased in the elderly if they are taking antibiotics or mineral oil over prolonged periods of time (Roe, 1986).

For the healthy elderly who are not receiving medications which inhibit vitamin K synthesis, absorption, or utilization, there is presently little evidence to suggest that the requirement for the vitamin is higher than in younger people. If they are eating a varied diet containing green vegetables, there is no evidence to suggest that there is a need for a vitamin K supplement.

Vitamin E. Vitamin E has been proposed as an antioxidant that can retard or prevent the aging process. Supporters of this theory believe that aging occurs mainly as a result of oxidative reactions in the body. They believe that in the process of lipid peroxidation there is an accumulation of cytotoxic free radicals and age-related pigments, such as lipofuscin, which are formed as a result of lipid auto-oxidation (Tappel et al., 1973). However, although vitamin E deficiency does increase the disposition of lipofuscin, vitamin E supplementation does not prevent lipofuscin accumulation, nor does it extend the lifespan of laboratory animals (Hayflick, 1985).

There are several isomers of vitamin E, including alpha-, beta-, gamma-, and delta-tocopherols. Of these forms, alpha-tocopherol is the most active. However, the American diet contains more gamma-tocopherol than alpha-tocopherol, and it has been shown that both isomers can contribute to the vitamin E activity of tissues (Aftergood and Alfin-Slater, 1978).

Vegetable oils, seeds, grains, and nuts are good sources of vitamin E. The 1980 RDA for vitamin E is 10 mg alpha-tocopherol equivalents for men and 8 mg alpha-tocopherol equivalents for women. In adults, particularly elderly adults, vitamin E deficiency is rare except in cases of severe malabsorption or in those subsisting for long periods of time on unsupplemented parenteral formulas (Binder, et al., 1965; Thurlow and Grant, 1982). There is presently no definitive evidence to suggest that the requirement for vitamin E increases in aging individuals.

Water-Soluble Vitamins

Thiamin. Thiamin is required as a coenzyme in reactions which are essential to the intermediary metabolism of cells. Cereal and cereal brans are the major natural food sources of thiamin, but in the United States, breads, other baked goods made with enriched flour, and breakfast cereals are fortified with thiamin. The absorption of thiamin from food may be reduced by concurrent heavy tea or alcohol consumption (Tanphaichitr and Wood, 1984).

Three forms of thiamin deficiency are distinguished: peripheral neuropathy ("dry beriberi"), cardiac beriberi, and the Wernicke-Korsakoff syndrome. In the United States, peripheral neuropathy and cardiac beriberi are rare. The Wernicke-Korsakoff syndrome (an organic brain syndrome, which is reversible in the acute phase) occurs mainly in alcoholics who are spree drinkers and who, during sprees, do not consume food. Alcoholics who develop the syndrome are likely to be Caucasian. Genetic variation in thiamin-dependent enzymes may decrease the susceptible individual's ability to utilize marginal amounts of dietary thiamin (Victor, Adams, and Collins, 1971; Blass and Gibson, 1977).

Thiamin intakes of most healthy, independent elderly in the United States are judged to be adequate, based on dietary recall. However, the elderly in the community and in geriatric facilities whose food intake is low have been found to be thiamin depleted. Alcohol abuse by the elderly is a risk factor for subclinical thiamin deficiency (Iber et al., 1982).

The 1980 RDA for individuals more than 51 years of age is 1.2 mg/day, but this RDA is not met by the elderly whose food intake is low. Further, up to 15 percent of the elderly population shows biochemical evidence of inadequate thiamin status using red cell transketolase activity as the index of thiamin nutriture. This finding is difficult to evaluate, since there is evidence that aging may affect this red cell enzyme assay (Markkanen, Heikinheimo, and Dahl, 1969).

Given that many elderly may now be increasing their energy expenditure through active exercise as a means of improving their fitness, they may concurrently increase their food-energy intakes to achieve weight maintenance. These changes in life-style may aid the elderly in meeting their thiamin requirements, provided that the increased food intake also provides more thiamin. However, it is as yet unknown whether exercise confers an increased need for thiamin in the elderly.

Riboflavin. Riboflavin in its active coenzyme forms, flavin mononucleotide (FMN) and flavin adenine dinucleotide (FAD), is required for oxidation-reduction reactions. Flavins are required for efficient energy utilization and in the metabolism of drugs. Rich food sources of the vitamin include milk, cheese, yogurt, and liver. Breads and many breakfast cereals are fortified with riboflavin.

Riboflavin deficiency (ariboflavinosis) is manifested by angular stomatitis, cheilosis, glossitis, and seborrheic dermatitis. Signs such as angular stomatitis are nonspecific and in the elderly may be caused by ill-fitting dentures or by drooling of saliva from the mouth. Unless the clinical signs that are suspected of being caused by riboflavin deficiency clear with administration of the vitamin, it cannot be proven that ariboflavinosis has been present (Roe, 1986).

The long-term riboflavin status of the elderly was studied by Rutishauser et al. (1979). These authors followed 23 adults and examined their riboflavin status in relation to intake for a period of 60 weeks. Determination of intake was from a record of food and beverages consumed for 1 year. Mean daily intakes of riboflavin were computed and found to be 1.2 ± 0.2 mg/day. At this level of intake, no clinical signs of riboflavin deficiency were present. There was considerable variability in riboflavin status within the group as reflected in the red cell glutathione reductase activity.

The RDA for riboflavin is 0.6 mg/1000 kcal/day for men and women, or 1.2 mg/day. The latter figure is based on a daily food-energy intake of 2000 kcal/day, which may not be consumed.

A special current concern that is under investigation is whether elderly having low food-energy intakes are at risk for riboflavin depletion. Also, since it has been shown that exercise increases the riboflavin requirements of young and middle-aged people, it is necessary to investigate whether this is also true in the elderly. Until this information is available, it is premature to reset the RDA for riboflavin for the older age groups.

Niacin. The niacin status of elderly people varies with economic status, being most adequate in the well-to-do and in those who habitually consume diets high in animal protein. Overt niacin deficiency with manifestations of pellagra is rare because of enrichment of bread and cereals with niacin. There is currently no scientific basis for recommending that the RDA for niacin should be increased (Garry et al., 1982).

Folic acid. Folate intakes of elderly populations have been shown to vary widely, and many studies have shown that elderly men and women may ingest less than the RDA from their diets (Vir and Love, 1979; Garry et al., 1982). There have also been studies of independently living and institutionalized elderly that have shown a high prevalence of mild folate deficiency. However, we have demonstrated that adequate folate nutriture can be maintained when healthy elderly ingest folate at the level of the RDA. Indeed, it is important to note that in elderly individuals who habitually consume readily available sources of folate, including fortified breakfast cereals and dark-green, leafy vegetables, erythrocyte folate levels are in the high range and similar to those of younger individuals with similar food habits (Weinberg, 1981). There is presently no justification for altering the RDA for folate.

Vitamin B$_6$. Many elderly men and women have low vitamin B$_6$ intakes. There is also some evidence that vitamin B$_6$ requirements increase with aging (Garry et al., 1982; Guilland et al., 1984). Methodological problems, however, exist in that (1) the vitamin B$_6$ content of some foods is unknown, (2) there is emerging evidence that the availability of vitamin B$_6$ may be different in foods of animal and vegetable protein, (3) the effects of exercise on vitamin B$_6$ requirements have not been computed, and (4) the biochemical assessment of vitamin B$_6$ nutriture is subject to misinterpretation. There is presently inadequate information to support any recommendation that the RDA for vitamin B$_6$ should be changed to meet the needs of the elderly.

Vitamin C. The marginal vitamin C status of some frail elderly people is related to the monotonous nature of their diets and to inadequate intake of citrus fruits and vegetables. However, currently many elderly whose vitamin C intake was previously low are consuming more of the vitamin because of fortification of fruit juices and other noncarbonated soft drinks. There is no definite evidence of a change in vitamin C absorption or metabolism with age, nor is there any evidence to suggest a need to increase the RDA for this vitamin (Kirk and Chieffi, 1953; Bowman and Rosenberg, 1982; Newton et al., 1985).

The Anti-oxidant Vitamins and the Reduction of Disease Risk in the Elderly

A broad range of disease processes, which are particularly prevalent in the elderly, including chronic inflammatory diseases, radiation damage, and cancer, involve reactive forms of oxygen which are generated by exposure to light and/or to chemicals in our diet or our external environment. Protection against oxidative damage, which has the potential for these long-range damaging effects may be afforded by anti–oxidant vitamins. Indeed, certain of these vitamins have been shown to actually stimulate the immune system which is suppressed in the aging process as well as by protein–energy malnutrition and in certain degenerative diseases occurring in the elderly.

Anti-oxidant vitamins have special potential in protecting the elderly against disease due to environmental agents which are carcinogenic. The vitamins and the vitamin-like compounds which fulfill such functions include the carotenoids, vitamin E, and vitamin C.

Certain carotenoids including beta-carotene and vitamin E have been shown capable of stimulating cellular immune function. This stimulation of the immune system was demonstrated in elderly men and women by measuring the percent of the various lymphocyte groups in the blood before and after giving this carotenoid. The beta-carotene stimulated those lymphocyte subpopulations which are associated with improved defense mechanisms. There was an increase in T–helper cells without any effect on T–suppressor cells. Daily doses of beta-carotene varied from 15–60 mg per day. The effects observed were dose dependent (Watson et al., 1991).

Vitamin E (tocopherol) levels in the plasma have been shown to be inversely related to gastrointestinal cancer risk (Knekt, 1988). Further, vitamin E stimulates cellular immune function in the elderly (Meydani et al., 1989).

Studies in normal people have shown that vitamin C given in large amounts is a nitrosation inhibitor; it reduces formation of nitrosamine–like compounds which are potentially carcinogenic (Tannenbaum et al., 1991).

MINERAL AND TRACE ELEMENT REQUIREMENTS

Calcium

Calcium requirements of the elderly may be greater than those of younger individuals. Evidences in support of the recommendation that the elderly should consume more calcium daily are the following:

1. Age-related bone loss is an accompaniment of the aging process, and these age-related changes in bone mass can be reduced or retarded by increased calcium intakes of older people.
2. Severe bone loss which occurs in some elderly people, particularly in elderly women, is the underlying cause of fractures, particularly hip fractures, which lead to chronic disability and high health care costs that must be reduced.
3. Calcium absorption decreases with age, and the age-related decrease in the efficiency of calcium absorption is particularly marked in women after menopause.
4. Because older people are less active and therefore subject to accelerated bone loss related to immobility, calcium requirements may be increased.
5. Human metabolic studies have shown that many elderly people are in negative calcium balance and that calcium balance can be achieved by increasing their intakes of calcium. It has been found that a level of 1.5 g/day achieves calcium balance (Heaney, Recker, and Saville, 1978; Heaney et al., 1982).
6. Epidemiological studies have indicated that by increasing calcium intake, the risk of hypertension may be reduced (McCarron, 1985).

Arguments against a recommendation that the calcium requirements of middle-aged and elderly people need to be increased are the following:

1. Age-related bone loss is a general phenomenon which is influenced in its severity by multiple factors, including genetic predisposition, level of activity, hormonal status, and several nutritional factors, e.g., the level of protein in the diet, the amount of dietary fiber ingested, calcium intake, vitamin D status, and fluoride intake. Therefore an increase in calcium intake would be unlikely to afford outstanding protection against the development of osteoporosis (Exton-Smith, 1985).

2. A general recommendation to increase calcium intakes in middle-aged and older women is not without health risk (Editorial, 1985). The risks which have been defined are based on the assumption that to achieve a desired daily intake of calcium people will take calcium supplements. Further, since the cheapest and most available calcium supplement is calcium carbonate, it is projected that the recommendation to increase calcium intake will be interpreted as a recommendation to take calcium carbonate supplements on a long-term basis. Risks of chronic ingestion of calcium carbonate in large amounts include the risk of the milk-alkali syndrome, which consists of chronic hypercalcemia and impaired renal function. It has been estimated that ingestion of 1 to 2 g of calcium per day can cause this problem in susceptible people. Additionally, if the calcium supplement is taken at mealtimes it could, because of its antacid effects, reduce the absorption of dietary folate and iron. There is also the risk of kidney stones in predisposed individuals.

Despite these risks, current information suggests that it may be advisable to encourage women, particularly postmenopausal women, to increase their calcium intakes. They should, however, attain their calcium needs from dietary sources of calcium, especially cheese, yogurt, or low-fat milk. If milk tolerance is impaired or if milk is disliked, calcium supplements should be taken under medical supervision and not at mealtimes.

Iron

Studies of independently living elderly populations, including those included in the NHANES I survey (Dallman, Yip, and Johnson, 1984), have indicated a low incidence of iron deficiency anemia. Iron stores tend to increase with age, and in the United States many elderly men and women consume more iron than the 10 mg/day which is the current RDA (Cook, Finch, and Smith, 1976; Lynch et al., 1982). When iron deficiency anemia develops in the elderly, it is most likely caused by bleeding, either because of chronic ingestion of aspirin or indomethacin or because of GI hemorrhage from a peptic ulcer, esophageal varices, or large bowel cancer.

Other risk factors for the development of iron deficiency in the elderly are long-term consumption of low-calorie diets; low intake of animal protein foods (particular meats); high consumption of tea, which reduces iron absorption; and achlorhydria, which occurs in about 10 percent of the elderly and which also may reduce iron absorption (Cook, Finch, and Smith, 1976; Lynch et al., 1982; Dallman, Yip, and Johnson, 1984; Alfin-Slater, 1984; Roe, 1985).

Since the recommended intake of iron seems to meet the needs of most healthy elderly, there does not currently seem to be any justification for an increase. However, it is extremely important for us to increase our awareness of elderly men and women who, because of poverty and loss of mobility, may be unable to obtain or prepare adequate food sources of iron. For these frail elderly, there is a need to provide congregate or home-delivered meals containing foods rich in iron.

Zinc

The recommended daily zinc allowance for adults is 15 mg daily. However, there is evidence that many men and women over 65 years of age consume less than this amount (Sandstead et al., 1982). Decreases in the intake of this trace element parallel decreases in food-energy intake that occur in the old elderly. Only about 30 percent of the zinc that is ingested is absorbed. In the elderly who follow recommendations to eat high-fiber diets, including bran, the absorption of zinc may be further decreased. It has been suggested that impaired cellular immune response and slow wound healing in the elderly may be related to zinc deficiency. However, loss of taste in the elderly is apparently not due to this cause. A need still exists to re-examine the zinc requirements of the elderly and to provide guidelines to elderly individuals on good sources of dietary zinc and on combining foods to optimize zinc absorption at mealtimes.

RECOMMENDED DIETARY ALLOWANCES

Recommended Dietary Allowances (RDAs) are defined as the levels of intake of essential nutrients that, on the basis of scientific knowledge, are judged by the Food and Nutrition Board to be adequate to meet the known nutrient needs of practically all healthy persons. The need to subdivide healthy elderly on the basis of age groups in order to set RDAs has been considered, but it seems premature to do this at this time since insufficient information is available on the needs of those who are healthy although very old. It is not appropriate to use the RDAs to define either the food-energy or nutrient needs of elderly who have acute or chronic diseases. For the purpose of setting RDAs, those 51 years of age or older are considered as the older age group in the population.

In the 10th edition of *Recommended Dietary Allowances* (1989), emphasis is placed on the food-energy needs of the elderly. On the basis of available evidence, the energy allowance of individuals above the age of 51 years is 1.5 × resting energy expenditure (REE). This assumes continued moderate physical activity, which is desirable. The average energy allowance for a man of reference size (77 kg) is 2300 kcal/day, while for women of reference size it is 1900 kcal/day. Strenuous physical activity will increase the food-energy needs of older as well as younger people. Included in this latest edition of the RDAs are the newly established RDAs for vitamin K and selenium, as well as a lowering of the RDAs for folate, vitamin B_6, vitamin B_{12}, and biotin.

TABLE 4-1   Complete 1989 RDAs for Those 51 and Older (Designed for the maintenance of good nutrition of practically all healthy people in the United States)

CATEGORY	AGE (YEARS) OR CONDITION	WEIGHT[b] (kg)	WEIGHT[b] (lb)	HEIGHT[b] (cm)	HEIGHT[b] (in)	PROTEIN (g)	FAT-SOLUBLE VITAMINS Vita-min A (μg RE)[c]	FAT-SOLUBLE VITAMINS Vita-min D (μg)[d]	FAT-SOLUBLE VITAMINS Vita-min E (mg α-TE)[e]	FAT-SOLUBLE VITAMINS Vita-min K (μg)
Males	51+	77	170	173	68	63	1,000	5	10	80
Females	51+	65	143	160	63	50	800	5	8	65

[a]The allowances, expressed as average daily intakes over time, are intended to provide for individual variations among most normal persons as they live in the United States under usual environmental stresses. Diets should be based on a variety of common foods in order to provide other nutrients for which human requirements have been less well defined. See text for detailed discussion of allowances and of nutrients not tabulated.
[b]Weights and heights of Reference Adults are actual medians for the U.S. population of the designated age, as reported by NHANES II. The median weights and heights of those under 19 years of age were taken from Hamill et al. (1979) (see pages 16–17). The use of these figures does not imply that the height-to-weight ratios are ideal.

Several factors are cited in the RDAs manual that influence the nutrient needs of some older people. These include the decreased ability of the aging skin to synthesize vitamin D, which makes a food source of vitamin D essential for elderly who do not go outdoors.

Among the water-soluble vitamins, it has been estimated that the folate needs of the elderly can be met by an intake of 135 mcg/day. This level of folate intake can maintain normal hematological status. The complete 1989 RDAs for those 51 years and older is shown in Table 4-1.

RELATIONSHIPS BETWEEN FOOD AND NUTRIENT INTAKE

Patterns of food intake determine nutrient intake. The diversity or variety of foods consumed has a profound influence on the nutrient quality of the diet. It can be generalized that a broad selection of foods from different food groups provides assurance against dietary deficiency of essential nutrients. Food groups that are generally recognized are (1) dairy products, (2) the "meat" group, or other protein-rich foods, (3) vegetables and fruits, and (4) cereal products. Elderly people should eat two servings daily of dairy products, one to two servings of the meat group, four servings of vegetables and fruits (which may include fruit juices), and four servings of cereals. Table 4-2 indicates foods which elderly adults should eat daily from the different food groups. Justification of this approach to dietary adequacy is that foods from the various food groups complement one another in supplying needed nutrients. Food sources of specific nutrients are indicated in Table 4-3 on page 84. When elderly people consume less than the recommended number of servings of food from the different food groups, the risk is that one or more nutrients may be consumed in less than optimal amounts. For example, elderly individuals who do not eat or

TABLE 4-1   (continued)

WATER-SOLUBLE VITAMINS							MINERALS						
Vita-min C (mg)	Thia-min (mg)	Ribo-flavin (mg)	Niacin (mg NE)[f]	Vita-min B₆ (mg)	Fo-late (μg)	Vitamin B₁₂ (μg)	Cal-cium (mg)	Phos-phorus (mg)	Mag-nesium (mg)	Iron (mg)	Zinc (mg)	Iodine (μg)	Sele-nium (μg)
60	1.2	1.4	15	2.0	200	2.0	800	800	350	10	15	150	70
60	1.0	1.2	13	1.6	180	2.0	800	800	280	10	12	150	55

[c]Retinol equivalents. 1 retinol equivalent = 1 μg retinol or 6 μg β-carotene. See text for calculation of vitamin A activity of diets as retinol equivalents.
[d]As cholecalciferol. 10 μg cholecalciferol = 400 ɪᴜ of vitamin D.
[e]α-Tocopherol equivalents. 1 mg d-α tocopherol = 1 α-ᴛᴇ. See text for variation in allowances and calculation of vitamin E activity of the diet as α-tocopherol equivalents.
[f]1 ɴᴇ (niacin equivalent) is equal to 1 mg of niacin or 60 mg of dietary tryptophan.

Source: Food and Nutrition Board, National Academy of Sciences—National Research Council Recommended Dietary Allowances,[a] Revised 1989.

TABLE 4-2   Recommended Daily Foods from the Four Food Groups

GROUP	FOOD	SERVINGS	HOUSEHOLD MEASURE
Dairy	Milk, skim	2	16 oz.
	-or-		
	American cheese +	1	1 slice
	Ice cream	1	1/2 cup
Meat	Chicken +	1	3 oz.
	Peanut butter	1	1 tbsp.
	-or-		
	Lean beef, lamb, or veal +	1	3 oz.
	Peas	1	1/2 cup
Vegetables and Fruits	Broccoli +	1	1/2 cup
	Tomatoes +	1	2 medium
	Orange juice	2	1-1/2 cups
	-or-		
	Carrots +	1	1/2 cup
	Spinach +	1	1/2 cup
	Cantaloupe +	1	1/2
	Orange juice	1	3/4 cup
Breads and Cereals	Bread, enriched +	3	3 slices
	Cold cereal, fortified	1	1/2 cup
	-or-		
	Bran muffin +	2	2
	Rice, enriched +	1	1/2 cup
	Bread, enriched whole wheat	1	1 slice

TABLE 4-3   Food Sources of Specific Nutrients

FOOD	NUTRIENTS
Milk	Protein, vitamins A, D, B_2, B_{12}, calcium
Cheese	Protein, vitamin B_2 and B_{12}, calcium
Ice cream	Vitamin B_{12}, calcium
Chicken	Protein, niacin, vitamin B_{12}, iron
Peanut butter	Protein, fat
Fish	Protein, iron
Peas	Protein, vitamin B_1, niacin, zinc
Broccoli	Pro-vitamin A, vitamin C, folacin, potassium
Tomatoes	Vitamin C
Orange juice	Vitamin C, potassium
Carrots	Pro-vitamin A
Spinach	Pro-vitamin A, vitamin C, folacin, vitamin K, iron, potassium
Cantaloupe	Vitamin C, potassium
Bread, enriched whole wheat	Carbohydrate, vitamins B_1, B_2, niacin, magnesium
Cereals, fortified	Carbohydrate, vitamins A, C, B_1, B_2, niacin, folacin, B_6 (+ fiber)
Bran muffins	Carbohydrate, B vitamins (+ fiber), vitamins B_1, B_2, niacin, magnesium
Rice, enriched	Carbohydrate, thiamin

drink dairy products are likely to consume too little calcium, vitamin D, and riboflavin for their needs.

Those who do not eat green vegetables or fruits may be at risk of not obtaining enough folacin, vitamin C, beta-carotene, and potassium for their needs.

Although omission of dairy foods, green vegetables, and fruit from the daily diet can be accepted as an index of a poor-quality diet, alternate means of satisfying nutrient needs are now available. One may take vitamin-mineral mixtures in physiological doses or a formula-type nutrient supplement. If an elderly individual will drink a small volume of milk per day, important nutrient requirements can be supplied by eating one or two servings of fortified cereal with the milk. A caution for dietitians advising the elderly on intake of foods fortified with folic acid: such foods should not be recommended until the elderly person has had a complete blood count with measurement of red cell indices. If a macrocytic anemia is discovered, serum vitamin B_{12} should be determined. No elderly person should be receiving daily folic acid supplements unless vitamin B_{12} deficiency (caused by pernicious anemia) has been excluded.

Alternate means of supplying nutrient requirements to the elderly to meet the RDA are shown in Table 4-4. The aim of this table is to demonstrate that nutrient needs can be supplied by carefully selected nutrient-rich foods or by semisynthetic formula foods. However, when foods included in the diet have a low nutrient-to-calorie ratio, more foods and more food items are required to cover nutrient needs.

TABLE 4-4   Alternate Means of Supplying Daily Nutrient Needs

A. LOW CALORIE MENU OF MANY NUTRIENT-RICH FOODS	B. HIGH CALORIE MENU WITH FEW NUTRIENT-RICH FOODS
RECOMMENDED	NOT RECOMMENDED

Breakfast

Orange juice, 1 glass	Apple juice, 1 glass
Cereal, 3/4 oz.	Frozen waffles, 2
Milk, skim, 1 glass	Syrup, 2 tbsp.
	Margarine, 2 tsp.
	Whole milk, 1 cup

Lunch

Grilled cheese sandwich, 1 (whole wheat bread, 2 slices, American cheese, 1 slice)	Chicken noodle soup, 1 can
	Saltine crackers, 8
	Cake, marble, 1 slice
Banana, 1	

Dinner

Chicken, 3 oz.	Beef pot pie, 1
Spinach, 1/2 cup	Broccoli, 1/2 cup
Potato, baked, 1 small	Sherbet, 1/2 cup
Margarine, 1 tbsp.	Cookies, 5
Orange, whole, 1 med.	

Snack

Milk, skim, 1 glass	Salted roast peanuts, 1/4 cup
	Milk chocolate bar, 2 oz.
	Whole milk, 1 cup

Number of foods

10	14

Total Kcal

1200	2600

RDA

Meets or exceeds in all specified nutrients if cereal is fortified.	Low in protein, vitamins A, D, C, B_1, B_2, niacin, folacin, calcium, and potassium if milk and broccoli are omitted. High in sodium.

C. SEMISYNTHETIC LIQUID DIET

Full liquid diets containing nutrients $\geq$ RDA can be supplied by Ensure (Ross), formulated to give 2000 kcal in 2 quarts. Indications for use of Ensure as a total liquid diet are when solid food cannot be swallowed. Single cans of Ensure can be given as a nutritional supplement when the diet is inadequate to meet nutrient requirements.

Particular risks associated with unwise food selection, storage, and preparation by the elderly are:

1. Too few different foods selected to supply nutrient needs
2. Food-energy intake unrelated to actual needs
3. Destruction of vitamins because of prolonged food storage, light exposure, prolonged cooking of foods in a large volume of water, addition of soda, microwave cooking, or overcooking for soft texture
4. Low fiber intake

DIETARY GUIDELINES FOR THE ELDERLY

Dietary guidelines for the population, including the elderly, are summarized in the National Research Council's monograph *Diet and Health* (1989). These guidelines are as follows:

1. Reduce total fat intake to 30 percent or less of total calories.
2. Every day eat five or more servings of a combination of vegetables and fruits, especially green and yellow vegetables and citrus fruits.
3. Increase intake of complex carbohydrates to 55 percent of total calories. Include cereals which provide good sources of dietary fiber.
4. Maintain a moderate protein intake.
5. Balance food intake and physical activity to maintain appropriate body weight.
6. Do not consume alcohol.
7. Limit total daily intake of salt.
8. Maintain adequate calcium intake.
9. Avoid taking dietary supplements in excess of the RDA during any one day.

QUESTIONS

Circle all correct answers (there may be more than one correct answer to each question).

1. Food energy needs are reduced with advancing age. The major reason is that:
   a. old people cannot digest much food
   b. old people conserve body heat better than young people
   c. sick older people recover more quickly on a restricted diet
   d. if a person is taking medicines, he or she should eat less food
   e. decreased physical activity is associated with decreased energy production
2. Needs for vitamin D are increased by:
   a. frequent colds
   b. decreased sunlight exposure

c. consumption of a low cholesterol diet
d. decreased physical activity
e. intake of certain drugs

3. In 1989, Recommended Dietary Allowances were given for specific age ranges among the elderly for:
   a. zinc
   b. vitamin D
   c. folacin
   d. thiamin
   e. food-energy

4. Protein requirements could change with age. Present evidence indicates that the protein requirements of healthy elderly are:
   a. less than those of younger persons
   b. equal to those of younger persons
   c. greater than those of younger persons

5. Prevalent conditions among the elderly that we know can alter nutrient needs are:
   a. decline in renal function
   b. congestive heart failure
   c. malabsorption
   d. chronic intake of medications
   e. dryness of the skin

REFERENCES

AFTERGOOD, L., and R. B. ALFIN-SLATER, "Effect of administration of alpha- and gamma-tocopherol on tissue distribution and red cell hemolysis in rats," *Int. J. Vitam. Nutr. Res.* 48 (1978), 32–37.

ALFIN-SLATER, R. B., "Aging: a condition or a disease?" in *Nutrition in Gerontology*, eds. J. M. Ordy, D. Harman, and R. B. Alfin-Slater. New York: Raven Press, 1984, pp. 323–30.

BAUERNFEIND, J. C., *The Safe Use of Vitamin A: A Report of the International Vitamin Consultative Group*. New York: The Nutrition Foundation, 1980.

BAUERNFEIND, J. C., and W. M. COURT, *Critical Review of Food Technology*. Boca Raton, FL: CRC Press, Inc., 1974.

BENDICH, A., and J. A. OLSON, "Biological actions of carotenoids," *FASEB J.*, 3 (1989), 1927–32.

BINDER, H. J., et al., "Tocopherol deficiency in man," *New Eng. J. Med.*, 273 (1965), 1289–97.

BLASS, J. P., and G. E. GIBSON, "Abnormality of a thiamine-requiring enzyme in patients with Wernicke-Korsakoff syndrome," *New Eng. J. Med.*, 297 (1977), 1367–70.

BOWMAN, B. B., and I. H. ROSENBERG, "Assessment of the nutritional status of the elderly," *Amer. J. Clin. Nutr.*, 35 (1982), 1142–51.

CHENG, A. H. R., A. GOMEZ, J. G. GERGAN, T. C. LEE, F. MANCKEBERG, and C. O. CHICKEDEE, "Comparative nitrogen balance study between young and aged adults using three levels of protein intake from a combination of wheat-soy-milk mixture," *Amer. J. Clin. Nutr.*, 31 (1978), 12.

CHYTIL, F., "Vitamin A and skin," in *Biochemistry and Physiology of the Skin*, ed. L. A. Goldsmith. New York: Oxford University Press, 1983, pp. 1187–94.

COHN, S. H., D. VARTSKY, S. YASAMURA, A. SAWITSKY, I. ZANZI, A. VASWANI, and K. J. ELLIS, "Compartmental body composition based on total body nitrogen, potassium, and calcium," *Amer. J. Physiol.*, 239 (1980), 524.

COOK, J. D., C. A. FINCH, and N. J. SMITH, "Evaluation of the iron status of a population, *Blood*, 48 (1976), 449.

DALLMAN, P. R., R. YIP, and C. JOHNSON, "Prevalence and causes of anemia in the United States, 1976–1980," *Amer. J. Clin. Nutr.*, 39 (1984), 437.

DEVGUN, M. S., C. R. PATERSON, B. E. JOHNSON, and C. COHEN, "Vitamin D nutrition in relation to season and occupation," *Amer. J. Clin. Nutr.*, 34 (1981), 1501–04.

FOOD and NUTRITION BOARD *Diet and Health: Implications for Reducing Chronic Disease Risk*," Washington, DC: National Academy Press, 1989, pp. 42, 146–48, 264–65, 312, 317, 432, 445, 511.

DURNIN, J. V. G. A., "Dietary intake of the elderly," in *Current Achievements in Geriatrics*, eds. W. F. Anderson and B. Isaacs. London: Cassell, 1964.

Editorial, "Calcium tablets for hypertension?" *Ann. Intern. Med.*, 103 (1985), 946–47.

EXTON-SMITH, A. N., "Physiological aspects of aging: relationship to nutrition," *Amer. J. Clin. Nutr.*, 25 (1972), 853–59.

EXTON-SMITH, A. N., "Mineral metabolism," in *Handbook of the Biology of Aging*, eds. C. E. Finch and E. L. Schneider. New York: Van Nostrand Reinhold Co., 1985, pp. 511–39.

EXTON-SMITH, A. N., and P. W. OVERSTALL, *Geriatrics*. Lancaster, England: M.T.P. Press, Ltd., 1979.

FARRIS, W. A., and J. W. ERDMAN, "Protracted hypervitaminosis A following long-term low-level intake," *J. Amer. Med. Assoc.*, 247 (1982), 1317–18.

FOOD AND NUTRITION BOARD, National Academy of Sciences, National Research Council, *Recommended Daily Dietary Allowances*, 9th Ed. Washington, DC, 1980.

FOOD AND NUTRITION BOARD, NRC, *Recommended Dietary Allowances*, 10th Ed. Washington, DC: National Academy Press, 1989, pp. 30, 33–34, 59–60, 93, 95, 103, 111, 127, 153, 159, 162, 208, 249–250.

FORBES, G. B., and J. C. REINA, "Adult lean body mass declines with age: some longitudinal observations," *Metabolism*, 19 (1970), 653—63.

FRASER, D. R., "Regulation of the metabolism of vitamin D," *Physiol. Rev.*, 60 (1980), 551–613.

GARRY, P. J., J. S. GOODWIN, W. C. HUNT, E. M. HOOPER, and A. G. LEONARD, "Nutritional status in a healthy elderly population: dietary and supplemental intakes," *Amer. J. Clin. Nutr.*, 36 (1982), 319–31.

GERSOVITZ, M., H. N. MUNRO, J. UDALL, and V. R. GARRY, "Albumin synthesis in young and elderly subjects using a new stable isotope methodology: response to levels of protein intake," *Metabolism*, 29 (1975).

GERSOVITZ, M., K. MOTIL, H. N. MUNRO, N. S. SCRIMSHAW, and V. R. YOUNG, "Human protein requirements: assessment of the adequacy of the current recommended dietary allowance for dietary problems in elderly men and women," *Amer. J. Clin. Nutr.*, 35 (1982), 6.

GILLUM, H. L., A. F. MORGAN, and F. L. SAILER, "Nutritional status of the aging," *J. Nutr.*, 55 (1955), 655–70.

GUILLAND, J. C., B. BEREKSI-REGUIG, LEQUEU, D. MOREAU, J. KLEPPING, and D. RICHARD, "Evaluation of pyridoxine intake and pyridoxine status among aged institutionalised people," *Int. J. Vitam. Nutr. Res.*, 54 (1984), 185–93.

HARPER, A. E. "Recommended Dietary Allowances for the elderly," *Geriatrics*, 33 (1978), 73–80.

HATOFF, D. E., S. L. GERTLER, K. MIYAI, B. A. PARKER, and J. B. WEISS, "Hypervitaminosis A unmasked by acute viral hepatitis," *Gastroenterology*, 82 (1982), 124–28.

HAYFLICK, L., "The aging process: current theories," *Drug-Nutr. Interac.*, 4 (1985), 13–33.

HEANEY, R. P., R. R. RECKER, and P. D. SAVILLE, "Menopausal changes in calcium balance," *J. Lab. Clin. Med.*, 92 (1978), 953–63.

HEANEY, R. P., J. C. GALLAGHER, C. C. JOHNSTON, R. NEER, A. M. PARFITT, and G. D. WHEDON, "Calcium nutrition and bone health in the elderly," *Amer. J. Clin. Nutr.*, 36 (1982), 986.

HOSTETTER, T. H., "Progressive glomerular injury: roles of dietary protein and compensatory hypertrophy," *Pharmacol. Rev.*, 36 (1984), 1018.

IBER, F. L., J. P. BLASS, M. BRIN, and C. M. LEEVY, "Thiamin in the elderly: relation to alcoholism and to neurological degenerative disease," *Amer. J. Clin. Nutr.*, 6 (1982), 1067–82.

KIRK, J. E., and W. CHIEFFI, "Vitamin studies in middle aged and old individuals. I. The vitamin A, total carotene, and alpha and beta carotene concentration in plasma," *J. Nutr.*, 36 (1948), 315–22.

KIRK, J. E., and W. CHIEFFI, "Vitamin studies in middle aged and old individuals. XII. Hypovitaminemia C," *J. Gerontol.*, 8 (1953), 305–11.

KNEKT, P. SERUM "Alpha-tocopherol and the risk of cancer," Helsinki: Publications of the Social Insurance Institution, (1988), 1–148.

KRASINSKI, S. D., J. S. COHN, E. J. SCHAEFER, and R. M. RUSSELL, "Postprandial plasma retinyl ester response is greater in older subjects compared with younger subjects," *J. Clin. Invest.*, 85 (1990), 883–892.

LINDER, M. C., "Nutrition and metabolism of vitamins," in *Nutritional Biochemistry and Metabolism*, ed. M. C. Linder. New York: Elsevier North-Holland, Inc., 1985, pp. 102–10.

LYNCH, S. R., C. A. FINCH, E. R. MONSEN, and J. D. COOK, "Iron status of elderly Americans," *Amer. J. Clin. Nutr.*, 36 (1982), 1032.

MACLAUGHLIN, J. A., and M. F. HOLICK, "Photobiology of vitamin D_3 in the skin," in *Biochemistry and Physiology of the Skin*, ed. L. A. Goldsmith, New York: Oxford University Press, 1983, pp. 734–54.

MARKKANEN, T., R. HEIKINHEIMO, and M. DAHL, "Transketolase activity of red blood cells from infancy to old age," *Acta Haemat.* (1969), 148–53.

McCARRON, D. A. "Is calcium more important than sodium in the pathogenesis of essential hypertension?" *Hypertension*, 7 (1985), 657–67.

McKENNA, M. J., R. FREANEY, A. MEADE, and F. P. MULDOWNEY, "Hypovitaminosis D and elevated serum alkaline phosphatase in elderly Irish people," *Amer. J. Clin. Nutr.*, 41 (1985), 101–09.

METTLIN, C., "The development of research on the epidemiology of vitamin A and cancer," in *Diet, Nutrition, and Cancer: From Basic Research to Policy Implications*, eds. D. A. Roe and T. C. Campbell. New York: Alan R. Liss, Publisher, 1983, pp. 125–34.

MEYDANI, S. N., M. P. BARKLUND, S. LIU, M. MEYDANI, R. A. MILLER, J. G. CANNON, F. D. MORROW, R. ROCKLIN, and J. B. BLUMBERG, *Amer. J. Clin. Nutr.*, 52, (1990), 557–563.

MILLER, B. E., and A. W. NORMAN, "Vitamin D," in *Handbook of Vitamins: Nutritional, Biochemical, and Clinical Aspects*, ed. L. J. Machlin. New York: Marcel Dekker, Inc., 1984, pp. 45–97.

MULDOON, M. F., S. B. MANUCK, and K. A. MATHEWS, "Lowering cholesterol concentrations and mortality: a quantitative review of primary prevention trials," *Brit. Med. J.*, 301 (1990), 309–14.

MUNRO, H. N., "Major gaps in nutrient allowances: the status of the elderly," *J. Amer. Dietet. Assoc.*, 76 (1980), 137–40.

MUNRO, H. N., and A. V. EVERETT, "Introduction to mini-symposium on nutrition and aging" in *Nutrition in Health and Disease and International Development*. Proc. Symp. XII Int. Congr. Nutr., Aug. 1981, San Diego, eds. A. E. Harper and G. K. Davis. New York: Alan R. Liss, Publisher, Inc., 1981, pp. 677–85.

NEER, R., M. CLARK, V. FREDMAN, et al., "Environmental and nutritional influences on plasma 25 hydroxy-vitamin D concentration and calcium metabolism in man," in *Vitamin D: Biochemical, Chemical, and Clinical Aspects Related to Calcium Metabolism*, eds. A. W. Norman, K. Schaeffer, D. V. Herrath, et al. West Berlin: De Gruyter, 1977, pp 595–06.

NEWTON, H. M. V., M. SHELTAWY, A. W. M. HAY, and B. MORGAN, "The relations between vitamin D_2 and D_3 in the diet and plasma 25(OH)D_2 and 25(OH)D_3 in elderly women in Great Britain," *Amer. J. Clin. Nutr.*, 41 (1985), 760–64.

NORDIN, B. E. C., M. R. BAKER, A. HORSMAN, and M. PEACOCK, " A prospective trial of the effect of vitamin D supplementation on metacarpal bone loss in elderly women," *Amer. J. Clin. Nutr.*, 42 (1985), 47–474.

Nutrition and Health in Old Age. The Cross-Sectional Analysis of the Findings of a Survey made in 1972/3 for Elderly People Who Had Been Studied in 1967/8, Report by the Committee on Medical Aspects of Food Policy, Department of Health and Social Security Report on Health and Social Subjects #16. London: Her Majesty's Stationery Office, 1979.

OLSON, J. A., "Vitamin A," in *Handbook of Vitamins: Nutritional, Biochemical, and Clinical Aspects*, ed. L. J. Machlin. New York: Marcel Dekker, Inc., 1985, pp. 1–43.

RAFSKY, H. A., B. NEWMAN, and N. JOLLIFFE, "A study of the carotene and vitamin A levels in the aged," *Gastroenterology*, 8 (1948), 612–15.

ROE, D. A., *Drug-Induced Nutritional Deficiencies.* Westport, CT: AVI Publishing Co., 1976, pp. 99–100.

ROE, D. A., *Drug-Induced Nutritional Deficiencies*, 2nd Ed. New York: AVI Publishing Co., 1986.

RUTISHAUSER, I. H. E., et al., "Long term vitamin status and dietary intake of healthy elderly subjects. I. Riboflavin," *Brit. J. Nutr.*, 42 (1979), 33–42.

SANDSTEAD, H. H., L. K. HENRIKSEN, J. L. GREGER, A. S. PRASAD, and R. A. GOOD, "Zinc nutriture in the elderly in relation to taste acuity, immune response, and wound healing," *Amer. J. Clin. Nutr.*, 36 (1982), 10–46.

SMITH, E. L., *Vitamin B_{12}*, 3rd Ed. New York: John Wiley & Sons, Inc., 1965, p. 180.

STEEN, G. B., B. ISAKSSON, and A. SVANBERG, "Body composition at 70 and 75 years of age: a longitudinal population study," *J. Clin. Exp. Gerontol.*, 1 (1979), 185.

The Surgeon General's Report on Nutrition and Health. DHHS (PHS) Publ. No. 88-50210. Washington, DC, 1988, pp. 595–614.

SUTTIE, J. W., "Vitamin K," in *Handbook of Vitamins: Nutritional, Biochemical, and Clinical Aspects*, ed. L. J. Machlin, New York: Marcel Dekker, Inc., 1984, pp. 147–198.

SUTTIE, J. W., and R. E. OLSON, "Vitamin K," in *Present Knowledge in Nutrition*, 5th ed. Washington, DC: The Nutrition Foundation, 1984, pp. 241–59.

TANNENBAUM, S. R., J. S. WISHNOK, and C. D. LEAF, "Inhibition of nitrosamine formation by ascorbic acid," *Amer. J. Clin. Nutr.*, 53 (1991) 247S–250S.

TANPHAICHITR, V., and B. WOOD, "Thiamin," in *Present Knowledge in Nutrition*, 5th ed. Washington, DC: The Nutrition Foundation, 1984.

TAPPEL, A. L., et al., "Effect of antioxidants and nutrients on lipid peroxidation fluorescent products and aging parameters in the mouse," *J. Gerontol.*, 28 (1973), 415.

THURLOW, P. M., and J. P. GRANT, "Vitamin E and total parenteral nutrition," *Ann. N. Y. Acad. Sci.*, 393 (1982), 121–32.

UANY, R., N. S. SCRIMSHAW, W. M. RAND, and V. R. YOUNG, "Human protein requirements: nitrogen balance response to graded levels of egg protein in elderly men and women," *Amer. J. Clin. Nutr.*, 31 (1978), 779.

VESTAL, R. E., "Methodological problems associated with studies of drug metabolism in the elderly," in *Proc. First World Conf. Clin. Pharmacol. and Therap.*, London, Aug 3–9, 1980, ed. P. Turner. London: Macmillan Publishing Ltd., 1980.

VICTOR, M., R. D. ADAMS, and G. H. COLINS. *The Wernicke-Korsakoff Syndrome: A Clinical and Pathological Study of 245 Patients, 82 with Post-mortem Examinations.* Philadelphia: F. A. Davis Co., 1971.

VIR, S. C., and A. H. G. LOVE, "Nutritional status of institutionalized and non-institutionalized aged in Belfast, North Ireland," *Amer. J. Clin. Nutr.*, 32 (1979), 1933–47.

WATSON, R. R., R. H. PRABHALA, and P. M. PLEZIA, "Beta-carotene on lymphocyte subpopulations in elderly humans: evidence for a dose response relationship," *Amer. J. Clin. Nutr.*, 53, (1991), 90–94.

WATT, B. K., and A. L. MERRILL, *Composition of Foods—Raw, Processed, Prepared*, Rev. Agric. Handbook No. 8. Washington, DC: U. S. Department of Agriculture, 1963.

WEINBERG, S., "Folacin intake and status of independent-living elderly women." M. S. thesis, Cornell University, 1981.

WHITE, W. S., and D. A. ROE, "Effect of in vivo irradiation on plasma levels of vitamin A and carotenoids," *Fed. Proc.*, 45 (1986), 831.

WINTERER, J. C., W. P. STEFFEE, W. D. A. PERERA, R. UANY, N. S. SCRIMSHAW, and V. R. YOUNG, "Whole body protein turnover in aging men," *Exp. Gerontol.*, II (1976), 79–87.

YOUNG, V. R., W. D. PERERA, J. C. WINTERER, et al., "Protein and amino acid requirements of the elderly—an overview," in *Nutrition and Aging*, ed. M. Winick. New York: John Wiley & Sons, Inc., 1976, pp. 77–118.

YUSPA, Y. H., "Retinoids and tumor promotion," in *Diet, Nutrition and Cancer: From Basic Research to Policy Implications.* New York: Alan R. Liss, Publishers, Inc., 1983, pp. 95–109.

ZANNI, E., D. H. CALLAWAY, and A. Y. ZEZULKA, "Protein requirements of elderly men," *J. Nutr.*, 109 (1979), 513–24.

chapter 5

Factors Determining Food Intake

FOOD HABITS

Food Preferences

Cultural factors. In the elderly, as in younger people, food preferences are to a great extent determined by family traditions, by ethnicity,
and by religious or traditional beliefs (Le Gros Clark, 1968). Foods that are
familiar are liked best, and even the elderly whose food intake is limited by
health problems prefer dishes which they have enjoyed since early life.
Regional foods are appealing if they are considered to be staples, essential
components of a "good meal," or a meal accompaniment. In the United
States an example of regional staples would be corn bread and corn meal
muffins, which are commonly eaten in the Southern states. "Essential"
components of meals include eggs and toast for breakfast, soup and a
sandwich for lunch, and meat or fish for dinner. The elderly may prefer
dinner foods in the middle of the day. Appropriate accompaniments to
meals include tea, coffee, and jam for breakfast, milk for lunch, and
potatoes and gravy for dinner.

With aging, rigidity of food habits usually increases, and the familiar
food pattern is much sought after. Ethnicity will determine food habits if
the traditions of the foods have been preserved. The elderly working-class
Italians usually want their pasta, as well as the zuppa or polenta, which
remind them of a secure family life. When an elderly person has always
eaten foods of his or her country or origin, it is very difficult to win them

away from these foods, and they will become particularly unhappy if such foods are denied them when they are in the hospital or in an extended care facility

Religious custom may determine food choice. For example, the Orthodox Jew believes that only kosher food may be eaten. Food choice may also be determined by season, whether the season is religious or climatic (fish during Lent and soup in the winter). Prestigious foods might be selected whether or not they are appropriate to the person's health and needs; for example, white bread is usually preferred over whole wheat or rye. Folklore and tradition may determine the choice of food for invalids and it is for this reason that the ailing elderly may want chicken broth which is "strengthening."

Social factors. Food preferences are highly influenced by education. As previously indicated, elderly people usually prefer familiar foods. Uneducated people are likely to have only had the experience of a relatively small number of different foods, and their food choices are among the foods that they know well. More educated people are likely to have experienced many different foods and therefore may have broader ranges of likes and dislikes.

The desire to try new foods in later life is a reflection of cultural experience in earlier years. Elderly people, however disabled, will enjoy unusual foods if they have done so during their earlier years. The university professor who is 90 and has lived in France may prefer ripe Brie cheese over processed cheese, whereas a 90-year-old ex-factory worker who has neither education nor the experience of foreign travel might dislike Brie intensely and would select the processed cheese.

Nutrition education affects food choice in that elderly people who have a knowledge of the caloric value of foods and also of the nutrient composition of foods may prefer to eat foods that have a high nutrient-to-calorie ratio. Many people who want to adhere to a special diet, either self-imposed or prescribed by a physician, will follow the diet more closely if they have a knowledge of nutrition and are able to read and comprehend food labels.

Situational factors. In the elderly, situational factors have a large bearing on food preference and choice. If an elderly person has limited financial resources, food choice will be from cheaper foods. If the person lives a long distance from a store or has no transportation, and the store has no delivery service, then preference is for foods that can be easily carried and that can be stored without refrigeration. If there are no cooking arrangements, or if cooking arrangements in the individual's residence are inadequate, then food choice will be from among items that do not require cooking or which only require a simple preparation. If the individual is living alone or with one other person of a similarly advanced age, then food preference is for items that are sold in small packages. When larger packages are purchased, usually part of the package has to be thrown away or the purchaser has to eat the same food, perhaps a vegetable, on several nights in succession. If an elderly person is disabled, then constraints on food choice and preference are multiple, resulting in a need to select from foods that do not require preparation, do not have to be removed from cans, and do not have to be cooked in any way which requires special manual dexterity.

Food availability determines the food choice of elderly people who live in domiciliary care facilities or nursing homes. In these situations, food choice is from the menu supplied as well as from the diet prescribed.

Although food preferences of the elderly may be similar to those of the young, people who are undertaking geriatric care often believe that their elderly charges want only certain foods which they deem appropriate. Nursing personnel in facilities for the elderly will commonly state that the residents or patients "won't eat salad or raw fruit" when, in fact, they have not made the experiment of directly presenting these items in an attractive form.

Medical factors. When unpleasant symptoms are associated with the intake of specific foods or beverages, these tend to be avoided. For example, if milk, cereal products, or fats induce diarrhea, then selection will be from among other types of food. Taste loss or perversion of taste and smell which occur in certain elderly people may determine avoidance of some foods and preference for others. Iatrogenic (doctor-prescribed) diets limit food choice. If these are used additively by patients, food choice may be limited to a very few items, to an extent that may contribute to malnutrition (Clarke and Wakefield, 1975).

DETERMINANTS OF FOOD INTAKE

Hunger and Appetite

Hunger comprises the physiological sensations that indicate a need for food. *Repletion* is the term for the visceral sensations associated with having eaten enough to satisfy hunger. *Appetite* indicates the desire for food, including hunger, but also includes the appeal of food whether hunger is present or not. *Satiety* indicates that enough food has been eaten to satisfy both hunger and the desire for food. Often satiety is also associated with indicators of having had enough, such as distension or abdominal bloating.

Appetite may be disturbed or reduced by (1) food aversions and (2) anorexia.

Food aversion. Reduction in food intake by the elderly may occur when the eating situation is unpleasant or when eating causes distressing symptoms. Circumstances which reduce the desire to eat include:

1. *Unattractive surroundings.* Eating is less attractive when the surroundings are dark, because the food cannot be seen; when the room is noisy, because of the distracting effect of noise; when the room is cold, because the person is preoccupied with the need to get warm; when the room is excessively

hot, because of a feeling of faintness; and when the room is dirty or unkempt, because this suggests that the hygiene of the food may be in doubt and because the appeal of food is always reduced if it is served in an unattractive manner.

2. *Unpleasant company.* An elderly person is less likely to eat if others present, including family, household members, home health aides, nurses' aides, or nurses, are silly, impatient, inattentive, or abusive. In the hospital situation, they are less likely to eat when other patients are noisy or psychotic.

3. *Bad food service.* The elderly will eat less if food is monotonous, if portions are too small, or too large, if hot dishes are served cold, if vegetables are not drained, if food is not fresh, if food arrives late, if food ordered is not available, if food is unattractive in appearance, if foods on the menu are disliked, if dishes are unfamiliar, if no provision is made for special diets, and if food taboos are not recognized.

4. *Disturbances during meals.* Less food will be eaten if meals are served at unaccustomed times or are interrupted. In hospitals, meals may be interrupted when procedures are scheduled at mealtimes.

Food aversion is a term which denotes antipathy to one or more foods, unwillingness to eat, or dislike of eating. Food aversions arise under the following circumstances:

1. When food or the process of eating food produces an unpleasant sensation
2. When the sight or thought of certain foods or the taste or smell of certain foods evokes the memory of something unpleasant
3. When foods are believed to have some unpleasant property

In the elderly, the following food-related symptoms evoke food aversion:

1. Gastric distension leading to breathlessness, as it occurs in patients with congestive heart failure
2. Abdominal pain and gassy diarrhea, as found in patients with secondary lactose intolerance associated with malabsorption syndromes
3. Dysphagia (pain on swallowing) associated with cancer of the mouth, pharynx, or esophagus; operative conditions of the mouth, pharynx or esophagus; radiation therapy involving the pharynx or neck; and cancer chemotherapy (e.g., methotrexate), which can cause oral ulceration
4. Distortion of taste or smell, usually associated with metastatic or widespread cancer and/or radiation therapy or cancer chemotherapy
5. Nausea with or without vomiting, related to radiation therapy or chemotherapy (It is to be emphasized that food aversions arise when foods are associated with these unpleasant events, although eating those foods does not induce unpleasant sensations. Thus, for example, if chocolate chip ice cream has been eaten at a time when intravenous cancer chemotherapeutic drugs are or have just been administered, then chocolate chip ice cream will forthwith be disliked because of its association with severe nausea which was actually the result of the bolus drug administration [Shils, 1979; Carter, 1981].)

Eating aversion in the elderly may indicate severe psychiatric disturbance. Causes include:

1. Psychotic depression causing a complete disinterest in food
2. Confusional states, where the patient is unaware of time or place
3. Paranoia, where patients believe the food is poisoned
4. Dementia (e.g., Alzheimer's disease), where the patient is unwilling to swallow or has developed a gagging reflex (Exton-Smith, 1973)

Elderly patients, particularly those with severe chronic disabilities or terminal illnesses, may stop eating as an unspoken signal that they do not wish to go on living.

The feeding of patients who rebel against eating should be approached with great caution, because it is not uncommon for patients under these circumstances to inhale pieces of food that have been fed to them by an overzealous relative, attendant, or nurse.

Anorexia. Anorexia in the elderly is usually associated with acute or chronic physical disease. Acute diseases associated with anorexia are febrile conditions such as pneumonia (bacterial or viral) and gastroenteritis. Chronic diseases associated with anorexia are:

1. GI disease, whether or not it is associated with jaundice, e.g., alcoholic liver disease, primary or secondary carcinoma of the liver, or carcinoma of the head of the pancreas
2. Cardiovascular diseases, e.g., congestive heart failure
3. Respiratory diseases, e.g., emphysema with pulmonary decompensation
4. Chronic renal disease, e.g., chronic nephritis with uremia
5. Cancer (In the elderly, the most common cause of severe anorexia in a patient who has previously had a good appetite is cancer. When anorexia develops in the elderly without obvious cause, the physician should carry out full oncological screening. If a patient complaining of loss of weight is seen by the nutritionist and loss of appetite is admitted, it is necessary for this to be reported immediately to the physician so that the patient can be investigated to find out whether or not cancer is present.)

Other conditions associated with anorexia are:

1. *Intake of marginal diets* (diets low in protein or thiamin)
2. *Malnutrition.* Avitaminoses, including deficiencies of thiamin, niacin, folacin, and vitamin B_6, are associated with anorexia. Zinc deficiency as may occur in elderly patients with alcoholic cirrhosis causes anorexia in association with loss of taste.
3. *Postgastrectomy syndromes.* Elderly patients who have had partial or total gastrectomies frequently are anorectic and/or may display early satiety. Reasons for this include vitamin deficiencies, which are the result of combined low intake and malabsorption; dumping syndrome (which causes a fear of eating rather than true anorexia); and an early feeling of fullness because of the small size of the gastric remnant (Floch, 1981).

TABLE 5-1   Major Causes of Reduced Food Intake in the Elderly

Unattractive surroundings	Cirrhosis
Unpleasant company	Congestive heart failure
Bad food service	Pulmonary insufficiency
Mealtime disturbances	Chronic renal disease
Breathlessness	Cancer
Gastric distension	Malnutrition
Abdominal pain	Postgastrectomy syndromes
Gassy diarrhea	Incoordination
Dysphagia	Paralysis
Taste or smell perversion	Arthritis
Nausea and vomiting	Loss of consciousness
Depression	Drugs, e.g. digoxin or cancer
Confusion	chemotherapeutic agents
Paranoia	Restricted diets
Dementia	Alcohol abuse

4. *Drugs.* Therapeutic drugs used in short- and long-term therapy can induce severe anorexia. Anorexia may be inevitable, as with certain cancer chemotherapeutic drugs, and may be associated with high drug dosage, as with high level of digoxin, or may be associated with drug toxicity, i.e., hepatoxicity or nephrotoxicity (Roe, 1979). (See discussion of the effects of drugs in the elderly in Chapter 9.)

Causes of reduced food intake in the elderly are in Table 5-1.

DISEASES ASSOCIATED WITH DECREASED INTAKE OF FOOD

Diseases that are not associated with anorexia can nevertheless cause the patient to take in very little food (Floch, 1981). See Table 5.2 for a summary of diseases which lower food intake.

TABLE 5-2   Geriatric Diseases Which Lower Food Intake

DISEASE	MECHANISM
Congestive heart failure	Food-related breathlessness
Scleroderma	Mouth cannot be fully opened
Cancer of the esophagus	Painful swallowing and regurgitation
Stroke	Unconsciousness

Reasons are:

1. The patient cannot open the mouth or cannot open it adequately.
2. The patient cannot swallow.
3. The patient cannot retain food because of vomiting or regurgitation.
4. Food cannot be given by mouth because the patient is unconscious.

DISABILITIES WHICH REDUCE FOOD INTAKE

Severely disabled elderly people have reduced food intake unless they can obtain assistance with food preparation and/or with eating (Exton-Smith, 1973). Types of disability associated with low food intake are paralyses (as in stroke patients), dementia (as in patients with Alzheimers's disease), crippling (as in patients with arthritis), incoordination (as in patients with Parkinson's disease), and blindness, particularly if the loss of vision has developed in later life.

Feeder Dependency and Food intake

Intake of food may also be reduced in demented nursing home patients who need to be fed by nursing aides. Problems that contribute to low food intake and to resultant protein-energy malnutrition in these patients include the tendency of these patients to refuse food or to push food out of their mouths. There may also be problems that are due to a lack of persistence on the part of the feeder. In addition, feeders may also acquire the habit of diluting pureed food with water, with the mistaken idea that more food is thus consumed. Nursing home staff who are responsible for feeding patients with cognitive deficits should use both verbal and nonverbal encouragement to improve food intake (Eaton et al., 1986).

DENTAL STATUS AND FOOD INTAKE

Elderly people who are edentulous and without dentures, as well as some who have dentures, experience difficulty in chewing certain foods (Kohrs et al., 1978; Posner, 1979). Dietary habits of denture wearers are influenced by the age at which the denture was acquired, the condition of the denture, the presence or absence of oral mucosal damage because of an ill-fitting denture, and motivation to eat. Many healthy denture wearers and edentulous older people eat foods which we believe require mastication. It appears that loss of masticatory ability can be tolerated in these people without health risk. Foods such as roast meat may be swallowed in larger pieces or may be cut up before it is eaten. Swallowing unchewed pieces of meat does not result in seriously impaired digestion.

A more significant problem with respect to the quality of the diet of edentulous or partially edentulous patients with or without dentures is that less motivated individuals will deliberately avoid meats, crisp vegetables, raw fruits, and even crisp bread rolls, because they complain that they cannot chew these foods and therefore cannot eat them. The physical, mental, and emotional health of these people should be evaluated. Health professionals should be aware that food avoidance in the elderly may be a sign of depression, even if absence of teeth or unserviceable dentures have previously been blamed for change in food habit.

Elderly patients who are in nursing homes and who are not afforded adequate opportunities for oral hygiene after meals may deliberately avoid foods which stick to their teeth or to their dentures.

SPECIAL DIETS

Just as the elderly are the chief drug users, so they are the chief users of special diets. Their diets may be:

1. Obtained by physician's order either in the medical office or in an acute care hospital or nursing home
2. On the advice of a physician by telephone call or by home visit
3. From a dietitian
4. From a community nutritionist
5. From a public health nurse
6. From another health paraprofessional such as an Expanded Food and Nutrition Education Program (EFNEP) aide
7. From family or friends
8. Self-prescribed
9. From newspapers or magazines
10. From other media, including TV and radio

Common ailments and prescribed special diets are:

1. Congestive heart failure—low-sodium diet
2. Atherosclerotic heart disease—low-cholesterol diet
3. Hypertension—low-sodium diet
4. Obesity—low-calorie diet
5. Diabetes—low-calorie, low-sugar diet
6. Renal failure—low-protein diet
7. Cirrhosis—low-protein, low-sodium diet
8. Diverticulosis and diverticulitis—low-fat diet
9. Constipation—high-fiber diet
10. Hiatus hernia—low-bulk diet
11. Cholecystitis and cholelithiasis—low-fat, low-cholesterol diet
12. Colostomy—low-fiber diet

Since chronic diseases of several different organ systems frequently coexist in the elderly, diets may be superimposed. Superimposition of diets—on the advice of either a physician or other health professional, as a result of lay advice from one or more people, or because of the individual's own conviction of needs—is a major cause of low food intake and dietary inadequacy.

Special diets are a major cause of malnutrition in the elderly. Special diets can be nutritionally inadequate when:

1. Food-energy intake is too low.
2. The number of food sources of essential nutrients is too limited.
3. The diet is too unpalatable to be consumed.
4. Foods excluded contain nutrients not included in foods permitted.
5. The adverse nutritional effects of the diet add to nutritional deficiencies because of disease and/or drugs.

DRUGS AND FOOD INTAKE

Drugs may be hyperphagic, producing increased food intake, or hypophagic, causing decreased food intake (Roe, 1979). With certain drugs or drug groups, effects on appetite are highly influenced by situational factors.

Hyperphagic Agents

Antihistamines. The appetite in debilitated elderly people can be stimulated by giving cyproheptadine hydrochloride (Periactin), which is both an antihistamine and a serotonin antagonist. Increased hunger with the administration of cyproheptadine occurs mainly when anorexia previously existed. However, cyproheptadine may produce unwanted sleepiness as a side effect.

Psychotropic agents. Appetite-promoting effects of psychotropic drugs have been recognized, particularly in older psychiatric patients on prolonged high-dosage therapies. Phenothiazines such as chlorpromazine (Thorazine) improve appetite in agitated patients. Benzodiazepines, including chlordiazepoxide (Librium) and diazepam (Valium), stimulate appetite and increase food intake in certain older people. Although the tranquilizers given to disturbed psychotic patients often cause a marked increase in food intake so that patients become obese, these same drugs given to geriatric patients may have an opposite effect. When phenothiazines or benzodiazepines are given in high dosage to elderly patients whose rate of drug metabolism is slowed, somnolence and disinterest in food is common and may be responsible for lowered food intake.

Tricyclic antidepressants. Special drugs in the tricyclic antidepressant class are recognized as having a marked effect on the desire for food. Amitriptyline (Elavil) increases appetite and food intake and may cause marked weight gain. Patients receiving these drugs may have a craving for sweets. Combined tricyclic and monamine oxidase inhibitor antidepressants have been found to induce weight gain in patients with depressive illness. It is to be noted, however, that for the elderly use of antidepressant drugs may cause severe behavorial problems, and trycyclic antidepressants sometimes cause agitation which may interfere with eating.

Hypophagic Drugs

Cancer chemotherapeutic agents. Cancer chemotherapeutic agents may induce anorexia because of their effects on the GI tract. The effects on food intake are usually related to associated nausea and vomiting. Drugs which at the time of administration commonly cause anorexia are doxorubicin hydrochlor (Adriamycin), asparaginase (Elspar), cyclophosphamide (Cytoxan), daunorubicin (Cerubidine), carmustine (BICNU), methotrexate, and mithramycin (Mithracin).

Anorexia associated with the administration of these drugs may be of brief duration, or may be prolonged because of effects of the drug on the GI tract. The anorexia associated with cancer chemotherapeutic agents can and frequently does markedly reduce food intake such that weight loss occurs (Johns, 1979).

Chelating agents. In the elderly, D-penicillamine (Cuprimine) is used for the treatment of rheumatoid arthritis. The drug can produce loss of taste because of drug-associated zinc and copper deficiency. Penicillamine forms complexes with these metals which are then excreted in the urine.

Alcohol

Alcohol abuse in the elderly can cause anorexia (Roe, 1979). Causes of anorexia in elderly alcoholics are inebriation, gastritis, lactose intolerance, pancreatitis, hepatitis, cirrhosis, ketoacidosis, alcoholic brain syndromes, and withdrawal syndromes. Anorexia in alcoholics can also be caused by thiamin, zinc, or protein deficiencies. It has been found that among the elderly, those who are drinkers may tend to have lower food intake than age-matched nondrinkers, even in the absence of alcohol abuse.

Cardiac Glycosides

Digitalis and other related cardiac glycosides, in high dosage, cause anorexia, which is usually associated with nausea (Banks and Nayab, 1974). Vomiting may also occur. Digitalis cachexia can result from chronic digitalis overdosage, and the marked weight loss found in this condition can imitate cancer cachexia. Return of appetite occurs rapidly when the drug dosage is appropriately adjusted.

ACE-inhibitors

The angiotensin converting enzyme (ACE) inhibitor drug, captopril, which is used to treat hypertension in the elderly, causes loss of taste or distorted taste perception in 4 to 5 percent of patients. This change in the ability to taste food results in a loss of appetite. Other ACE inhibitor drugs, including enalapril and lisinopril, seldom produce these side effects (Breckenridge, 1988).

OVERREPORTING OF FOOD INTAKE BY ELDERLY RECEIVING APPETITE-REDUCING DRUGS

Elderly men and women who are consuming hypophagic drugs such as digitalis glycosides and captopril as well as elderly alcohol abusers over-report what they eat. Indeed, if receiving home-delivered meals, hospital meals, or nursing home diets, they will report what is provided to them as having been eaten (Roe, 1988).

QUESTIONS

Circle all correct answers (there may be more than one correct answer to each question).

1. Which of the following are true?
    a. Rigidity of food habits usually increases with aging.
    b. The elderly in nursing homes will not eat salads.
    c. Food preferences are influenced by food experiences.
    d. Appetite and hunger are synonymous.
2. Which of the following are true?
    a. People on cancer chemotherapy may develop food aversions.
    b. People on cancer chemotherapy may develop anorexia.
    c. Anorexia is associated with cancer.
    d. Anorexia is associated with cancer cure.
    e. Anorexia explains weight loss in the cancer patient.
3. Cross out the incorrect word(s) "do" or "do not" in the following sentences:
    a. Diseases associated with anorexia *do/do not* cause elderly patients to consume very little food.
    b. Edentulous elderly people who enjoy roast meat *do/do not* eat meat.
    c. Food avoidances in the elderly *do/do not* signify depression.
    d. Diets low in thiamin *do/do not* cause anorexia.
    e. Diets high in thiamin *do/do not* cause anorexia.
4. The two lists indicate special diets and their medical indications. Pair them correctly:
    a. low cholesterol   i.   cirrhosis
    b. low sodium   ii. congestive heart failure
    c. low protein   iii. diabetes
    d. low protein, low sodium   iv. atherosclerotic heart disease
    e. low calorie, low sugar   v.   renal failure
5. Malnutrition may arise from special diets that restrict which of the following foods?
    a. cookies
    b. calories

c. number of foods
d. cholesterol
e. protein

6. Demented patients may become malnourished for all except one of the following reasons:
   a. Because they are not fed adequate calories
   b. Because they reject food
   c. Because they are fed a diet that is too calorically dense
   d. Because they cannot buy or prepare food for themselves
   e. Because the food purees they receive are diluted with water

REFERENCES

BANKS, T., and A. NAYAB, "Digitalis cachexia," (letter), *New Eng. J. Med.*, 290 (1974), 746.

BRECKENRIDGE, A., "Angiotensin converting enzyme inhibitors," *Brit. Med. J.*, 296 (1988), 618–20.

CARTER, S. K., "Nutritional problems associated with cancer chemotherapy," in *Nutrition and Cancer Etiology and Treatment*, eds. G. R. Newell and N. M. Ellison. New York: Raven Press, 1981, pp. 303–17.

CLARKE, M., and L. M. WAKEFIELD, "Food choices and institutionalized vs. independent-living elderly," *J. Amer. Dietet. Assoc.*, 66 (1975), 600–04.

EATON, M., I. MITCHELL-BONAIR, and E. FRIEDMAN, "The effect of touch on nutritional intake of chronic organic brain syndrome patients," *J. Gerontol.*, 41 (1986), 611–16.

EXTON-SMITH, A. N., "Nutritional deficiencies in the elderly," in *Nutritional Deficiencies in Modern Society*, eds. A. N. Howard and I. McLean Baird. London: Newman Books, Ltd., 1973, p. 86.

FLOCH, M. H., *Nutrition and Diet Therapy in Gastrointestinal Disease*. New York: Plenum Publishing Corporation, 1981, pp. 151–61.

JOHNS, M. P., *Drug Therapy and Nursing Care*. New York: Macmillan, Inc., 1979, pp. 263–92.

KOHRS, M. B., R. O'NEAL, A. PRESTON, D. EKLUND, and O. ABRAHAMS, "Nutritional status of elderly residents in Missouri," *Amer. J. Clin. Nutr.*, 31 (1978), 2186–97.

LE GROS CLARK, F., "Food habits as a practical nutrition problem," *World Rev. Nutr. Dietet.*, 9 (1968), 56–84.

POSNER, B. M., *Nutrition and the Elderly*. Lexington, MA: Lexington Books, 1979.

ROE, D. A., *Alcohol and the Diet*. Westport, CT: AVI Publishing Co., 1979, pp 27–41.

ROE, D. A., "Interactions between drugs and nutrients," *Med. Clin. N. Amer.*, 63 (1979), 985–1007.

ROE, D. A., "Validation of Food Intake Recalled by Frail Elderly." Final Report submitted to New York State Dept. Health. Cornell University, Ithaca, NY, August 1988.

SHIL, M. E., "Nutritional problems induced by cancer," *Med. Clin. N. Amer.*, 63 (1979), 1009–25.

chapter 6

Assessment of Nutritional Status

Nutritional assessment of the elderly may have one or more different purposes depending on the questions being asked and on whether the assessment is of groups or individuals. Nutritional assessment of groups of elderly may be required in epidemiological studies, including cross-sectional or longitudinal descriptive studies which examine their status or change in status over time. Nutritional assessment of elderly groups may also be undertaken in cohort studies to determine the relative risk of disease or adverse disease outcome in those having or not having particular diets or food-chemical exposures. Further, nutritional assessment of groups of elderly may be an integral part of case control studies, in which the dietary characteristics of individuals with or without particular acute or chronic diseases are being explored. Although most commonly nutritional assessment of groups of elderly is for survey or surveillance purposes, it may also be carried out to provide information on the nutritional needs of the elderly to assess the outcome of nutritional intervention or to evaluate the impact of feeding programs. Goals and methods for nutritional assessment of elderly groups are summarized in Table 6-1.

Nutritional assessment of elderly individuals may be carried out with the objective of screening for nutritional disorders, nutritional diagnosis, diet or drug prescription, monitoring of the effects of nutritional intervention, determination of risk of adverse outcome, or teaching purposes. The goals and selected methods for the nutritional assessment of elderly individuals are summarized in Table 6-2.

TABLE 6-1   Goals and Selected Methods for Nutritional Assessment of Elderly Groups

GOALS	METHODS
Examination of nutritional disease prevalence	Cross-sectional descriptive survey
Study of change in nutrition or in the prevalence of nutritional disease	Longitudinal descriptive study
Investigation of the risk of disease or adverse disease outcome of persons having particular diets	Cohort study
Study of the dietary or nutritional antecedents of persons with or without particular diseases	Case control study
Controlled studies of nutritional requirements	Experimental study in a metabolic unit
Evaluation of community-feeding programs	Nutritional surveillance

The nutritional assessment of the elderly can be approached according to the needs of the caregiver(s) or program planners requiring the information. Physicians need to obtain a diagnostic nutritional assessment of their patients to determine if a nutritional deficiency or specific diet-related disease is present, to make a differential diagnosis, to measure the degree of nutritional depletion or excess, and to determine the need for nutritional intervention. They may also need nutritional assessment to determine the risks of surgery, to obtain a relative risk for drug-induced nutritional depletion or of a disease complication, or to determine the risk of premature death. Nurses need to carry out and use nutritional assess-

TABLE 6-2   Goals and Selected Methods for the Nutritional Assessment of Elderly Individuals

GOALS	METHODS
Determination of the presence or absence of common nutritional or diet-related diseases	Nutritional screening
Identification of types and degrees of malnutrition	Nutritional diagnosis
Diet prescription	Nutritional and medical assessment
Drug prescription	Assessment of the risk of drug-nutrient interaction
Determination of the risk of nutrition-associated complications	Subjective global assessment
Teaching	Bedside patient examination

ment to make patient care plans. Pharmacists need to use nutritional assessments so that they can advise elderly patients or their caregivers on when and how to take drugs. Dietitians need to make and use nutritional assessments to plan diets and the nutritional support of patients using tube-feeding methods. Paraprofessional caregivers need to use simple nutritional assessment methods to monitor their patients. Program planners need nutritional assessments of the elderly to develop or assess the impact of community-feeding programs.

When the goals of nutritional assessment are identified and the purposes for which the information is required are defined, the assessment may have one or more of the following components:

1. Clinical
2. Dietary
3. Anthropometric
4. Hematological
5. Biochemical
6. Immunological
7. Diagnostic
8. Therapeutic
9. Prognostic

Each component requires selection of acceptable and feasible methods that (1) answer the needs of the user of the information, (2) develop measurement skills, (3) ensure quality control, (4) provide a means to determine the reliability and validity of the tests, and (5) acknowledge the constraints inherent in application of that method of assessment to an elderly individual or population (Clark and Blackburn, 1983).

CLINICAL ASSESSMENT

The aims of the clinical assessment of nutritional status are:

1. To find whether the elderly individual has had symptoms or signs which causally explain an observed change in nutritional status
2. To discover whether this individual has had health problems or diagnosed disease or disabilities or is receiving drugs which could causally explain these changes in nutritional status
3. To determine whether this individual has signs present which are diagnostic of nutritional disease
4. To determine whether these signs are reversed by selective and specific nutritional intervention

Components of clinical assessment include:

1. Medical history (The patients' descriptions of medical problems related to nutritional disease are shown in Table 6-3.)
2. Assessment of disability in relation to foraging and feeding skills

TABLE 6-3   Medical Problems and Diagnoses Related to Nutritional Disease

PATIENT'S DESCRIPTION (OR DESCRIPTION BY RELATIVE)	DIAGNOSIS IN MEDICAL RECORD
Loss of flesh	Cachexia (chronic protein-energy malnutrition)
Cancer	Neoplastic disease (organ or site and type specified ± metastases)
Sore tongue/sore mouth	Glossitis or stomatitis due to ariboflavinosis, pellagra, ill-fitting dentures, candidiasis, radiation therapy, cancer chemotherapy or drug reaction
Can't swallow or keep food down	Plummer-Vinson syndrome; systemic sclerosis; carcinoma of the pharynx or esophagus
Disease of the bowels ("Food goes right through me," "Blood in my bowel movements," or "Stoppage of the bowels")	Gluten-sensitive enteropathy; inflammatory bowel disease; carcinoma of the colon or rectum; diverticular disease; late effects of gastrectomy or intestinal bypass or resection
Liver disease	Alcoholic cirrhosis
Bleeding problems	Scurvy; vitamin K deficiency due to anticoagulants
Poor (tired) blood	Anemia (nutritional)
Skin disease	Exfoliative dermatitis; pemphigus; pemphigoid; pellagra; other nutritional dermatoses
Hormone problem, low-thyroid	Obesity; myxedema; thyrotoxicosis
Heart disease	Congestive heart failure; alcoholic heart disease; hypertensive heart disease; atherosclerotic heart disease
Chest disease	Emphysema; chronic bronchitis; cor pulmonale
Stroke/paralysis	Hemiplegia; cranial nerve paralysis; peripheral neuropathy; Parkinson's disease

3.   Physical examination to determine if signs indicative of nutritional deficiency or excess are present. (Signs of nutritional deficiency and excess are shown in Tables 6-4 and 6-5.)

In the elderly, clinical assessment presents special challenges because both symptoms and signs which may be indicative of nutritional disease can also be the result of non-nutritional causes. For example, cracks at the corners of the mouth may occur in patients with riboflavin deficiency, but in the elderly, cracks at the corners of the mouth can be caused by drooling of saliva. Again, easy bruising can be caused by vitamin K deficiency, particularly in individuals who are taking anticoagulants, or by scurvy, but a much more common cause is aging of the skin with attendant skin fragility (Verbov, 1974).

Symptoms and signs commonly found in the elderly which can have both nutritional and non-nutritional etiologies are listed in Table 6-6 on

TABLE 6-4   Signs of Nutritional Deficiency

NUTRIENT	CLINICAL SIGNS
Ascorbic acid	Perifollicular hemorrhages, bleeding gums, subperiosteal and joint hemorrhage, impaired wound healing (scurvy)
Biotin	Alopecia, seborrhoeic dermatitis, neuritis
Calcium	Rickets/osteomalacia, tetany
Carnitine	Muscle weakness
Chloride	Hypochloremic alkalosis, heat collapse, loss of consciousness, death
Chromium	Glucose intolerance
Cobalamin (vitamin B_{12})	Megaloblastic anemia, ataxia, sensory neuropathy, optic atrophy, confusional state
Copper	Low neutrophils, hypochromic anemia, scurvy-like bone disorder in infants
Essential fatty acids	Scaly dermatitis
Folic acid (folate)	Megaloblastic anemia, megaloblastic defect of mucous membranes
Iodine	Goiter, cretinism
Iron	Microcytic hypochromic anemia, Plummer-Vinson syndrome, koilonychia
Magnesium	Tremor, tetany, convulsions
Niacin	Phototoxic dermatitis, diarrhea, depression/confusion (pellagra)
Phosphate	Weakness, congestive heart failure, hemolytic anemia, osteomalacia
Potassium	Muscular weakness, cardiac arrythmia, digitalis intoxication, glucose intolerance, renal impairment
Protein	Hypoalbuminemia, edema
Pyridoxine	Neuritis, exfoliative dermatitis, hypochromic/sideroblastic anemia, seizures
Riboflavin	Angular stomatitis, cheilitis, glossitis, seborrhoeic dermatitis, corneal vascularization (ariboflavinosis)
Sodium	Confusion, dry tongue, low intraocular tension, low urine volume, hypotension, coma, death
Thiamin (vitamin B_1)	Cardiac failure, polyneuritis (beriberi), Wernicke-Korsakoff syndrome
Vitamin A	Night blindness, xerophthalmia, sterility, follicular hyperkeratosis
Vitamin D	Epiphyseal enlargement, bowing of legs, muscle weakness, tetany (rickets and osteomalacia)
Vitamin E	Hemolytic anemia
Vitamin K	Ecchymoses and GI, urinary, and CNS hemorrhage
Zinc	Growth retardation, sexual immaturity, dermatitis, loss of taste, impaired cellular immune function, delayed wound healing

TABLE 6-5 Clinical Features of Hypervitaminoses: Acute and Chronic Effects, Risk Factors, and Toxic Dose

VITAMIN	ACUTE EFFECT OF PHARMACOLOGICAL TOXIC DOSE	SYMPTOMS AND SIGNS OF CHRONIC VITAMIN OVERLOAD	RISK FACTORS	TOXIC DOSE (CHRONIC DAY DOSE)
Vitamin A	Nausea and vomiting, exfoliation	Dry skin, partial alopecia, loss of eyebrows, anorexia, bone pain, jaundice, hepatomegaly, ascites	Rx for cutaneous disease, viral or alcoholic liver disease	Normal adults, ≥50,000 IU; adults with liver disease, ≥25,000 IU
Beta-carotene	—	Carotenemia	Rx beta-carotene for cancer prevention	>30 mg
Vitamin D	Anorexia	Headache, confusion, polyuria, hypercalcemic anemia	Sarcoidosis	Infants >5,000 IU; adults ≥100,000 IU
Vitamin E	—	Purpura	Intake of coumarin anticoagulants	≥800 IU
Vitamin K	—	—	—	—
Niacin	Flushing	Hepatic dysfunction, hyperglycemia, peptic ulcer, acanthosis nigricans	—	>1 g
Pyridoxine	—	Sensory neuropathy	Rx for carpal tunnel syndrome or premenstrual tension	>2 g

(Continued)

TABLE 6-5   Clinical Features of Hypervitaminoses: Acute and Chronic Effects, Risk Factors, and Toxic Dose (*Continued*)

VITAMIN	ACUTE EFFECT OF PHARMACOLOGICAL TOXIC DOSE	SYMPTOMS AND SIGNS OF CHRONIC VITAMIN OVERLOAD	RISK FACTORS	TOXIC DOSE (CHRONIC DAY DOSE)
Vitamin C	—	Diarrhea, hyperoxaluria, renal calculi	Oxalate urolithiasis	>4 g
Folic acid	—	—	Seizures on phenytoin	>5 mg
Sodium	Edema	Hypertension	Genetic, renal, and cardiac factors	Acute, >30 g salt/day; chronic, depends on disease
Potassium	GI ulcers, vitamin B_{12} malabsorption	Renal failure	Renal factors	Acute, >20 g KCl/day; chronic, depends on disease
Magnesium	Laxative effect	Hypotension, coma	Renal factors	Acute, <15 g $MgSo_4$/day
Zinc	Nausea, vomiting, chills	—	—	Depends on anion
Iron	Nausea, vomiting, GI bleeding	Hemochromatosis	Genetic factors	Acute, >300 times requirement
Selenium	Vascular collapse	Alopecia, loss of nails, dermatitis	—	Acute, >100 times requirement
Iodine	Iodism	Iodine goiter	Hypersensitivity	>2 mg/day unless allergic

TABLE 6-6 Symptoms and Signs with Nutritional and Non-nutritional Etiologies in the Elderly

SIGNS AND SYMPTOMS	NUTRITIONAL ETIOLOGY	NON-NUTRITIONAL ETIOLOGY
Night blindness	Vitamin A deficiency	Cataract
Congestive heart failure	Beriberi	Late effect of rheumatic, coronary, or alcoholic heart disease
Angular stomatitis	Ariboflavinosis	Oral candidiasis, drooling
"Phototoxic" dermatitis	Pellagra	Actinic reticuloid, thiazide photosensitivity
Peripheral neuropathy	Vitamin B_6 deficiencies (drug induced)	Diabetic neuropathy
Purpura	Scurvy, vitamin K deficiency	Purpura, vasculitis, senile skin changes

page 111. As can be easily appreciated, taken alone without attendant history or evaluation of other clinical or laboratory findings, these apparent indicators of malnutrition are not diagnostically specific. Indeed, even if the presenting health complaints, medical history, and physical examination suggest nutritional disease, it is necessary to support the diagnosis (1) by laboratory findings, (2) by the finding that the condition resolves with specific nutritional intervention, or (3) if the condition does not respond promptly to nutritional intervention, by the finding that a secondary cause of malnutrition is present (e.g., metastatic cancer).

Other problems in the clinical assessment of nutritional status in elderly individuals include (1) failure to complain because the condition is accepted as one of the problems of aging; (2) multiplicity of disease symptoms, only some of which may have a nutritonal causation; and (3) mental confusion. A further constraint on nutritional diagnosis is that the elderly person's description of his or her problem may not be understood because of the use of archaic terms, local word usage, ethnic terms, or a language with which the interviewer is not familiar. Physicians and nurses who are interviewing and examining elderly patients need to be reminded that malnutrition is most commonly disease related and caused by cancer, alcohol abuse, late complications of bowel surgery, chronic drug therapies, or special diets.

ORAL ASSESSMENT

The need to assess the oral status of the elderly is critical to the overall assessment of their nutritional status, since the presence of oral disease may degrade the adequate intake of nutrient dense foods. Indeed, foods that need to be chewed, such as conventionally prepared meats, fruits, and vegetables, may not be tolerated by the elderly with stomatitis or oral ulceration. In addition coronal dental caries and/or periodontal disease associated with loose or absent teeth may limit the kinds of foods that are eaten. It has also been found that elderly with ill-fitting dentures should avoid certain foods, such as meats, that need to be chewed, as well as high fiber foods which may get stuck between the denture and the roof of the mouth (Carlos and Wolfe, 1989).

Adequate assessment of the condition of the oral mucosa is necessary to diagnose such nutritional deficiencies such as ariboflavinosis, pellagra, folate deficiency, and zinc deficiency. Oral assessment of the elderly requires the services of a geriatric dentist, who has the specialized training

TABLE 6-7 Screening Instrument for Oral Status of the Elderly

Question 1: Do you have any difficulty in eating food as usually prepared?
Yes No

Question 2: Do you have a difficulty in chewing meats or hard vegetables?
Yes No

Question 2a: [For those responding yes to question 2]: Is your chewing difficulty related to not having teeth?
Yes No

Question 2b: [For those responding no to question 2a]: Is your chewing difficulty due to trouble with your own teeth?
Yes No

Question 2c: [For those responding no to questions 2a and 2b]: Is your chewing difficulty due to poorly fitting dentures?
Yes No

Question 2d: [For those responding no to questions 2a–2c, inclusive]: Is your chewing difficulty due to a sore mouth?
Yes No

Question 3: Do you have difficulty in swallowing food?
Yes No

Check all conditions present from the following list:

1. Edentulous (does not have denture)
2. Edentulous (has denture, not worn)
3. Ill fitting dentures   ____ upper   ____ lower
4. Severe dental decay
5. Swollen gums
6. Glossitis (red tongue without papillae)
7. Ulcers in the mouth
8. Stomatitis (white patches, blisters, or erosion of the oral mucosa)
9. Dry mouth
10. Oral prosthesis
11. Unable to open mouth
12. Hemiplegia or other paralytic disease involving face
13. Has dentures but not wearing them
14. Ulcers in the mouth

and experience necessary. However, oral screening using simplified methods to define the presence or absence of oral or dental problems can be carried out by a clinical nutritionist if use is made of a screening record form as shown in Table 6-7.

DIETARY ASSESSMENT

Dietary assessments of the elderly are carried out for the following reasons:

1. To chart food consumption patterns of individuals or groups
2. To examine changes in food intake patterns over time
3. To give presumptive evidence of food-energy and nutrient intake
4. To obtain actual food-energy and nutrient intakes
5. To investigate episodes of microbiological or chemical food poisoning
6. To assess the feeding practices of hospitals and geriatric care institutions
7. To assess the nutritional quality of the food supplied by congregate and home-delivered meal programs

Qualitative or semiquantitative dietary assessment may be made from records of food purchases, dietary history interview, or food frequency records. Records of food purchases are of particular value in that habitual purchase of very few foods provides a proxy indicator of nutritional risk. Whether or not a record of food purchases is a valid indicator of the quality of the diet depends on whether (1) these purchases are the sole source of food for that person and (2) the food is actually consumed by that person rather than being shared by others, thrown away, or fed to pets. When frail elderly who are at nutritional risk are living alone, their food purchases may be made by relatives, friends, homemakers, or home health aides. To obtain records of food purchases, the cooperation of the person buying the food is necessary, since the method depends on keeping accurate shopping lists. Simple computations which can be made from shopping lists include enumeration of the total number of different foods purchased, the division of the foods purchased into food groups, estimation of the diversity of the diet, and food expenditures. The enumeration of the total number of foods purchased is particularly useful in the nutritional surveillance of the frail or housebound elderly where the aim is to monitor select indicators of nutritional risk over time and across geographical areas so that home-delivered meal programs can be better targeted to meet real demand. When nutritional surveillance is being carried out, shopping list information should be combined with demographic data (Carl, 1980).

In dietary history interviews of the elderly, a short diet questionnaire is preferable. Such diet questionnaires can be used to examine both the current pattern of food intake and change in the pattern of food intake over time. A particular value of this method is to find out about meal patterns, days an individual may go without food, number of hot meals per week, and whether or not nutritionally important foods are omitted from the diet. A practical use of this information is to design therapeutic diets which are acceptable to the elderly patient because they conform with the usual eating pattern. A methodological advantage is that the questionnaires can be administered by community workers who are not nutritionists. Disadvantages are that the individual may mislead the interviewer by suggesting that his or her diet is better or worse than it actually is because of a desire to show an ability to cope with food-related activities or, conversely, a desire to obtain food assistance.

Food frequency records may be qualitative or semiquantitative (Figures 6-1 and 6-2). For example, they may contain questions on how often a glass of milk is drunk or a slice of bread is eaten. For certain food items, such information is useful in assessing dietary quality, but when an attempt is made to assess intake of alcoholic beverages in this manner, information is only likely to be accurate for moderate or nondrinkers (Roe, 1979).

Quantitative dietary assessment of the elderly may be made using recalls, diet records and histories, household surveys of food consumption or disappearance, observation of actual food consumed, tray weigh-back, and analysis of diet replicates (Campbell and Dodds, 1976; Karkeck, 1984).

Dietary Assessment in the Community

The purpose of assessment is to find out what an individual is eating now, what he or she has eaten in the past, recent changes in the diet, and how many nutrients are consumed. Dietary assessment may involve qualitative or quantitative methods. Qualitative methods include (1) a short dietary quiz and (2) a food frequency questionnaire.

Qualitative methods are used to screen the diets of independently living elderly for possible nutritional deficiencies or excesses and to determine their pattern of food intake. Information can be obtained on what foods are eaten or not eaten, how often particular foods are consumed, and how many foods are consumed. Food frequency questionnaires can also be used to examine the diversity of the diet. In the elderly the quality of the diet is directly related to the number of different foods eaten or to the diversity of the diet. Semiquantitation of food frequency questionnaires can be achieved, e.g., when questions are asked on how often a *glass* of milk is drunk or a *slice* of bread is eaten.

In the elderly, food frequency questionnaires are best administered by either a dietitian or other nutritionist or by a health professional such as a physician or nurse.

The advantages of using food frequency questionnaires are that they do not require recordkeeping, that they do not require an extended time commitment, and that they can be administered by a non-nutritionist.

In the last three years, semiquantitative methods have been developed and tested that permit evaluation of eating patterns and the changes in these eating patterns over time. Speed of data collection and analysis can be achieved in evaluating the elderly as well as in evaluating younger

FOOD ITEM	FREQUENCY*	USUAL METHOD OF PREPARATION USED**
Milk	Examples: 1	f dried, reconstituted
Cheese	3	b
Yogurt	0	
Ice cream	0	
Eggs	3	b
Dried beans	0	
Peas		
Peanut butter		
Meat		
Fish		
Poultry		
Liver		
Bread		
Rice		
Pasta		
Tortillas		
Cereal < Hot Cold		
Potatoes		
Vegetables < Green Yellow		
Citrus fruit and Fruit iuices		

*0 = never
1 = once a day or more
2 = several times a day
3 = once a week
4 = once a month

**a = raw
b = cooked
c = fresh (fruit/vegetable)
d = frozen
e = canned
f = other (state)

FIGURE 6-1   Qualitative Food Frequency Questionnaire.

subjects by using precoded questionnaires from which information can be input directly into a PC or PC-compatible microcomputer (Willett et al., 1985; Block et al., 1986).

The quality of the data obtained, however, still requires critical review. Particular problems that may reduce the validity of the dietary information obtained from frail elderly include the following:

FOOD ITEM	FREQUENCY*	AMOUNT EATEN**	USUAL METHOD OF PREPARATION USED***
Example: Milk	1	6 oz. cup	canned, diluted
Bread	2	1 slice	f toasted

*0 = never   **Glass   ***a = raw
 1 = once a day or more   (size)   b = cooked
 2 = several times a day   Cup   c = fresh (fruit/vegetable)
 3 = once a week   Slice   d = frozen
 4 = once a month   Number   e = canned
                                                   f = other (state)

FIGURE 6-2   Semiquantitative Food Frequency Questionnaire.

1. The number of days for which food-frequency data is requested may be insufficient. If the number of days requested is too few, there is a risk that the average diet per month may appear to be lower in certain nutrients, such as carotenoids, folate, potassium, and magnesium, than is actually true.
2. Estimates by the respondents of their intake may be more or less than they actually ingest. Errors made in either direction are influenced by the elderly person's education, recent memory, and knowledge of what foods are used in the preparation of various menu items.
3. The person providing the information may be a surrogate. If so, this person may or may not be able to report faithfully about what the elderly person eats. The accuracy of reports depends on the accuracy of the surrogate's powers of observation and also on the amount of time the surrogate spends in the elderly person's home (Block and Hartman, 1989; Samet, 1989).

The information given is not useful unless the respondent retains memory of food intake and is cooperative. Another disadvantage is that actual intake levels of food-energy and nutrients are not obtained.

A diet questionnaire or short diet quiz is shown in Figure 6-3. Diet questionnaires or short diet quizzes examine the pattern of food intake and find out what foods are omitted from the diet. Diet quizzes are essential when it is necessary to prescribe a regimen of medication using drugs which may be influenced by intake of food or beverages. Diet questionnaires which address the pattern of food intake are also appropriately used in situations when therapeutic diets are being prescribed or modified.

The advantages of short dietary questionnaires are that they can be administered by non-nutritionists, that they require only moderate patient cooperation, that they require only limited memory, and that the patient does not have to keep records. The disadvantages are that no information is obtained on amounts of food consumed and that information given may be misleading if the patient provides false information because of a desire to please the questioner or in self-defense, e.g., when an alcoholic indicates that he or she has a good diet.

Quantitative dietary assessment may be made using twenty-four–hour recall of food intake, diet record, diet history, individual or household survey, observation of actual food consumed, and diet analysis (analysis of diet replicates).

Recalls. The 24-hour diet recall has been widely used in individual and group dietary assessment. Food intake may be recorded on a form such as that illustrated in Figure 6-4. Use of 24-hour food records to

FIGURE 6-3 A Sample Dietary Questionnaire.

		Yes	No
Do you drink milk?		☐	☐
If yes, whole milk	☐		
2% milk	☐		
skim milk	☐		
other	☐		

Specify ______________________________

____

Please indicate which of the following foods you eat and how often.

	never or hardly ever (less than once a week)	sometimes (not daily but at least once a week)	every day or nearly every day
Cheese, yogurt, ice cream	☐	☐	☐
Eggs	☐	☐	☐
Dried beans, peas, peanut butter	☐	☐	☐
Meat, fish, poultry	☐	☐	☐
Bread, rice, pasta, grits, cereal, tortillas, potatoes	☐	☐	☐
Fruits or fruit juices	☐	☐	☐
Vegetables	☐	☐	☐

If you eat fruits or drink fruit juices every day or nearly every day, which ones do you eat or drink most often? (Not more than three.)

____

____

If you eat vegetables every day or nearly every day, which ones do you eat most often? (Not more than three.)

____

____

	Yes	No
Do you usually eat anything between meals?	☐	☐

If yes, name the 2 or 3 snacks (including bedtime snacks) that you have most often.

_____

_____

Do you or the person who prepares your meals have use of a		
working stove	☐	☐
refrigerator	☐	☐
piped water	☐	☐
Do you take vitamins or iron?	☐	☐

If yes, how often? _____

What kind? _____

Do you take other nutrient supplements?

Sustacal ☐

Ensure ☐

Wheat germ ☐

Bone meal ☐

Kelp ☐

Other (state) _____

Are you on a special diet?   Yes ____ No ____   If yes, what is the reason?

low salt; specify type of diet ☐ _____

weight reduction; specify type ☐ _____

diabetic; specify type of diet ☐ _____

Other; specify reason for diet and type of diet ☐ _____

Who recommended the diet? _____

Do you eat meals in a congregate meal site?   Yes ___ No ___ If yes, no. meals/wk. ___

Do you have meals delivered to your home?   Yes ___ No ___ If yes, no. meals/wk. ___

FIGURE 6-3   A Sample Dietary Questionnaire. (Continued)

evaluate the diet of an aged person is seldom advisable because valid information requires excellent memory and responsibility of the respondent for her or his own food preparation or cooperation from a household member or home helper who has been responsible for the preparation of

We want you to tell us all you have eaten or have drunk for the last 24 hours.
Start by telling us what you ate most recently.

DATE	TIME	FOOD/BEVERAGE ITEM	AMOUNT	DESCRIPTIONS*
SAMPLE:				
9/9/82	*8 am*	*Coffee, doughnut*	*1 coffee,* *1 doughnut*	*Black with sugar*
9/8/82	*10 pm*	*Cookies* *Ginger ale*	*3* *1 glass*	*Chocolate chip* *Canada Dry*
9/8/82	*6 pm*	*Soup* *Toast*	*1 cup* *2 slices*	*Campbell's chicken* *noodle* *Pepperidge Farm,* *white*
9/8/82	*Noon*	*Coffee* *Waffles* *Syrup* *Butter*	*2 cups* *2* *2 tbsp.* *2 tsp.*	*Black* *Frozen* *Vermont Maple*

*Columns may be added for "where eaten" and "who prepared."

FIGURE 6-4   Record of 24-hour Food Recall.

the respondent's food and has actually been able to observe what has been consumed.

Diet records. An excellent means of obtaining dietary information from very cooperative elderly patients who have been fully instructed on how to make these records are 3-, 5-, and 7-day diet records. Usually in the elderly, diet diaries that exceed 3 days' length are not dependable. If the weekend diet differs from that of other days, it is appropriate to use a weekend day, as well as week days, in the diet record. In all diet records the respondent is requested to write down the time of day when a food or beverage is consumed, the name of that food or beverage, its composition, and the amount eaten or drunk. A representative set of instructions for keeping a diet diary and a recording sheet is shown in Figures 6-5 and 6-6.

Interpretation and analysis of information supplied in the diet record has to be done by a trained nutritionist or dietitian. However, it is necessary that the nutritionist give oral instructions to the person making the diet record on exactly how the record should be prepared. The use of food models is also advised in demonstrating to the individual how to indicate amounts of food by household measures. When the diet record is handed

---

INSTRUCTIONS FOR RECORDING 3-DAY FOOD DIARY

---

1. This diary is to be kept for three consecutive days (e.g., Tuesday, Wednesday, Thursday).

2. Please write down everything that you put in your mouth (food, drink, nutrient supplements, vitamins, etc.). For each day use a separate sheet–you may need more than one sheet for the same day.

3. Record under the headings provided:

   Time–approximate time of day food is eaten

   Where Eaten–was it at home, dining hall, daughter's house, etc.

   Food Item–a detailed description of foods eaten

   List name of food or beverage

       brand name whenever possible

       type–fresh, canned, dried, frozen

       list approximate ingredients and amounts in mixed dishes (e.g. stews)

   Amount Eaten–approximate measure–

       by cup (or portion of a cup, e.g., one-half cup)

       and/or by tablespoon or teaspoon

       and/or dimensions (size), in inches

   Use the measuring cups and spoons and ruler to help you here.

   Method of Preparation–please indicate how the foods were prepared/cooked,

       i.e., boiled, steamed, fried, poached, broiled, toasted, grilled, baked, microwaved, or fresh/raw.

   Who Prepared–Did you prepare the meal? (self) or a friend, family member, etc?

   Do not forget to measure and record added milk, cream, and sugar, and also any alcohol-containing beverages, i.e. brandy, whiskey, wine, beer, etc.

FIGURE 6-5   Instructions for 3-day Food Diary.

in, it has to be checked for completeness, and the respondent may be questioned when it seems likely that meals or parts of meals have been omitted or where detail on the amount of food has been omitted. Completed diet records are analyzed by using food composition tables such as the U.S. Department of Agriculture (USDA) Handbook 8 or 456 or by using computerized food composition data bases such as the Ohio State Data Base (Watt and Merrill, 1963; Adams, 1975; Herzler and Haever, 1977). When each day's food intake has been analyzed for food energy content and content of those nutrients which are of specific interest and importance, then an average may be taken of each day's food energy and nutrient content, and this is then expressed as a percent of RDA (Food and Nutrition Board, 1989).

In the elderly, advantages of the diet record as a means of nutritional assessment include the fact that more than 1-day's food intake is obtained and that the diet record can be used as a means to obtain information on intake and regularity of intake of both nutrient supplements, including vitamins, minerals, or mineral-vitamin mixtures, as well as alcoholic beverages and medications. Records of alcoholic beverage consumption are commonly underestimated in patients who are alcohol abusers. The disad-

NAME   *Jane Brown*

DAY _2_   DATE   *August 3, 1982*

TIME	WHERE EATEN	FOOD ITEM	AMOUNT EATEN	METHOD OF PREPARATION	WHO PREPARED
12:30 PM	home	Roast beef sandwich w/Milbrook white bread	2 slices	toasted	self
"	"	Roast beef	3 slices; about 3 oz.	roasted	"
"	"	iceberg lettuce	1 leaf	fresh	"
"	"	Kraft mayonnaise	1 tsp.		"
"	"	Low fat milk	1 cup		
"	"	peach, fresh	1 med.	fresh	
6 PM	daughter's house	chicken thigh	1 thigh	fried	daughter
"	"	white rice	1/2 cup	boiled	"
"	"	carrots, frozen	1/2 cup	boiled	"
"	"	lettuce salad: romaine lettuce	2 leaves	fresh	"
"	"	cucumber slices	3 slices 1/4 in. thick	"	"
"	"	red wine	1/2 cup		homemade
"	"	Saralee chocolate cake, frosted	2" slice	bought	bought
8:30 PM	home	whole milk with brandy: milk	8 oz. milk	warmed	self
		brandy	2 tbsp.		
"	"	Lorna Doone cookies	3 whole	bought	

FIGURE 6-6   Example of 3-day Food Diary.

vantage of the diet record method in the elderly is that it is necessary that the respondent be responsible for food preparation or that the food preparer keep the diet record. The quality of diet records is related to education. Diet records necessitate writing capability and/or understanding of the use of a tape recorder. The diet record method cannot be utilized unless a nutrition professional is available to interpret the data supplied.

Diet histories. Diet histories must be obtained by a trained dietitian. These histories give information on long-term dietary habits and current diet (Burke, 1947). Qualitative and quantitative data are obtained. The elderly individual must be fully cooperative and have an intact memory. Diet histories can be of use in the home or in a domiciliary care facility.

Individual or household survey. Foods available to the individual or household can be determined by interview coupled with examination of foods present in the home. The usefulness of this method depends upon the identification of the nutritional risk to the elderly of a limited quantity or low quality of food. If an elderly individual is living with other family members or household members, examination of foods available in the home will not necessarily provide insight into the food available to or consumed by the elderly individual. On the other hand, when an elderly person is living alone or with another elderly person, a survey of food in the home can offer important information on foods available to and eaten by that individual. It is, of course, important to ascertain from the interview whether or not any meals are eaten away from the home, e.g., at a congregate meal site, a restaurant, or at the home of another person.

Observation of actual diet consumed. Measurement of food ordered, purchased, or prepared does not always give a realistic picture of food consumed. Food may be stored, discarded, shared with family, friends, or pets, or left as plate waste. To find out what an elderly person actually eats, records should be made from direct observation of meals prepared for consumption and plate waste. Actual intake can then be assessed by the difference.

Diet analyses. Cooperative elderly individuals can be instructed to collect a replicate diet. Over 24-hour periods, duplicate samples of *all* foods consumed and beverages ingested are put into plastic jars. It is preferable that beverages are put into separate containers from solid foods. The food and beverage collections are refrigerated. At the end of the 24-hour period, the collection vessels are picked up by the nutritionist. The total diet is homogenized in a gallon blender with distilled water. The total homogenate is weighed, and weighed aliquots of the homogenate are then subjected to nutrient analysis. Samples can be analyzed wet or after freeze-drying. If the quantity of a particular nutrient in the aliquot is determined, then the amount of that nutrient in the total diet can be calculated.

Diet analyses are best combined with 3-day diet records, with the food collections being made on the third day.

Assessment of Food Purchasing and Eating Patterns of Independently Living Elderly

An assessment of the food-purchasing pattern of an elderly person may be carried out for one or more of the following reasons:

1. To find out whether the individual has economic problems that limit their ability to buy food.
2. To find out if the individual can get to the food store on a regular basis without assistance.
3. If food shopping is reported as difficult, to determine if this is due to transportation difficulties, impaired mobility, impaired vision, physical distress, or confusion.
4. To determine whether the individual is buying foods for himself or herself that are of adequate variety and nutrient content to meet nutrient needs.
5. To determine if the individual understands the types of foods that should be purchased to meet a special diet prescription.
6. To monitor changes in the ability to buy food that may be indicative of a need for shopping assistance or the provision of home-delivered meals.
7. To find out if the individual is obtaining meals at a congregate meal site.
8. For homebound elderly, to find out whether home-delivered meals are being provided and, if so, whether enough meals are being provided to meet the individual's needs.

In order to obtain concise information on the ability of an elderly person to get food for himself or herself, it is recommended that a nutrition questionnaire be employed (Simko et al., 1989).

The aims of this method are to utilize records of food purchases by individuals to determine the nutritional quality of diets (Carl, 1980).

The assumption is made that food purchases are only for the elderly person who lives alone, that shopping lists are available for a period of at least 28 days, and that the individual whose food-energy and nutrient intake is being examined does not have access to foods which do not appear on the shopping lists.

Food purchases for housebound elderly individuals living alone may be made by relatives, friends, or shopping aides. The cooperation of the person who is responsible for the food shopping must be obtained unless a local agency for the elderly, which supplies shopping aides, keeps the shopping lists in their files.

Purchases of all food items on each shopping list will be determined. Data to be collected by a nutritionist or public health nurse should include food item, weight or liquid measure, and cost. Total food purchases for a 28-day period can then be summed and averaged to yield weekly or daily food available to the person. The nutrient content of the available food can then be computed using USDA Handbook 456 or coded for use with the Ohio State University computerized data base (Adams, 1975; Herzler and Haever, 1977).

The RDA for the individual 51 years and older is obtained for calories and the following 16 nutrients: protein, carbohydrate, fat, calcium, phosphorus, iron, zinc magnesium, vitamin A, thiamin, riboflavin, niacin, vitamin C, vitamin B_6, vitamin B_{12}, and folacin (Food and Nutrition Board, 1989). However, for the magnesium, vitamin B_6, and folacin content of foods, there is a need to utilize data provided by Freeland and Cousins (1976); Murphy, Willis, and Watt (1975); U.S. Department of Agriculture

(1969); and Perloff and Butrum (1977). The percent of the RDA for food-energy and these nutrients can be calculated if the food purchases are expressed as nutrients obtained per day.

Simple computations which can also be obtained from shopping list information are the division of purchased foods into food groups and the total number of different foods purchased. The total number of foods purchased in an elderly housebound population has been found to be related to the nutritional quality of the diet. Nutrients consumed per dollar expended can also be determined.

The value of the shopping list method for the determination of the nutritional quality of the diet in elderly housebound people is limited, in that food waste is not measured and information is not obtained on foods that are not eaten during the period of food purchase inventory. Use of this method is being evaluated in circumstances where a food survey of the elderly in a community is being carried out under circumstances in which access to private homes is limited.

The combination of shopping list food surveys with demographic information is important. Information on the age range and income bracket of the target population group can be obtained from housing authorities or from census tract data (Carl, 1980).

Dietary Assessment in Institutions

The goal is to assess the nutritional adequacy of diets provided in institutions, including domiciliary care facilities, intermediate care homes, and nursing homes. To evaluate the nutritional adequacy of food served, one must calculate the amount of food served and determine the difference between the amounts of food purchased as of a known date before the food inventory and the amounts of food remaining in the facility on the day of the inventory.

Repeated food inventories are required when the nutritional adequacy of the diet of the institution is to be monitored. The period of the food inventory must be constant. It is recommended that a 28-day inventory be employed, because shorter inventories used in computations of the nutritional adequacy of institutional food have been shown to overstate the quality of the food (Davies and Holdsworth, 1979).

The number of patients and residents is then determined, and the food-energy and nutrients available to the persons in the two groups are calculated. Nutrients for which calculations should be performed include protein, calcium, phosphorus, magnesium, zinc, vitamin A, thiamin, riboflavin, niacin, ascorbic acid, vitamin B_6, vitamin B_{12}, and folacin.

The RDA for men and women over the age of 51 years should be used for these calculations.

To calculate nutrient requirements, the RDA for each nutrient per man or woman should be calculated and then multiplied by the number of persons of each sex in the facility. The products are then added together. This figure represents the total RDA for calories and 14 selected nutrients for all residents in the facilities for 1 day.

To assess the nutritional adequacy of the food served, the percentage of the RDA is calculated by dividing the total nutritive quality of all the food served by the RDA for each nutrient and multiplying by 100.

To compute the nutrient composition of the food issued, it is recommended that a computerized data base, such as the Ohio State University program, be employed. Limitations of this data base include missing values for several of the key nutrients, including magnesium, zinc, folacin, vitamin B_{12}, and vitamin B_6.

Nutritionists who are computing the nutritional quality of geriatric institutionalized food are advised to keep a file on new and reliable tables of nutrient values and to modify the data base to supply presently missing values by selective additions as new information is published.

Assessment of Feeding Practices in Geriatric Care Facilities

The aims of this type of study are to determine the degree of nutritional risk for the residents, to determine resident satisfaction with the food service, and to assess whether modification in the system would be carried out (Allington et al., 1980).

The questionnaires are prepared for the administrator, the food service manager or dietitian, the cook, and the residents. Questions addressed to the administration pertain to the method of food purchase, food expenditure, staffing pattern and staff responsibilities, and the nutritional assessment of patients and patient care plans. Questions addressed to the food service manager, dietary aide, or dietitian relate to their knowledge of nutrient requirements of the elderly, menus for staff and residents and menu rotation, special diets, standardization of recipes, arrangements made for feeding or assisted self-feeding of residents, monitoring of plate waste, and food hygiene.

Questions for the cook relate to the use of recipes and cooking methods other than those stipulated by the food service manager and the use of food preparation methods which cause nutrient destruction.

Questions to the residents relate to satisfaction or dissatisfaction with the food, foods missed, foods enjoyed or disliked, satisfaction with portion size, frequency and times of meals, and whether food suggestions made by residents are heeded.

All questionnaires should ask certain consistent questions pertaining to the food service.

From the completed questionnaires, the nutritionist investigator should be able to assess the quality of the dietary service to the facility. Answers to the following questions should be analyzed using composite information obtained from the four questionnaires:

1. Is the staff (nursing, kitchen, dining room, etc.) adequate in number and qualifications?
2. Are food costs appropriate to patient and staff needs?
3. Do the staff members eat different foods than the residents?

4. Do patient care plans specify diet and dietary changes, with reasons?
5. Does the food service manager understand food groups, nutrients supplied by particular foods, and nutrient requirements of elderly persons?
6. Are the patients weighed? How often?
7. Is patient food consumption monitored?
8. What are the methods of food storage?
9. What health screening is required for kitchen staff and others concerned with feeding patients?
10. How are dishes and utensils washed?
11. How are vegetables prepared?
12. Are salads served?
13. How often is milk served?
14. How often is citrus fruit juice served?
15. How often are fortified breakfast cereals served?
16. Is the menu monotonous?
17. Do special diets conform to recommended therapeutic guidelines?
18. Do patients complain that meals are inedible?
19. What foods do patients say they long for?
20. Are patients dissatisfied with menu changes made in response to their suggestions?
21. Is there disagreement in the answers to questions between the administration, the food service manager, the cook, and the residents?

When dietary assessment of the elderly is carried out, the assumption is that the diet of the individual or group being assessed meets a standard of adequacy. The standard may be arbitrary, or based only on a general assumption of need, or may be according to guidelines provided by the national body that sets recommended dietary intakes.

Standards of adequacy based on assumption of need include:

1. *Meals per day.* The need is for at least one hot meal per day.
2. *Food groups per day.* The need is for four groups—e.g., milk, meat or protein-rich alternate food, cereal, and fruit or vegetable.
3. *Food sources of specific nutrients.* The need is for nutrient-dense foods.

Standards of adequacy based on national guidelines for health include:

1. *Recommended Dietary Allowances (RDA).* The assumption is that the elderly's food-energy requirements are lower than those of younger adults but, with few exceptions, their nutrient requirements are similar (Harper, 1978).
2. *National dietary goals.* In the United States these are (U.S. Department of Agriculture, 1980):

a. To consume only as much food-energy as is expended
b. To increase consumption of complex carbohydrates
c. To reduce consumption of refined and processed sugars
d. To reduce fat consumption to 30 percent of total food-energy
e. To reduce saturated fat consumption to 10 percent of total energy intake
f. To reduce cholesterol consumption to 300 mg or less per day
g. To limit intake of sodium by reducing intake of salt to 5 g or less per day
h. To reduce consumption of alcohol

3. *Guidelines for special diets.* An example would be diabetic diets.
4. *Dietary standards for nursing homes.* In the United States these are (Social Security Administration, 1974):

a. That at least three meals per day or their equivalent must be served with not more than 14 hours between the evening meal and breakfast
b. That a bedtime nourishment should be offered to all patients
c. That foods must be prepared by methods to conserve their nutritional value
d. That therapeutic diets be prescribed by the physician
e. That menus be planned and followed to meet the nutritional needs of the patients and that the menus be approved by a registered dietitian
f. That the dietary staff be free of communicable disease
g. That food be procured from approved sources and stored, prepared, distributed, and served under sanitary conditions

Most of the dietary standards and recommendations for the elderly are subject to qualification. Qualifications are needed because of the heterogeneity of the population with respect to nutritional needs and ignorance of precise requirements. However, practical guidelines can be set for the diets of most elderly people. The following guidelines can be used to evaluate the adequacy of the diet in surveys and surveillance programs, in communities, and in clinical practice:

1. All men and women should be able to get food each day.
2. All independently living elderly, including those who are homebound, should be able to get at least seven hot or main meals per week.
3. All independently living men and women should be able to buy or get twelve or more nutrient-rich foods per week.
4. All men and women should be able to satisfy their fluid needs.
5. Food-energy intakes should be adjusted for level of activity and need for weight maintenance or modification.
6. Food sources of all essential nutrients should be consumed daily. (Food sources of specific nutrients are shown in Table 6-8.)
7. Daily foods should be from the four food groups. (Recommended daily foods from the four food groups are shown in Table 6-9.)

TABLE 6-8   Rich Food Sources of Specific Nutrients

NUTRIENT	MAJOR FOOD SOURCES
Protein	Milk, cheese, meat, fish, eggs
Complex carbohydrates	Bread, breakfast cereals, rice, pasta
Vitamin A	Sweet potatoes, carrots, greens, winter squash, cantaloupe, milk, liver
Thiamin	Pork, fortified breakfast cereals
Riboflavin	Milk, buttermilk, cheese, liver
Niacin	Enriched bread, fortified breakfast cereals, liver, chicken, tuna
Folate	Fortified breakfast cereals, broccoli, spinach
Ascorbic acid	Citrus fruits and fruit juices
Vitamin B_6	Liver, stuffed peppers, fortified breakfast cereals
Vitamin B_{12}	Meats, fish, eggs, cheese
Sodium*	Ham, corned beef, hot dogs, cold cuts, bacon, olives, pickles, ketchup, canned soups
Potassium	Spinach, collard greens, potatoes, bananas, oranges, orange juice
Calcium	Milk, cheese, yogurt
Magnesium	Enriched breakfast cereals, chocolates

*Need to restrict in hypertensives and those with congestive heart failure.

8. Healthy elderly should consume diets which meet both the RDA and national dietary goals. (The 1989 RDA are shown in Table 6-10.)
9. Elderly men and women on special diets should follow the guidelines of the approved national association such as the American Diabetes Association in so far as these apply.
10. Elderly on drugs should eat at intervals that are appropriate so that there is no meal interference with drug absorption. (Drugs to be taken with food or fasting are shown in Table 6-11).

In summary, in dietary assessment of the elderly, care must be taken to consider not only the aims of the assessment but also the capabilities of the elderly population or individual and the skills of the recorder.

TABLE 6-9   Daily Foods from the Four Food Groups for the Elderly

FOOD GROUPS	DAILY FOODS
Dairy	Milk (2% or 1%), cheese, yogurt
Cereals	Whole wheat bread, bran muffins, fortified breakfast cereals
Meat	Chicken, turkey, fish, lean beef or veal
Vegetables	Carrots, squash, peas, broccoli, spinach

TABLE 6-10   Recommended Dietary Allowances for the Elderly[a]

	MALES	FEMALES
Age	51 +	51 +
Weight (kg)	77	65
Weight (lb)	170	143
Height (cm)	173	160
Height (in)	68	63
Protein (g)	63	50
Vitamin A (μg RE)[b]	1000	800
Vitamin D (μg)[c]	5	5
Vitamin E (mg a-TE)[d]	10	8
Vitamin K (μg)	80	65
Vitamin C (mg)	60	60
Thiamin (mg)	1.2	1.0
Riboflavin (mg)	1.4	1.2
Niacin (mg NE)[e]	15	13
Vitamin B_6 (mg)	2.0	1.6
Folacin (μg)[f]	200	180
Vitamin B_{12} (μg)	2.0	2.0
Calcium (mg)	800	800
Phosphorus (mg)	800	800
Magnesium (mg)	350	280
Iron (mg)	10	10
Zinc (mg)	15	12
Iodine (μg)	150	150
Selenium (μg)	70	55

[a]The allowances are intended to provide for individual variations among most normal persons as they live in the United States under usual environmental stresses. Diets should be based on a variety of common foods to provide other nutrients for which human requirements have been less well defined.
[b]Retinol equivalents. 1 RE = 1 μg retinol or 6 μg β-carotene.
[c]As cholecalciferol. 10 μg cholecalciferol = 400 IU of vitamin D.
[d]α-Tocopherol equivalents. 1α-TE = 1 mg d-α-tocopherol.
[e]Niacin equivalents. 1 NE = 1 mg niacin or 60 mg dietary tryptophan.
[f]The folacin allowances refer to dietary sources as determined by *Lactobacillus casei* assay after treatment with enzymes (conjugases) to make polyglutamyl forms of the vitamin available to the test organ.
Adapted from Food and Nutrition Board, National Academy of Sciences, *National Research Council Recommended Daily Dietary Allowances,* 10th Ed. (Washington, DC, 1989).

TABLE 6-11   Drugs Commonly Taken by the Elderly Which Are Best Absorbed in the Fasting Condition or After Food

DRUGS BEST TAKEN FASTING		DRUGS BEST TAKEN AFTER FOOD	
Penicillin V	Nafcillin	Griseofulvin	Labetolol
Penicillin G	Cephalexin	Nitrofurantoin	Hydralazine
Amoxicillin	Tetracycline	Propranolol	Chlorothiazide
Ampicillin	Isoniazid	Metoprolol	
Pivampicillin	Rifampin		

ANTHROPOMETRIC ASSESSMENT

Anthropometric assessment of the elderly may be limited to reported height and weight or may include measurements of arm and leg lengths, midarm circumference, abdominal circumference, and skinfolds. In surveys, as well as in surveillance of the elderly, particularly of the frail elderly in their own homes, it has been found that reported height and weight are highly correlated with real height and real weight. Correlations of reported and actual weights and heights of a homebound sample are shown in Table 6-12. The heights of these people, as measured, are less than the reported heights. It can be surmised with some supporting evidence that this is because these elderly are reporting their maximal height before they lost height through age-related bone loss. In a study of the elderly in a geriatric institution in which the men were all veterans, it was found that reported heights were similar to their heights as shown in their service discharge records.

An elderly person's height can be measured with a tape or with an anthropometer if that individual can stand upright against a wall. If a tape is used, it should be fixed to the wall, and a flat board or ruler should be placed on the individual's head. Measurement of height may be impossible in the frail elderly because the individual cannot stand upright against the wall, and it is certainly inaccurate when the individual is kyphotic. Further, the feasibility of height measurements is related to the individual's ability to stand unaided unless the measurer has someone to assist. Other problems relating to height measurements include the need to wear shoes with heels of unequal height, lower leg amputations, unsteadiness, and abnormal movements. If the individual is confined to bed or unable to stand but is not kyphotic, the crown-to-heel length may be substituted for the height measurement, but this requires that head and food boards be available, as in the measurement of the length of an infant (Figure 6-7).

A further difficulty having to do with height measurements is that these measurements cannot be used to create data on body mass index (weight/height^2) because of the variable height loss with age. Various proxy measures of height have been proposed, including arm span, ulnar length, fibular length, and knee height. Simple equations and nomograms have been provided by Chumlea, Roche, and Steinbargh (1985) for estimating the stature of elderly men and women from knee height and age. Knee height can be determined with the patient either in the sitting or in the recumbent position. Knee height is highly recommended as a proxy measure for stature because of high correlation with actual stature, ease of measurement by health professionals, and low interobserver error.

TABLE 6-12   Relationship between Reported and Actual Heights of Homebound Elderly

	REPORTED (MEAN)	ACTUAL (MEAN)	SPEARMAN RANK CORRELATION COEFFICIENT
Height (inches)	66	63	0.79
Weight (pounds)	148	139	0.95

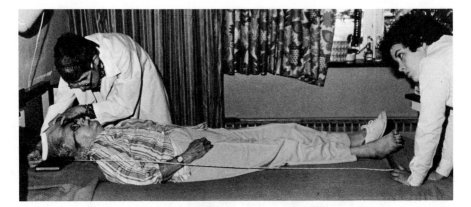

FIGURE 6-7   Crown-to-heel height measurement of bedridden patient. (Note that two persons are required to make this measurement—one to place the head against a board and the other to position the feet.)

Weight is best measured on a calibrated beam-type scale with a digital readout, but weight may also be obtained using a bathroom scale. (The bathroom scale needs to be checked between measurements for accuracy using an object of known weight.) The weighing of individuals who cannot stand unaided should be on a scale with a broad base, on which a chair of known weight can be placed. For bedridden patients, weighing requires the use of a hoist with beam-type calibrated scale or a bed scale (Figure 6-8). Although it may be possible to assess the change of weight of individuals by frequent weighing on the same scale, creating weight data for geriatric care institutions is limited by the high incidence of amputees. Fatness or leanness can be assessed by girth, or circumferential, measurements or by measurement of skinfolds. Since fat distribution may be of prognostic significance, with accumulation of upper abdominal fat having an adverse effect on mortality and fat deposition around the thighs having no such adverse prognosis, it has been recommended that these circumferential measurements be made. Indeed, Andres, Bierman, and Hazzard (1985) suggest a simple measurement of girth around the waist and hips and the recording of the ratio between the waist and hip circumferences.

However, the prognostic use of these measurements is limited in that they are not usually carried out at present in nutritional surveys either of the elderly or of younger populations. For purposes of monitoring changes in body mass over time and detecting wasting in the frail elderly, it is recommended that midarm circumference be measured. This measure is highly correlated with body mass index. (The Spearman rank correlation coefficient of midarm circumference with body mass index for the institutionalized elderly is 0.69 for men and 0.89 for women.) The measurement can be accurately obtained by health paraprofessionals and by nurses and nutritionists working with impaired elderly individuals in the community.

In the elderly, fatness is best assessed from measurements of triceps

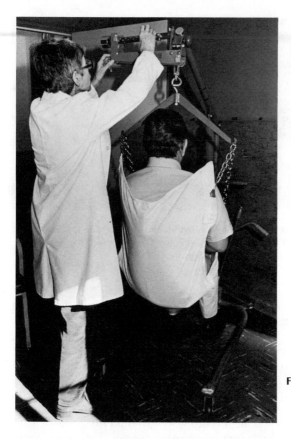

FIGURE 6-8   Patient Lifter and
Beam Scale Used
to Weigh Elderly
Patients.

skinfold thickness (Figure 6-9). Thickness can be measured by use of Lange
or Harpenden calipers or by use of plastic calipers that are available from
Ross Laboratories or McGaw. The validity of skinfold measurements by
plastic calipers has been examined by Leger, Lambert, and Martin (1982),
and they found that both types of plastic adipometers yielded valid results.
However, skinfold measurements by nurses and clinical nutritionists are
subject to interobserver error, especially if training is inadequate.

When either midarm circumference or triceps skinfold measurements are being made, the midpoint of the arm is determined with a nylon
tape measure as halfway between the tip of the acromion process of the
shoulder and the olecranon process of the elbow. This point is marked with
a pen, and the circumference and fatfold thickness are obtained at this
level on the arm. From the combined measurements, the arm muscle area
can be computed as in the following formula:

Arm muscle area (cm^2) =
$$\frac{[\text{Arm circumference} - \pi \times \text{Triceps skinfold (mm)}]^2}{400 \ \pi}$$

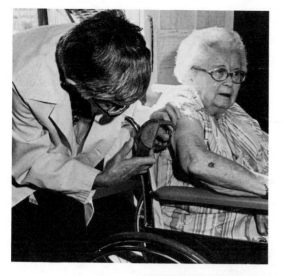

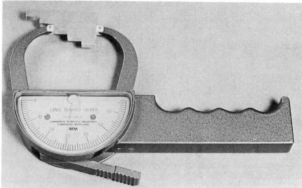

FIGURE 6-9 Measurement of Triceps Skinfold Thickness with Lange Skinfold Calipers.

The arm muscle area and diameter are measures of lean body mass (Table 6-13). Although it is usual to measure midarm circumference and triceps skinfold using the left arm, choice of arms in the elderly may be determined by neuropathology and particularly by late effects of stroke with unilateral wasting. Other problems having to do with measurement of triceps skinfold in the elderly include sagging skin, increased compressibility of the fat folds on the back of the arm, difficulty in making the measurement in a recumbent or noncooperative patient, and high interobserver error. Serial measurements of triceps skinfold thickness carried out by the same trained nutritionist, nurse, or physician will provide valuable information on fatness or change in fatness over time. Weight-for-height-for-age values for the elderly are shown in Table 6-14.

Reference values for other anthropometric "norms" in the elderly

TABLE 6-13 Midarm Muscle Area for U.S. Adults (Data Collected during HANES I, 1971 to 1974)

AGE GROUP (YEARS)	MEN (cm²) (MEAN ± SEM)	WOMEN (cm²) (MEAN ± SEM)
55–64	62.2 ± 0.2 (n = 598)	42.3 ± 0.2 (n = 669)
65–74	57.7 ± 0.1 (n = 1657)	41.2 ± 0.1 (n = 1822)

TABLE 6-14 Assessment of Weight-for-Height-for Age in Persons 65 Years and Older

HEIGHT IN INCHES	WEIGHT IN POUNDS
MEN	
62	148
63	146
64	147
65	155
66	160
67	167
68	169
69	172
70	181
71	188
72	183
73	190[a]
74	194[a]
WOMEN	
57	130
58	133
59	137
60	138
61	144
62	146
63	149
64	152
65	153
66	162
67	173
68	168

[a]Estimated values obtained from linear regression equations. Note: Examined persons were measured without shoes. Clothing weight ranged from 0.20 to 0.62 lb., which was not deducted from weights shown.

Adapted from *Weight by Height by Age for Adults 18–74 Years: U.S., 1971–74*, DHEW Publ. No. (PHS) 79-1656, Sept. 1979.

have been reported based on the data from the First Health and Nutrition Examination Survey (NHANES I) (Bishop, 1984). Estimates of obesity are available from the U.S. Department of Health and Human Services (DHHS) (1983).

It is important to recognize that there are no national statistics based on anthropometric measurements of elderly who are over 74 years of age and that when such information is reported in tables, it is based on extrapolations. For direct information on the anthropometric measurements of the very old, we must presently rely on smaller surveys such as that carried out by Yearick (1979).

For data on changes in anthropometric measurements of the elderly over time, reference should be made to the British and Swedish longitudinal studies (Nutrition and Health, 1979; Noppa et al., 1980). Risk assessment may be determined from anthropometric data in the elderly. However, it is important to understand that in this population the anthropometric indicators of morbidity and premature death are disease specific.

ASSESSMENT OF BODY COMPOSITION

The methods used for the assessment of changes in body compositions due to aging or geriatric nutritional disease include serial measurements of body water, body fat, and bone density. These measurements are now possible because of the development of special instrumentation. Of the methods available, those appropriate to clinical settings include single and dual photon absorptiometry for bone density measurements (Heymsfeld et al., 1989) and bioelectric impedance techniques for the measurement of fat and fat-free mass (Chulmea and Baumgartner, 1989). The bioelectrical impedance method would seem to offer several advantages in the measuring of elderly patients in nursing homes since the apparatus is portable and the technique requires little patient cooperation. However, in practice, its use is limited because for valid measurements it is necessary that body water and electrolyte levels remain constant (Lukaski, et al., 1986).

ASSESSMENT OF PHYSICAL ACTIVITY
AND ENERGY EXPENDITURE

In order to be able to make an accurate assessment of the food-energy needs of the elderly, it is necessary to obtain valid estimates of physical activity and energy expenditure. Complex retrospective activity questionnaire responses are notoriously inaccurate and are entirely inappropriate for elderly people with memory problems. A simple check list on usual activity over several 5 to 7 day periods may be useful to gauge whether the healthy elderly individual is sedentary or moderately active. Oxygen consumption and heart rate monitoring are useful methods for the assessment of activity patterns and of energy expenditures for the healthy elderly. But difficulties may arise from the use of a face mask and with electrode contact with the skin (Shephard, 1989). The doubly labeled water technique for measuring the total energy expenditure is the best method for use with the elderly if the necessary supplies, equipment, and personnel are available (Livingstone et al., 1990).

HEMATOLOGICAL ASSESSMENT

In the elderly, as in other age groups, hematological assessment can be used to screen for malnutrition. Characteristic changes occur in the morphology of the red and white cell series, in the hemoglobin level, in packed red cell mass, and in the computed red cell indices in nutritional anemias. The extent to which these changes can be used in the diagnosis of nutritional deficiency depends not only on the duration of the deficiency but also on whether or not confounding factors are present. For example, confounding factors that limit our ability to assess the severity of anemia include dehydration and polycythemia caused by chronic obstructive lung disease.

To screen for anemia, it is necessary to determine the packed cell volume (hematocrit reading as percent of a defined volume of blood) and the hemoglobin level (grams of hemoglobin per deciliter). A high hematocrit reading is frequently indicative of dehydration, and when found, should necessitate a repeat packed cell volume and hemoglobin determination after the patient has been adequately hydrated.

To diagnose a nutritional anemia, a complete blood count is required, and supportive evidence is usually needed, not only from examination of the morphology of the hemopoietic precursor cells in the bone marrow but also from selective biochemical assessment of nutritional status and from monitoring the response to nutrients that are hematinics. Normal or acceptable values for hemoglobin, packed cell volume, red cell (erythrocyte) count, total white cell (leukocyte) count, leukocyte differential count, and red cell indices are shown in Table 6-15. In the very old, sex-related differences in hemoglobin values are diminished, and it may be appropriate to use similar reference values for both sexes. Further, the high prevalence of low hemoglobin values found in the NHANES I survey has suggested the need to use lower hemoglobin values in the elderly to assess whether anemia exists (Russell, 1983). However, since present evidence for developing new hematological norms for the elderly rests on evidence obtained both from independently living and institutionalized elderly in whom a pathological cause of anemia may exist, it seems wiser to use similar ranges of acceptable values for the young, middle-aged, and the old. It has further been pointed out by Htoo, Kotkoff, and Freedman (1979) that if new hematological values were accepted for the elderly, this might increase the risk of missing a true anemia.

Common nutritional anemias in the elderly include iron deficiency (Kalchthaler and Rigor Tan, 1980), folate deficiency, and vitamin B_{12} deficiency (Chanarin, 1969). However, the common causes of these anemias are different in the elderly from those encountered among younger

TABLE 6-15   Acceptable Values for Hemoglobin, Hematocrit, Red Cells and White Cells, and Leukocyte Differential Count

DIFFERENTIAL COUNT		NORMAL HEMATOLOGICAL VALUES (M = MALE; F = FEMALE)		
CELL	ADULT (%)	TEST		NORMALS
Neutrophil	50–60	WBC	M	7.8 ± 3
Band	0–1	× 10³	F	7.8 ± 3
Eosinophil	1–3	RBC	M	5.4 ± 0.7
Basophil	0–1	× 10⁶	F	4.8 ± 0.6
Monocyte	4–10	Hgb	M	16 ± 2
Lymphocyte	25–40	g	F	16 ± 2
		Hct	M	47 ± 5
		%	F	42 ± 5
		MCV	M	87 ± 7
		μ³	F	90 ± 9
		MCH	M	29 ± 2
		μμg	F	29 ± 2
		MCHC	M	34 ± 2
		%	F	34 ± 2

people. In the elderly, the hematological changes of chronic iron deficiency are most often caused by blood loss resulting from intake of aspirin or NS AIDS, hemorrhage from a peptic ulcer or carcinoma of the colon, or use of anticoagulants. Because of the urgent need for intervention in these drug- and disease-related disorders, it is important to emphasize that no time should be wasted in assessing the iron intake of an elderly person with evidence of iron deficiency anemia until these and other causes related to blood loss have been excluded.

Folate deficiency in the elderly is most commonly caused by low intake of dietary folacin, but may also be caused by a malabsorption syndrome or drugs. In the past, when diagnosis of folate deficiency was on the basis of lowering of serum folate values, a high prevalence of folate deficiency was reported in the elderly (Girdwood, Thomson, and Williamson, 1967). However, a diagnosis based on serum or plasma folate values may be erroneous in the elderly, who commonly take aspirin, because aspirin causes an acute lowering of plasma folate which is unattended by other evidence of a folate deficiency anemia (Lawrence, Lowenstein, and Eichner, 1984).

The common causes of vitamin B_{12} deficiency in the elderly are pernicious anemia and late effects of gastrectomy or ileal resection, which lead to a severe reduction in vitamin B_{12} absorption (Chanarin, 1969). With respect to hematological assessment, the central question is whether changes in the cell of the hematopoietic system that are characteristic of the nutritional anemias are modified by aging or by age-related disorders. Although maturational defects of the red and white cell series are characteristic of the anemias associated with folate and vitamin B_{12} deficiency, there is no evidence that these maturational defects change with age or that the life span of the red or white cells is reduced in the elderly. However, there is evidence that events occurring in the brief life of a red cell mimic those occurring in the aging of other cells (Ganzoni, Oakes, and Hillman, 1971). On the other hand, the morphological changes, including macro-cytosis and ovalocytosis, which are characteristic of folate and vitamin B_{12} deficiency, can occur in the elderly in anemias which are not caused by deficiency of either of these vitamins. Macrocytosis without ovalocytosis, which is termed round macrocytosis, occurs in myxedema, myeloma, and alcohol-related disorders of the bone marrow, all of which may be common in elderly patients. Ovalocytosis without macrocytosis may occur in the myelophthisic anemias that are also frequently seen in the elderly (Colman, 1981).

Guidelines for the hematological investigation of nutritional anemias in the elderly are as follows (Colman, 1981):

1. Establish that morphological changes are present in the peripheral blood smear.
2. Determine whether macrocytosis or megaloblastosis is present.
3. Investigate the nature of the macrocytosis (whether caused by iron deficiency) or the megaloblastosis (whether caused by folate or vitamin B_{12} deficiency).
4. Diagnose and treat the underlying disorder.
5. Monitor the hematological responses to treatment.

BIOCHEMICAL ASSESSMENT

Biochemical assessment of nutritional status may be employed to deter-mine the level of recent intake of specific nutrients, to estimate nutrient stores in body fluids (plasma or serum) or in the tissues (blood cells or liver), to obtain functional measures of nutritional adequacy or deficiency, and to determine nutritional risk (Sauberlich, Skala, and Dowdy, 1974). In the development of nutritional deficiency, biochemical changes precede clinical signs of deficiency. However, biochemical assessment is used to confirm or refute nutritional diagnoses that are based on clinical, dietary, anthropometric, or hematological assessment. Limitations on using bio-chemical assessment as a means of establishing nutritional diagnoses in the elderly are:

1. Age-related changes in biochemical parameters
2. Ignorance of normative values for older age groups
3. Inadequate laboratory facilities in geriatric institutions
4. Problems in collecting samples, e.g., 24-hour urine samples from incontinent patients
5. Impaired absorptive function for the test substance
6. Decreased renal clearance of the test substance

7. Drug interference with biochemical assay
8. Difficulty in separating cause and effect

Plasma albumin concentrations are reduced with aging, and therefore a moderately decreased mean plasma albumin level for an elderly population cannot be construed as caused by protein deficiency (Miller, Adir, and Vestal, 1978). The biochemical standards by which acceptability of laboratory values is judged are mainly derived from younger subjects. Further, in the elderly, biochemical parameters of vitamin status may or may not correlate well with dietary intake. A high correlation between folate intake, as computed from 3-day records or direct analyses, and plasma folate values has been found in a healthy elderly group (Weinberg, 1983). On the other hand, it has been shown that biochemical parameters of vitamin B_6 do not correlate well with intake of this vitamin in the hospitalized elderly (Vir and Love, 1978).

Evidence strongly suggests that failure to establish a good correlation between vitamin intake and status in the elderly in hospitals or institutions may be caused by confounding variables, such as the effects of disease or drugs that can impair vitamin nurriture.

Very few geriatric institutions have laboratories that are capable of biochemical assessment of vitamin or mineral status. In most of these institutions, the practice is to send routine blood samples to area laboratories for biochemical profiles and specific vitamin assays, particularly serum folate or vitamin B_{12}. Little effort is made to ensure quality control in the assays, and there is a remarkable paucity of tests carried out, perhaps owing in part to an effort to reduce costs and to the mistaken idea that it is better not to bother the elderly patients by drawing a blood sample. Collection of 24-hour urine samples is impossible without catheterization in the incontinent patient and in the patient who is incapable of emptying his or her bladder by voluntary means. Knowledge of this fact mitigates against the employment of load tests or other urinary assessment methods for the determination of vitamin or mineral status. However, at present, there are many alternate blood tests, and these may be more specific and sensitive indicators of vitamin or mineral depletion.

A real concern is that drugs taken by the elderly patient may interfere with the test procedure or may cloud interpretation of the test results. The medical and nursing staffs of geriatric institutions and the physicians caring for elderly in the community should have references available that will enable them to avoid false positive and negative tests because of drug interference. Drug interference with the assessment of nutritional status has been discussed by Roe (1981) and Hansten (1973).

The interpretation of biochemical test results is also made more difficult in the elderly by the problem of deciding whether a nutritional deficiency found is causing a particular functional deficit or vice versa. For example, a positive association has been found by Goodwin, Goodwin, and Garry (1983) between vitamin nurriture and cognitive functioning, but it is not clear whether mentally sharp elderly eat better or whether better nutrition aids the memory.

Biochemical tests for the assessment of nutritional status are summarized in Table 6-16. Drugs interfering with the biochemical assessment of nutritional status are shown in Table 6-17.

TABLE 6-16   Biochemical Assessment of Nutritional Status

	ACCEPTABLE	LOW	DEFICIENT
Plasma retinol (μg/100 ml)	>20.0	10–20.0	<10.0
Serum folate (ng/ml)	>6.0	3–6.0	<3.0
Red cell folate (ng/ml)	>150	100–150	<100
Serum vitamin B$_{12}$ (pg/ml)	>200	100–200	<100
Serum vitamin B$_6$ (ng/ml)	>4.0	3–4.0	<3.0
Red cell vitamin B$_6$ (ng/ml)	14.0	12–14.0	<12.0
Serum ascorbic acid (mg/100 ml)	>0.30	0.20–0.29	<0.20
Leukocyte ascorbic acid (mg/100 ml)	>15	8–15	<8
Red cell transketolase TPPE %	<15	16–20	>20
Red cell glutathione reductase AC	>1.2	1.2–1.4	>1.4
Calcium (mg/dl)	8.5 = 10.5 (2.12 = 2.62 mmol/l)	—	—
Phosphate (mg/dl)	2.5 = 4.5 (0.8 = 1.4 mmol/l)	—	—
Serum albumin (g/dl)	3.8 = 4.4	—	—

TABLE 6-17   Drugs Interfering with the Biochemical Assessment of Nutritional Status

STATUS ASSESSMENT	SPECIFIC ASSAY	DRUGS INTERFERING
Vitamin D, calcium	Serum calcium (plasma)	Thiazides
Thiamin	Erythrocyte transketolase	5-Fluorouracil, furosemide
Folate	Serum folate (plasma)	Aspirin, alcohol, antibiotics, folic acid antagonists
Vitamin A	Plasma carotenoids	Mineral oil, canthaxanthine

IMMUNOLOGICAL ASSESSMENT

Delayed hypersensitivity skin tests for microbial and fungal antigens are used to examine cellular immune function. Negative responses to intradermal recall antigens, or anergy, are a common finding in severe protein-energy malnutrition (Chandra, 1981). Positive outcome of nutritional intervention can be assessed by return of positive responses. However, whereas malnutrition is the most frequent cause of secondary immunodeficiency and of negative skin tests, factors other than malnutrition, including old age and cancer, can cause anergy (Howard and Meguid, 1981). Therefore, when skin tests are used to monitor response to nutritional intervention in elderly patients, failure for the tests to become positive should not necessarily be accepted as being caused by inadequate treatment.

DIAGNOSTIC ASSESSMENT

The proof of a nutritional diagnosis is still often established by administration of a nutrient that is believed to be deficient in the diet or in the patient. Selective intervention may indeed be an effective diagnostic measure, provided that interpretation of the outcome is appropriate and safe. Too many small nutritional surveys of the elderly have claimed a response to vitamin administration as proof of a previous deficiency when, in fact, other factors, such as response to disease treatment, could explain the response. Further, the response was so delayed that there is no true temporal relationship between the giving of a nutrient supplement and the happy outcome.

Means to establish nutritional diagnoses by intervention are summarized in Table 6-18.

TABLE 6-18 Means to Establish Nutritional Diagnoses by Intervention

PRESENTING SYMPTOMS OR SIGNS	SUSPECTED DIAGNOSIS	INTERVENTION
Megaloblastic anemia (without neurological signs)	Folate deficiency	Administer 2 μg vitamin B_{12} intramuscularly daily for 7 days; get reticulocyte count daily; if *no* response, give 5 mg folic acid daily for 10 days
Angular stomatitis	Riboflavin deficiency	Administer 5 mg riboflavin twice daily for 14 days
Purpura	Scurvy	Exclude drug cause; check for thiazides and anticoagulants; get CBC and platelet count; give 300 mg ascorbic acid daily for 7 days

Safety is paramount in determining vitamin deficiencies by intervention in such a manner and sequence as not to interfere with a causative assessment. Thus, in determination of the nutritional cause of a megaloblastic anemia, it is essential to give vitamin B_{12} before giving folic acid to avoid the pitfall of seeing a hematological response to folic acid as evidence for a folate deficiency.

PROGNOSTIC ASSESSMENT

Nutritional indicators of prognostic importance have been identified. For example in a study carried out in Nottingham, England, it was found that weight, midarm circumference, triceps skinfold thickness, plasma albumin, plasma retinol binding, protein, and plasma retinol were lower in elderly patients who died soon after the tests were performed. However, these were the same patients who were clinically classified as wasted and who had poor appetites or cancer (Kemm and Allcock, 1984). Further, a prognostic nutritional index may be obtained by a combination of anthropometric, biochemical, and immunological assessment in a hospitalized population. However, it has been questioned whether these provide better prognostic tools than a skilled clinical classification of malnutrition (Detsky et al., 1984). Although there are not enough physicians or clinical nutritionists who are able to make a nutritional diagnosis with accuracy, completeness, and prognostic significance in the elderly, the established clinical and laboratory methods used in younger people should be retained.

QUESTIONS

Circle all correct answers (there may be more than one correct answer to each question).

1. The following instruments and methods are used in nutritional assessment of the elderly. Indicate appropriate applications.
   a. Lange calipers
   b. knee height
   c. packed red cell volume
   d. 3-day food record (diary)
   e. skin tests

2. Distinguish between the following *symptoms* and *signs* of malnutrition
   a. feeling of walking on cotton
   b. loss of appetite
   c. dependent edema
   d. glossitis
   e. pain on swallowing
   f. koilonychia

    g. diarrhea
    h. ataxia
    i. loss of memory
    j. pallor (conjunctival)

3. Which of the following statements are *correct?*
   a. The best method for obtaining information on the food intake of the elderly is a 24-hour food recall.
   b. Elderly men and women are unable to complete 3-day records.
   c. The advantage of using food frequency questionnaires is that they do not require record-keeping.
   d. Diet histories must be obtained by a trained dietitian.
   e. To find out what an elderly patient actually eats, records should be obtained from the hospital food service department.

4. Iron deficiency can be determined by use of which three of the following tests?
   a. plasma retinol
   b. plasma ferritin
   c. red cell folacin
   d. red cell protoporphyrin
   e. serum iron

5. Which of the following statements is correct?
   a. The blood picture in folacin and vitamin B_{12} deficiency is similar.
   b. The blood picture in folacin and vitamin B_{12} deficiency is entirely different.

6. Indicate which of the following statements are true.
   a. Activity diaries are useful to assess the energy expenditure of patients in skilled nursing facilities.
   b. There are no feasible methods to measure energy expenditure in the impaired elderly.
   c. Stature can be computed from knee height using nomograms.
   d. The bioelectrical impedance method for the measurement of body composition is particularly useful in edematous patients.

REFERENCES

ADAMS, C. F., *Nutritive Value of American Foods in Common Units*, Agric. Handbook No. 456, Washington, DC: U.S. Department of Agriculture, 1975.
ALLINGTON, J. K., M. E. MATTHEWS, V. K. JOHNSON, and N. E. JOHNSON, "A short method to ensure nutritional adequacy of food served in nursing homes: 1. Identification of need; 2. Development of a model food plan," *J. Amer. Dietet. Assoc.*, 76 (1980), 458–70.

ANDRES, A., E. L. BIERMAN, and W. R. HAZZARD, *Principles of Geriatric Medicine.* New York: McGraw-Hill Book Co., 1985, pp. 311–18.

BISHOP, C. W., "Reference values for arm muscle area, arm fat area, subscapular skinfold thickness, and sum of skinfold thicknesses for American adults," *J. Parent. Ent. Nutr.,* 8 (1984), 515–22.

BLOCK, G., and A. M. HARTMAN, "Issues in reproducibility and validity of dietary studies," *Amer. J. Clin. Nutr.,* 50 (1989), 1133–38.

BLOCK, G., A. M. HARTMAN, C. M. DRESSER, et al., "Data-based approach to diet questionnaire design and testing," *Amer. J. Epidemiol.,* 124 (1986), 453–69.

BURKE, B. S., "The dietary history as a tool in research," *J. Amer. Dietet. Assoc.,* 23 (1947), 1041–46.

CAMPBELL, V. A., and M. L. DODDS, "Collecting dietary information from groups of older people," *J. Amer. Dietet. Assoc.,* 51 (1976), 29.

CARL, J. W., *Food Purchases of Housebound Elderly.* M.N.S. Thesis, Cornell University, Ithaca, NY, 1980.

CARLOS, J. P., and M. D. WOLFE, "Methodological and nutritional issues in assessing the oral health of aged subjects," *Amer. J. Clin. Nutr.,* 50 (1989), 1210–18.

CHANARIN, I., *The Megaloblastic Anemias.* Oxford: Blackwell Scientific Publications, Ltd., 1969, pp. 457–74.

CHANDRA, R. K., "Immunodeficiency in undernutrition and overnutrition," *Nutr. Rev.,* 39 (1981), 225.

CHUMLEA, W. C., and R. N. BAUMGARTNER, "Status of anthropometry and body composition data in elderly subjects," *Amer. J. Clin. Nutr.,* 50 (1989), 1158–66.

CHUMLEA, W. C., A. F. ROCHE, and D. MUKHERJEE, *Nutritional Assessment of the Elderly through Anthropometry.* Columbus, OH: Ross Laboratories, 1984.

CHUMLEA, W. C., A. F. ROCHE, and M. L. STEINBAUGH, "Estimating stature from knee height for persons 60–90 years of age," *J. Amer. Geriat. Soc.,* 33 (1985), 116–20.

CLARK, N. G., and G. L. BLACKBURN, "Nutritional assessment of the institutionalized," in *Nutrition in the Young and in the Elderly,* eds. E. W. Haller and G. I. Cotton. Lexington, MA: Collamore Press, 1983, pp. 11–23.

COLMAN, N., "Laboratory assessment of folate status," *Clin. Lab. Med.,* 1 (1981), 775–96.

DAVIES, L., and M. D. HOLDSWORTH, "A technique for assessing nutritional 'at risk' factors in residential homes for the elderly," *J. Human Nutr.,* 33 (1979), 165–69.

DETSKY, A. S., J. P. BAKER, R. A. MENDELSON, S. L. WOLMAN, D. E. WESSON, and K. N. JEEJEEBHOY, "Evaluating the accuracy of nutritional assessment techniques applied to hospitalized patients: methodology and comparisons," *J. Parent. Ent. Nutr.,* 8 (1984), 154–59.

EVANS, H. K., and D. J. GINES, "Dietary recall method comparison for hospitalized elderly subjects," *J. Amer. Diet. Assoc.,* 85 (1985), 202–05.

FOOD AND NUTRITION BOARD, NATIONAL ACADEMY OF SCIENCES, *National Research Council Recommended Daily Dietary Allowances,* 10th Ed. Washington, DC, 1989.

FREELAND, J. H., and R. J. COUSINS, "Zinc content of selected foods," *J. Amer. Dietet. Assoc.,* 68 (1976), 526–529.

GANZONI, A. M., R. OAKES, and R. M. HILLMAN, "Red cell aging in vivo," *J. Clin. Invest.,* 50 (1971), 1373–78.

GIRDWOOD, R. H., A. D. THOMSON, and J. WILLIAMSON, "Folate status in the elderly," *Brit. Med. J.,* 2 (1967), 670–72.

GOODWIN, J. S., J. M. GOODWIN, and P. J. GARRY, "Association between nutritional status and cognitive functioning in a healthy elderly population," *J. Amer. Med. Assoc.*, 249 (1983), 2917–39.

HANSTEN, P. D., *Drug Interactions. Part II. Drug Effects on Clinical Laboratory Test Results*, 2nd Ed. Philadelphia: Lea & Febiger, 1973, pp. 257–453.

HARPER, A. E., "Recommended dietary allowances for the elderly," *Geriatrics*, 33 (1978), 73–80.

HERZLER, A. A., and L. M. HAEVER, "Development of food tables and uses with computers," *J. Amer. Dietet Assoc.*, 70 (1977), 20.

HEYMSFELD, S. B., J. WANG, S. LICHTMAN, et al., "Body composition in elderly subjects: A critical appraisal of clinical methodology," *Amer. J. Clin. Nutr.*, 50 (1989), 1167–75.

HOWARD, L., and M. M. MEGUID, "Nutritional assessment in total parenteral nutrition," *Clin. Lab. Med.*, 1 (1981), 611–30.

HTOO, M. S. H., R. L. KOTKOFF, and M. L. FREEDMAN, "Erythrocyte parameters in the elderly: an argument against new geriatric normal values," *J. Amer. Geriat. Soc.*, 27 (1979), 548.

KALCHTHALER, T., and M. E. RIGOR TAN, "Anemia in institutionialized elderly patients," *J. Amer. Geriat. Soc.* 28 (1980), 108–13.

KARKECK, J. M., "Assessment of the nutritional status of the elderly," *Nutr. Support Serv.*, 4 (1984), 23–33.

KEMM, J., and J. ALLCOCK, "The distribution of supposed indicators of nutritional status in elderly patients," *Age and Aging*, 13 (1984), 21–28.

LAWRENCE, V. A., J. E. LOEWENSTEIN, and E. R. EICHNER, "Aspirin and folate binding: in vivo and in vitro studies of serum binding and urinary excretion of endogeneous folate," *J. Lab. Clin. Med.*, 103 (1984), 944–48.

LEGER, L. A., J. LAMBERT, and P. MARTIN, "Validity of plastic skinfold caliper measurements," *Hum. Biol.*, 54 (1982), 667–75.

LIVINGSTONE, M. B. E., A. M. PRENTICE, W. A. COOWARD, et al., "Simultaneous measurement of free living energy expenditure by the doubly labeled water method and heart rate monitoring," *Amer. J. Clin. Nutr.*, 52 (1990), 59–65.

LUKASKI, H. C., W. W. BOLUNCHUK, C. B. HALL, et al., "Validation of tetrapolar bioelectrical impedance method to assess human body composition," *J. Appl. Physiol.*, 60 (1986), 1327–32.

MILLER, A. K., J. ADIR, and R. E. VESTAL, "Tolbutamide binding to plasma proteins of old and young human subjects," *J. Pharm. Sci.*, 67 (1978), 1192–93.

MURPHY, E. W., B. W. WILLIS, and B. K. WATT, "Provisional tables on the zinc content of food," *J. Amer. Dietet. Assoc.*, 66 (1975), 345–55.

NOPPA, H. M., M. ANDERSSON, G. BERGTSSON, et. al., "Longitudinal studies of anthropometric data and body composition: the population study of women in Göteborg, Sweden," *Amer. J. Geriat. Soc.*, 33 (1980), 155–62.

Nutrition and Health in Old Age: The Cross-Sectional Analysis of the Findings Made in 1972/3 of Elderly People Studied in 1967/8, Report by the Committee on Medical Aspects of Food Policy, Department of Health and Social Security Report on Health and Social Subjects #16. London: Her Majesty's Stationery Office, 1979.

PERLOFF, B. P., and R. R. BUTRUM, "Folacin in selected foods," *J. Amer. Dietet. Assoc.*, 70 (1977), 161–72.

Roe, D. A., *Alcohol and the Diet*. Westport, CT: AVI Publishing Co., 1979, pp. 149–59.

ROE, D. A., "Drug interference with the assessment of nutritional status," *Clin. Lab. Med.*, 1 (1981), 647–64.

RUSSELL, R., *The Problem of Evaluating Nutritional Status of the Elderly.* Chapel Hill, NC: Publications Department, Institute of Nutrition, University of North Carolina, 1983.

SAMET, J. M., "Surrogate measures of dietary intake," *Amer. J. Clin. Nutr.* 50 (1989), 1139–44.

SAUBERLICH, H. E., J. H. SKALA, and R. P. DOWDY, *Laboratory Tests for the Assessment of Nutritional Status.* Cleveland: CRC Press, Inc., 1974.

SHEPHARD, R. J., "Assessment of physical activity and energy needs," *Amer. J. Clin. Nutr.*, 50 (1989), 1195–1200.

SIMKO, M. D., C. COWELL, and M. S. HREHA, Eds. *Practical Nutrition: A Quick Reference Guide for the Health Practitioner.* Rockville, MD: Aspen Publications, Inc., 1989, pp. 291–92.

SOCIAL SECURITY ADMINISTRATION, "Skilled nursing facilities: standards for certification and participation in Medicare and Medicaid programs," *Federal Register,* 39, 12 (Jan. 1974), 2237.

TRULSON, M. F. and M. B. McCANN, "Comparison of dietary survey methods," *J. Amer. Diet. Assoc.,* 35 (1959), 672.

U.S. DEPARTMENT OF AGRICULTURE, "Pantothenic acid, vitamin B_6, and vitamin B_{12} in foods," *U.S.D.A. Home Econ. Res. Rep.,* No. 36, 1969.

U.S. DEPARTMENT OF AGRICULTURE/U.S. DEPARTMENT OF HEALTH, EDUCATION, AND WELFARE, *Dietary Guidelines for Americans (Joint Statement).* Washington, DC: U.S. Government Printing Office, 1980.

U.S. DEPARTMENT OF HEALTH, EDUCATION, AND WELFARE, "Weight by height by age for adults 18–74 years: U.S., 1971–74." DHEW Publ. No. (PHS) 79–1656. Sept. 1979.

U.S. DEPARTMENT OF HEALTH AND HUMAN SERVICES, "Obese and overweight adults in the United States," Data from the Natl. Health Survey Series 11, No. 230, DHHS Publ. No. (PHS) 83-1680. Hyattsville, MD: National Center for Health Statistics, Feb. 1983.

VERBOV, N. J., *Skin Diseases in the Elderly.* London: Wm. Heinemann Medical Books, Ltd., 1974, pp. 24–176.

VIR, S. C., and A. H. G. LOVE, "Vitamin B_6 status of the hospitalized aged," *Amer. J. Clin. Nutr.,* 31 (1978), 1383–91.

WATT, B. K., and A. L. MERRILL, *Composition of Foods—Raw, Processed, Prepared,* Rev. Agric. Handbook No. 8, Washington, DC: U.S. Department of Agriculture, 1963.

WEINBERG, S., *Folacin Intake and Status of Independently-Living Elderly Women.* M.S. Thesis, Cornell University, Ithaca, NY, 1983.

WHEELER, M. S., *Dietary Methodology for Valid Measurement of Mean Daily Potassium and Magnesium Intake in Homebound Elderly Individuals.* M.N.S. Thesis, Cornell University, Ithaca, NY, 1984.

WILLETT, W. C., L. SAMPSON, M. J. STAMPFER, et al., "Reproducibility and validity of a semiquantitative food frequency questionnaire. *Amer. J. Epidemiol.,* 122 (1985), 51–65.

YEARICK, E. S., "Nutritional status of the elderly: anthropometric and clinical findings," *J. Gerontol.,* 33 (1979), 657–62.

chapter 7

Nutritional Deficiencies

Nutritional deficiencies in the elderly can result from short-term or long-term ingestion of a diet which is inadequate in food-energy or lacking in one or more specific nutrients. Under physiological conditions, a diet is deficient if it does not meet the needs of most healthy individuals of a particular age group. Since the nutritional needs of most elderly people differ from the needs of younger people (including the middle-aged) for which the RDA are set, and since the elderly differ one from another in their food-energy and nutrient requirements, dietary adequacy for the elderly is better defined as a diet which, for a given individual, prevents malnutrition and cannot be improved by additions or modifications in the levels of food-energy and nutrients supplied.

Diets which lead to development of nutritional deficiency are (1) monotonous, (2) low in food energy, (3) restrictive, and (4) low in nutrient-calorie ratio.

Variety or dietary diversity will increase the quality of the diet, as will calorie adequacy. Conversely, the fewer the number of foods eaten, the greater the risk that sources of essential nutrients will be excluded or will be inadequate. Diets high in sweets or which include heavy daily intake of alcoholic beverages satisfy the hunger needs of the elderly without providing needed nutrients.

In the United States, diets of the elderly are often deficient in folacin. Diets low in food-energy are also low in iron. Elderly persons not consuming milk will have inadequate intakes of calcium, vitamin D, and riboflavin.

DISEASES

Acute and chronic diseases are likely to reduce food intakes because of associated loss of appetite (Exton-Smith and Overall, 1979; Hodkinson, 1980). Acute diseases and injuries which convey a nutritional risk are shown in Table 7-1. In the presence of acute disease, intake of food is likely to be markedly reduced or to cease altogether. At the same time, catabolic effects of disease increase nutrient requirements. Nutritional needs for wound healing after injury or surgery can magnify nutrient deficits. In elderly surgical patients, protein-energy malnutrition is frequently found both in the pre- and postoperative periods. Pre- and postoperative causes of malnutrition in the elderly are shown in Table 7-2.

   Chronic diseases which are associated with malnutrition in the elderly are listed in Table 7-3. Types of nutritional deficiency commonly associated with these diseases are indicated, together with etiological factors. Chronic disease processes lead to malnutrition by impairment of food intake or retention, by causing maldigestion and malabsorption, by increasing renal

TABLE 7-1   Acute Diseases and Injuries of the Elderly Associated with Anorexia

Acute bronchitis
Pneumonia (viral or bacterial)
Other bacterial infections
Other viral infections
Oral candidiasis (yeast infections of the mouth)
Generalized dermatitis or other dermatoses with severe itching
Acute confusional psychoses
Acute cholecystitis
Burns
Fractures
Intestinal obstruction

TABLE 7-2   Pre- and Postoperative Causes of Malnutrition

PREOPERATIVE	POSTOPERATIVE
Pain	Intravenous fluids
Vomiting	No food allowed by mouth
No food allowed by mouth	Catabolic effects of surgery
Alcoholic binge prior to hospitalization	Lack of nutritional support
Intravenous fluids	Deficiencies of formula feeds (enteral or
Burn losses	parenteral)
	Short bowel syndrome
	Postgastrectomy syndromes

TABLE 7-3   Chronic Diseases Associated with Malnutrition in the Elderly

Congestive heart failure	Arthritis
Cancer	Organic brain syndromes
Chronic nuerological diseases with	Psychotic depression
paralysis	End-stage renal disease
Alcoholic cirrhosis	Maldigestion/malabsorption syndromes,
Chronic bronchitis and emphysema	e.g., chronic pancreatitis, radiation
	enteritis

losses of nutrients, and this condition is also brought about by decreasing the efficiency of nutrient utilization (Roe, 1979).

DRUGS

Drug groups and individual drugs that cause malnutrition are shown in Table 7-4. The drugs listed are all in common use by geriatric patients living at home or in hospitals or extended care facilities. Several drugs which can lead to malnutrition may be taken by patients on multiple-drug regimens (Roe, "Interactions," 1979; Roe, 1981). It is also significant that drugs used for different pharmacological purposes can have additive effects in producing nutrient depletion. Thus, whereas laxatives and most diuretics increase potassium depletion, taken together they can induce a potassium deficiency if the potassium intake is insufficient to meet drug-imposed, as well as physiological, requirements.

Nutritional deficiencies caused by the use of common drugs are shown in Table 7-5.

TABLE 7-4   Common Drugs Which Cause Malnutrition in the Elderly

DRUG USE	DRUG
Cardiac disease	Digitalis
Hypertension	Thiazides (e.g., hydrochlorothiazide)
	Furosemide
	Ethacrynic acid
	Triamterene
Arthritis	Aspirin
Gout	Indomethacin
	Colchicine
Indigestion (Antacids)	Magnesium and aluminum hydroxide
Constipation (Laxatives)	Mineral oil, phenolphthalein
Insomnia/anxiety (Sedatives)	Barbiturates

TABLE 7-5 Nutritional Deficiencies Caused by Common Drugs Taken by the Elderly

DRUG AND DRUG GROUP	DEFICIENCY

1. Cardiac glycosides
    Digitalis
	Anorexia → protein-energy
	    malnutrition
	Zinc and magnesium deficiency

2. Diuretics	Thiazides → Potassium, zinc, and magnesium Furosemide depletion Ethacrynic acid Triamterene → Folacin deficiency

3. Anti-inflammatory drugs
    Aspirin
    Indomethacin
    Colchicine
	GI Blood loss → iron deficiency
	Malabsorption of fat soluble and water soluble
	    vitamins

4. Antacids (antacid abuse)	Phosphate depletion; osteomalacia
5. Laxatives (laxative abuse)	Mineral oil → Deficiency of vitamins A, D, and K Phenolphthalein (Potassium deficiency) Multiple nutrient deficiencies due to malabsorption Folacin and vitamin D deficiency

MULITFACTORIAL CAUSES

Although it can be generalized that in the elderly malnutrition is caused by the combined effects of poor diet, disease, and drugs, in practice, if malnutrition is subdivided into the categories of protein-energy malnutrition, avitaminosis, and mineral deficiencies, causative factors can be seen to have differing importance. Thus, protein-energy malnutrition is most likely to be caused by acute and chronic disease; avitaminoses are usually caused by a deficient diet; and mineral deficiencies are mainly caused by the effects of drugs. In each of these types of malnutrition, multiple causation is frequent, but the relative importance of any one etiological factor is different.

PROTEIN-ENERGY MALNUTRITION

Protein-energy malnutrition in the elderly, as in younger persons, may be acute or chronic.

Acute Protein-Energy Malnutrition (PEM)

Acute PEM develops in previously well-nourished or obese people when they are on a starvation regimen while undergoing the catabolic stress of infection, injury, or surgery (Butterworth and Weinsier, 1980). Acute PEM occurs in hospitalized patients whose previous nutritional status may have been satisfactory but who are denied access to food. Alternatively, acute PEM can develop in patients who cannot eat because of disease-related causes. Signs of acute PEM are apathy, weakness, edema, delayed wound healing, intolerance of anesthesia, susceptibility to adverse drug reactions, and impaired cellular immune function. Diagnosis is by history, by clinical examination and identification of edema, including wound edema; by hematological studies showing lymphocytopenia; by biochemical determinants, including the finding of hypoalbuminemia; and by skin tests showing a lack of allergic responses to standard antigens, including candida and mumps antigens.

Chronic Protein-Energy Malnutrition

Chronic PEM is synonymous with *cachexia*. Cachexia usually results from low food intake, secondary to anorexia. In the elderly, common causes of cachexia are cancer (particularly disseminated neoplastic disease), chronic neurological disease associated with paralysis, end-stage hepatic or renal disease, and high-dosage digitalis therapy. Very low food intake is a frequent occurrence in the demented elderly, not only because food may be refused or pushed out of the mouth but also because of a lack of feeder skills. Cachexia in feeder-dependent elderly in nursing homes is becoming increasingly recognized (Pinchovski-Devin and Kaminski, 1987). Although cachexia is mainly caused by reduced energy and protein intake, additional causal factors are catabolic effects of disease and excessive losses of nutrients by malabsorption or through protein-losing enteropathy.

Signs of cachexia are emaciation, loss of subcutaneous fat, loss of lean body mass, brittleness of the hair, ridged or banded nails, and crazy-pavement dermatosis of the lower legs. Acute PEM may be superimposed on cachexia.

Protein Malnutrition

Severe protein malnutrition is the result of excessive protein losses as produced by extensive burns; by bullous (blistering) dermatoses (pemphigoid or pemphigus); by protein-losing enteropathy, which may occur with cancer; or by renal disease with massive albuminuria. The latter may develop in the elderly with inorganic mercury intoxication, secondary to administration of mercurial diuretics. Severe protein malnutrition causes edema, hypoalbuminemia, and failure of wound healing.

Fat-Soluble Vitamin Deficiencies

Vitamin D deficiency. In the elderly the disease osteomalacia, which is caused by a vitamin D deficiency, develops in people who are house-bound or institutionalized and not exposed to sunlight (Lawson et al., 1979). Etiological factors which frequently coexist are low dietary intake of vitamin D and chronic intake of drugs such as barbiturates and phenytoin which interfere with the hydroxylation of vitamin D in the liver. Causes of vitamin D deficiency in the elderly are summarized in Table 7-6.

TABLE 7-6   Causes of Vitamin D Deficiency in the Elderly

1. Environmental
   a. Lack of exposure to sunlight
   b. Wearing of heavy clothing and/or use of light barriers
2. Dietary
   a. Lack of intake of milk or other dietary sources of vitamin D
3. Malabsorption
   a. Gluten-sensitive enteropathy—senile type
   b. Postgastrectomy
   c. Resection of small intestine
   d. Pancreatic insufficiency
   e. Drugs causing malabsorption
      i. Laxative abuse—mineral oil, phenolphthalein
      ii. Cholestyramine
   f. Geriatric intestinal mucosal atrophy
   g. Biliary obstruction
      i. Intrahepatic
      ii. Extrahepatic
   h. Radiation enteritis—chronic
4. Impaired hepatic 25-hydroxylation of vitamin D
   a. Cirrhosis
   b. Geriatric effect
5. Increased catabolism of vitamin D due to drugs
   a. Phenytoin (Dilantin)
   b. Phenobarbital
   c. Glutethimide
6. Impaired 1-hydroxylation of vitamin D metabolites in the kidney
   a. Chronic renal failure
   b. Geriatric effect
   c. Diphosphonates
7. Phosphate depletion
   a. Antacid abuse (phosphate binding)
   b. Malabsorption syndromes
   c. Hyperparathyroidism
   d. Hemodialysis
   e. Total parenteral alimentation
   f. Metabolic acidosis
   g. Fanconi syndrome—adult type

Symptoms and signs of osteomalacia in the elderly are:

1. Pain related to the back, chest, and limbs that is worsened by sudden movement, muscle strain, weight-bearing, and pressure
2. Bone tenderness elicited by pressure
3. Skeletal deformities, including loss of height, kyphosis, scoliosis, pigeon chest, and bowing of long bones
4. Muscle weakness involving proximal limb muscles

5. Waddling gait secondary to muscle weakness
6. Paresthesias, muscle cramps, and tetany secondary to severe hypocalcemia

Diagnostic test for osteomalacia are:

1. *Radiological examination.* Findings are decreased skeletal radiodensity indicative of demineralization and pseudofractures (Looser's zones, which are symmetrical radiolucent bands at the ends of long bones and in the ribs, pubic bones, and scapulae). Osteoporosis frequently coexists with osteomalacia.
2. *Bone biopsy.* Findings are osteoid seams and undermineralization.
3. *Biochemical tests.* In geriatric patients there is hypophosphatemia with or without hypocalcemia. Alkaline phosphatase is usually increased. Total urinary hydroxyproline is elevated. Serum parathyroid hormone (PTH) may be elevated in the early stages of the disease. Serum 25-hydroxycholecalciferol may be lowered. Biochemical findings alone are not diagnostic, but biochemical tests may corroborate diagnosis and indicate causal mechanisms.
4. *Therapeutic intervention.* Administration of vitamin D or a vitamin D metabolite or exposure to ultraviolet light will relieve symptoms, heal radiological changes, and reverse abnormal biochemical findings. Cure may require treatment of causal pathology on discontinuation of drugs.

Vitamin A deficiency. Overt vitamin A deficiency is very uncommon in the elderly in the United States. Subgroups such as elderly alcoholics and the elderly with malabsorption syndromes may be at risk. Alcohol and vitamin A metabolisms' are competitive. Vitamin A absorption is impaired by certain drugs, including mineral oil and cholestyramine.

Mild to moderate vitamin A deficiency is usually symptom free. Patients may complain of difficulty in finding their way about at night or difficulty in adapting to the light in darkened rooms. Night blindness can be identified by dark adaptation tests. Improvement in dark adaptation follows administration of vitamin A. Night blindness in elderly alcoholics is caused by vitamin A or zinc deficiency.

Diagnostic tests for vitamin A deficiency include (1) measurement of plasma retinol, (2) performance of dark adaptation tests, and (3) administration of vitamin A in therapeutic doses (Garry, 1981).

Vitamin K deficiency. Vitamin K deficiency in the elderly can be caused by drugs or disease (Roe, 1976).

Drugs causing vitamin K deficiency are:

1. Coumarin anticoagulants (vitamin K antagonists)
2. Broad-spectrum antibiotics (tetracycline or cephalosporins)
3. Cholestyramine

Diseases causing vitamin K deficiency are:

1. Alcoholic cirrhosis
2. Other severe liver disease

Low dietary intake of vitamin K per se will not cause a vitamin K deficiency because vitamin K_2 is synthesized by bacteria in the large intestine. Massive intake of vitamin E can precipitate vitamin K deficiency in patients on coumarin anticoagulant drugs. Patients who are on anticoagulant drugs and barbiturates may become vitamin K deficient when the barbiturates are discontinued. This is because the stimulation by barbiturates of the anticoagulant drug metabolism is removed and anticoagulant drug effects are prolonged. Vitamin K deficiency may also develop in patients on anticoagulant drugs whose vitamin K intake is low and who, at the same time, are given oral broad-spectrum antibiotics which inhibit vitamin K_2 synthesis.

Vitamin K deficiency is manifested by hemorrhage. Hemorrhage into the skin is called purpura. Purpura is common in vitamin K deficiency, but in the elderly may be caused by changes in the skin. Oozing hemorrhage may occur from wound sites, from hemorrhoids, into the GI tract, or from other sites of trauma.

Diagnostic tests for vitamin K deficiency are:

1. Measurement of prothrombin time and related indices (Prothrombin times are prolonged in vitamin K deficiency.)
2. Discontinuation of anticoagulant drugs
3. Administration of vitamin K by oral or parenteral routes

Water-Soluble Vitamin Deficiencies

Vitamin B_{12} deficiency. In the elderly a vitamin B_{12} deficiency is commonly caused by lack of gastric intrinsic factor (IF), which causes vitamin B_{12} malabsorption. Gastric intrinsic factor is lacking in pernicious anemia (Addison's anemia). A late effect of partial or total gastrectomy is inadequate production of IF, and this also causes vitamin B_{12} deficiency. Table 7-7 offers a classification of causes of vitamin B_{12} deficiency. Other frequent causes of vitamin B_{12} deficiency in the elderly are vitamin B_{12} malabsorption caused by ileal disease or ileal resection (Hoffbrand, 1971). Rarely prolonged intake of a vegetarian diet is the cause of vitamin B_{12} deficiency.

Symptoms of vitamin B_{12} deficiency can be divided according to etiology. Symptoms associated with anemia are:

1. Weakness
2. Dyspnea

Gastorintestinal symptoms are:

1. Sore tongue or mouth
2. Anorexia
3. Nausea
4. Gastric discomfort

TABLE 7-7   Causes of Vitamin B$_{12}$ Deficiency in the Elderly

1. Malabsorption
   a. due to lack of gastric intrinsic factor
      i. Addison's disease (pernicious anemia)
      ii. Partial gastrectomy
      iii. Total gastrectomy
   b. due to loss of ileal absorption site
      i. Regional enteritis
      ii. Radiation enteritis
      iii. Ileal resection
   c. due to drugs
      i. Colchicine
      ii. Neomycin
2. Diet
   Vegan diet (rare cause)

5. Flatulence
6. Abdominal pain
7. Episodic diarrhea

Neurological symptoms are:

1. Burning pains in limbs
2. Tingling of fingers and toes
3. Numbness, cold, or tightness of skin
4. Difficulty in walking
5. Unsteadiness
6. Incontinence

Physical signs are:

1. Pallor
2. Lemon-yellow color of skin
3. Tachycardia
4. Hypotension
5. Systolic murmur
6. Loss of position and vibration sense, particularly in lower limbs
7. Ataxia (worse when eyes are closed)
8. Depression
9. Memory impairment
10. Visual impairment
11. Abnormal tendon reflexes (positive Babinski sign)

Diagnostic tests are:

1. By history, symptoms, and physical signs
2. By presence of megaloblastic anemia with megaloblasts in the bone marrow and peripheral blood
3. Serum vitamin B_{12} levels in deficient range
4. Schilling test results indicative of vitamin B_{12} malabsorption
5. Resolution of anemia and of all symptoms, including neurological symptoms following injection of vitamin B_{12}

Folacin deficiency. Folacin deficiency is reported as the most common nutritional deficiency in the elderly (Hurdle and Williams, 1966; Chanarin, 1973). Causes include low intake caused by avoidance of rich food sources of the vitamin such as liver, green leafy vegetables, and breakfast cereals which are fortified with folic acid. Folacin deficiency is prevalent in elderly alcoholics because of grossly inadequate diets, malabsorption, loss of folacin into the stomach (Ménétrier's disease), and impaired metabolism or storage of folacin coenzymes in the liver. Drugs taken by the elderly which cause folacin deficiency include phenytoin (Dilantin), phenobarbital, cholestyramine, sulfasalazine, and methotrexate (Roe, 1982). Folacin deficiency may be caused by disease-associated malabsorption syndromes. A full list of causes of folacin deficiency in the elderly is shown in Table 7-8.

Clinical features of folacin deficiency include megaloblastic anemia, which always occurs in severe folacin deficiency and is identical with that found in vitamin B_{12} deficiency. An organic brain syndrome may also occur

TABLE 7-8   Causes of Folacin Deficiency in the Elderly

Malabsorption of Folacin
   Gluten-sensitive enteropathy (senile type)
   Tropical sprue
   Radiation enteritis
   Alcoholic enteritis
   Inflammatory bowel disease
   Cholestyramine
   Sulfasalazine

Hyperexcretion and Malutilization of Folacin
   Cirrhosis
   Congestive heart failure
   Ménétrier's disease (loss of folacin into the stomach)
   Methotrexate ⎫
   Triamterene   ⎬ Folacin antagonists
   Trimethoprim ⎭
   Phenytoin
   Phenobarbital
   Glutethimide

and is characterized by mental confusion and loss of memory which is different from the neurological manifestations of vitamin B_{12} deficiency. Diagnostic tests for folacin deficiency are:

1. Complete blood count, including red cell indices
2. Examination of stained blood films
3. Determination of plasma and red cell folacin
4. Hemopoietic response to folacin supplementation

Differentiation of folacin deficiency from vitamin B_{12} deficiency is essential because therapeutic doses of folic acid will not prevent progression of the neurological signs of vitamin B_{12} deficiency, which can only be halted or resolved by vitamin B_{12} injections. It is therefore important to exclude the diagnosis of vitamin B_{12} deficiency before administering therapeutic doses of folic acid to patients with megaloblastic anemia.

Riboflavin deficiency. The causes of riboflavin deficiency are low intake and malabsorption, particularly in patients with laxative abuse or disease-induced chronic diarrhea with malabsorption. Impaired synthesis or liver storage of flavin coenzymes occurs in elderly alcoholics with liver disease (Nichoalds, 1981).

Clinical features of riboflavin deficiency include (1) angular stomatitis; (2) glossitis (purplish or beefy tongue, which may be sore or burning); and (3) dermatitis localized to the face, particularly the nose, nasolabial folds, and skin in front of the ears; and dermatitis of the scrotum. In both sexes the dermatitis may be generalized with a tendency to localization in skinfolds. Skin changes are particularly widespread in elderly persons with ariboflavinosis. In the elderly the most common causes of angular stomatitis (cracks at the corners of the mouth) are an edentulous condition or ill-fitting dentures and not riboflavin deficiency (Dreizen, 1974).

Diagnosis is by erythrocyte glutathione reductase assay. Measurement of riboflavin excretion in the urine as a diagnostic test is not recommended in the elderly. Whereas in younger persons riboflavin excretion is related to riboflavin intake, in the elderly, daily riboflavin excretion in the urine may be difficult to measure because 24-hour urine samples cannot be obtained. Further, riboflavin excretion may be high in riboflavin-deficient elderly patients because of potentiation of urinary losses of this vitamin by catabolic disease, infection, ingestion of broad-spectrum antibiotics, or accidental boric acid ingestion. Corroboration of the diagnosis is by administration of riboflavin, which will clear the dermatitis and mucosal changes (Exton-Smith, 1973).

Thiamin deficiency. In geriatric patients the major cause of thiamin deficiency is alcohol abuse. Classical beriberi is rare, and the usual manifestation of thiamin deficiency in elderly alcoholics is the Wernicke-Korsakoff syndrome. Whether or not the Wernicke-Korsakoff syndrome will occur in alcoholics is determined by genetic predisposition. Genetic predisposition occurs in those who have abnormal (mutant) transketolase enzyme. Thiamin deficiency has been reported in elderly patients with gastric carcinoma and in hemodialysis patients.

The Wernicke-Korsakoff syndrome occurs in alcoholics with a long-standing problem who have been on prolonged drinking sprees and are not eating (Roe, "Alcohol," 1979). Onset is rather abrupt. In the acute phases of the disease (Wernicke's encephalopathy), ocular signs occur, with drooping of the eyelids (ptosis), small pupils (miosis), paralysis or partial paralysis of muscles controlling upward gaze, and nystagmus. Ataxia and muscle weakness are common. Since the disease is usually first recognized following sudden discontinuation of alcohol ingestion, symptoms associated with alcohol withdrawal may confuse the clinical picture. Apathy, listlessness, indifference, disorientation, drowsiness, and a semicomatose state are usually present. Korsakoff's psychosis, the late stage of the disease, is associated with confabulation (making up of events to fit memory gaps), severe memory loss, loss of perceptual function, and an inability to perform simple tasks without supervision (Victor, Adams, and Collins, 1971). Beriberi presents with signs of peripheral neuritis or congestive heart failure. Heart disease in elderly alcoholics is more likely to be caused by the toxic effects of alcohol than beriberi (Douglas Talbott, 1975).

The diagnosis of thiamin deficiency is made by history of alcohol abuse, by determination of erythrocyte transketolase, and by administration of thiamin. Wernicke's encephalopathy is reversible by megadosages of thiamin, with recommended doses of 100 to 200 mg thiamin given intravenously, followed by doses of 50 to 100 mg orally. Signs of Korsakoff's psychosis tend to improve with administration of high dosages of thiamin, but reversal of clinical signs is incomplete (Riggs and Boles, 1944).

Vitamin B_6 deficiency. Vitamin B_6 deficiency can be caused by drugs which are vitamin B_6 antagonists. In the elderly, chronic intake of isoniazid (isonicotinic acid hydrazide, INH), cycloserine, L-dopa, or penicillamine can cause vitamin B_6 deficiency, both because complexes of the vitamin with the drug are excreted in the urine and because these drugs may inhibit activity of pyridoxal kinase, which converts vitamin B_6 to its active form, pyridoxal phosphate (Roe, 1976).

Alcohol abuse can lead to a functional vitamin B_6 deficiency because of ethanolic inhibition of pyridoxal kinase (Lumeng and Li, 1974).

Dietary deficiency of vitamin B_6 sufficient to cause symptoms is rare. However, calculation of vitamin B_6 intakes of hospitalized aged suggests that dietary intakes of vitamin B_6 by many older persons are deficient (Vir and Love, 1977).

Signs of vitamin B_6 deficiency include dermatitis, which may be generalized, peripheral neuritis; depression; and sideroblastic anemia. Sideroblastic anemia indicates a condition in which iron is not utilized optimally for heme synthesis and instead is deposited within red cell precursor cells.

Diagnosis is (1) by history and clinical findings, (2) by determination of erythrocyte glutamic pyruvic transaminase before and after *in vitro* stimulation with pyridoxal phosphate, and (3) by determination of serum vitamin B_6 and pyridoxal phosphate (Hampton, Chrisley, and Driskell,

1977). In drug-induced vitamin B_6 deficiency or alcohol-induced vitamin B_6 deficiency, normalization of laboratory tests as well as resolution of clinical signs may require high doses of vitamin B_6.

Vitamin C (ascorbic acid) deficiency. The major cause of ascorbic acid deficiency in the elderly is an inadequate dietary intake of the vitamin. Dietary deficiency of ascorbic acid occurs with exclusively milk diets or with diets lacking in fruit, green vegetables, and potatoes (Hodges et al., 1969).

High doses of salicylates (aspirin) may cause vitamin C depletion (Coffey and Wilson, 1975).

Signs of vitamin C deficiency may be rather nonspecific in elderly people. For example, mental confusion can occur with vitamin C deficiency or from other causes. Similarly, vitamin C deficiency may present with lassitude and fatigue. Signs of scurvy include purpura, subperiosteal hemorrhages, bleeding from the gums, and delayed wound healing, which are common complaints in the elderly and do not offer diagnostic clues. Healing of bed sores is also slowed. Skin changes other than purpura may occur, including follicular hyperkeratosis.

Diagnosis is by history, by physical examination, and by determination of serum, leukocyte, and platelet ascorbate. Diagnosis is confirmed by cure with administration of ascorbic acid in therapeutic dosages (Vir and Love, 1978).

Deficiencies of Major Minerals and Trace Elements

Phosphate depletion. Phosphate depletion may occur in geriatric patients receiving antacids as self-prescribed treatment for flatulence, indigestion, or other symptoms referable to the GI tract. It may also occur when phosphate-binding antacids are prescribed in end-stage renal disease or when such antacids are used as prophylaxis against steroid-induced peptic ulcer. Further, phosphate depletion is particularly liable to occur in patients with steroid-related or alcohol-related ulcer disease (Lotz, Zisman, and Bartter, 1968).

Symptoms of phosphate depletion are those suggestive of myopathy with severe muscle weakness. Muscle weakness is usually of proximal muscles. Fatigue, malaise, and bone pain caused by osteomalacia may be present. Diagnostic tests are biochemical with demonstration of hypophosphosphatemia, hypophosphaturia, hypercalciuria, and normocalcemia (Fitzgerald, 1978). Symptoms are relieved by stopping antacids and by administration of phosphate.

Potassium deficiency. Potassium deficiency is common in the elderly. Causes are dietary and disease- and drug-related (Judge et al., 1974).

Low potassium intakes in the elderly are caused by reliance on carbohydrate foods and avoidance of food sources rich in potassium, particularly vegetables, fruits, and milk.

Major causes of potassium deficiency include prolonged vomiting or diarrhea and diabetic acidosis. In hospital patients, potassium deficiency may occur with starvation or with intravenous alimentation if care is not taken to maintain electrolyte balance.

Potassium deficiency in the elderly is often drug induced. Excessive losses of potassium into the urine occur with use of diuretics, including thiazide diuretics, furosemide, and ethacrynic acid. Abuse of laxatives and cathartics can also cause potassium depletion. Prolonged or high-dosage intake of corticosteroid hormones also causes potassium deficiency and hypokalemia (Roe, 1981). Table 7-9 summarizes causes of hypokalemia (low serum potassium).

It is important to note that patients on reduced potassium intakes may be the same patients who are taking potassium-depleting drugs or who have diseases which contribute to potassium depletion. Hypokalemia is a cause of digitalis-related arrhythmias.

Symptoms of potassium deficiency are weakness, anorexia, nausea, vomiting, listlessness, apprehension, sometimes diffuse pain, drowsiness, stupor, and irrationality. However, hypokalemia can exist without any abnormal clinical findings. When symptoms of hypokalemia are present, the most common finding is profound muscle weakness. Electrocardiographic changes are also characteristic (Nardone, McDonald, and Girard, 1978).

Diagnosis is from determination of serum or red cell potassium levels and electrocardiogram. Symptoms are relieved by administration of potassium salts. It is to be noted, however, that potassium toxicity can occur from ingestion of concentrated potassium chloride solution, which can induce small bowel ulceration. No toxicity is associated with increasing the level of potassium in the diet.

Magnesium deficiency. Magnesium deficiency is most frequently seen in elderly patients with gastrointestinal diseases, leading to malabsorption in patients with hyperparathyroidism, bone cancer, hyperaldosteronism, diabetes mellitus, and thyrotoxicosis. Alcoholics may become magnesium depleted because of high renal losses and low intake (Rude and Singer, 1981).

TABLE 7-9   Causes of Hypokalemia

1. Deficient diet
2. Gastrointestinal potassium wasting
3. Renal potassium wasting due to disease
4. Drug-induced potassium wasting
   a. diuretics including organomercurial thiazides, ferrosemides, and ethacrynic acid
   b. antibiotics including carbenicillin and penicillin
   c. liquorice and extracts of liquorice
   d. laxatives
   e. corticosteroids
   f. nephrotoxic drugs

Drugs which may induce magnesium depletion include digitalis and oral diuretics.

Diet per se is not a cause of magnesium deficiency, but intake may be reduced to zero when patients are not allowed any food and are maintained on intravenous dextrose-saline.

Clinical signs of magnesium deficiency are neuromuscular in type, including generalized seizures, vertigo, muscle weakness, tremors, depression, irritability, and psychotic behavior.

Diagnosis is by measurement of serum magnesium and by response of patients to magnesium salt supplementation.

Zinc deficiency. Zinc deficiency in the elderly is caused by the combined effects of diet, disease, alcohol, and therapeutic drugs. Diet-related factors include low intake of zinc-rich foods, and high intakes of foods that reduce zinc availability, including high phytate-containing cereals such as oatmeal and high-fiber foods such as bran cereals. When elderly surgical patients are on prolonged intravenous feeding or are maintained on chemically defined diets, zinc intake is negligible unless zinc salts have been added to the formula (Underwood, 1977; Pulmissaro, 1974; Greger and Sciscoe, 1979).

Disease states leading to zinc deficiency include all catabolic disorders associated with muscle wasting as well as hepatic and renal disease. Alcohol abuse may be associated with zinc deficiency because of low zinc intake, malabsorption, and hyperexcretion of zinc in the urine. Acute zinc deficiency in the alcoholic is likely to occur when malnourished patients who have been on drinking sprees are admitted to the hospital for surgical procedures and are given intravenous dextrose-saline only.

Drugs which cause zinc deficiency in the elderly are diuretics and digitalis glycosides, which increase renal losses of zinc.

Signs of zinc deficiency include symmetrical dermatitis, which begins on the hands and spreads over the arms and to the lower limbs before appearing on the trunk. The skin lesions are crusted and fissured. Loss of taste is characteristic of zinc deficiency. However, loss of taste in the aged may result from other causes, including the aging process itself. Wound healing is delayed after injury or surgery. Depression occurs in some zinc-deficient patients (Jacob, 1981).

Diagnosis is by measurement of zinc in hair and serum and by resolution of the signs of deficiency when zinc supplements are administered. In malnourished elderly who have depressed cellular immune function, it has been shown that administration of 50 mg of zinc daily for a period of 8 weeks may improve immune function. This was demonstrated by the observation of a change from an anergic response to a normal response with regard to delayed hypersensitivity skin tests (Chandra, 1984).

Iron deficiency. Iron deficiency is common in the elderly. A major cause is blood loss (Bowering, Sanchez, and Irwin, 1976). Blood loss is caused by hemorrhage from malignant tumors in the gastrointestinal tract, bleeding esophageal varices in portal hypertension with cirrhosis, bleeding

TABLE 7-10 Infrequent Nutritional Deficiencies in the Elderly

NUTRITIONAL DEFICIENCY	CLINICAL SIGNS
Niacin	Pellagra (light sensitivity, diarrhea, depression, mental confusion)
Essential fatty acid	Scaly dermatitis

peptic ulcer, or hemorrhage outside the GI tract. High intake of aspirin or non-steroidal, anti-inflammatory drugs for relief of arthritic pain, can induce capillary bleeding in the stomach or intestine, which, over time, can lead to severe iron deficiency anemia (Boardman and Hart, 1967; Leonards and Levy, 1973).

A low intake of iron is correlated with a low intake of food-energy (average iron intake equals 6 mg/1000 kcal). An inadequate intake of heme iron is associated with low animal protein consumption. High intake of tea impairs iron absorption, as does deficient intake of vitamin C.

Signs of iron deficiency include nonspecific signs of anemia such as pallor, weakness, and breathlessness. In the Plummer-Vinson syndrome (Patterson-Kelly syndrome), iron deficiency is associated with dysphagia (painful swallowing). The painful swallowing in this condition is related to a precancerous condition of the pharynx, which may be associated with very prolonged iron deficiency. Patients with this condition may develop pharyngeal or esophageal cancer.

Screening tests of anemia include hemoglobin and hematocrit determination. Diagnosis of iron deficiency is from complete blood counts, including red cell indices; examination of stained blood films and bone marrow; and serum iron, erythrocyte protoporphyrin, and serum ferritin values. The anemia will respond to iron supplements, e.g., ferrous sulfate, when iron absorption is normal and when the primary disease or drug cause of the anemia is removed (Sayers, 1981).

Causes and signs of less common nutritional deficiencies to be found occasionally in elderly persons are shown in Table 7-10.

QUESTIONS

Circle all correct answers (there may be more than one correct answer to each question).

1. Diets associated with the development of nutritional deficiencies in the elderly have one or more of the following characteristics:
   a. low cholesterol
   b. low fiber
   c. low in nutrient-calorie ratio
   d. high alcohol
   e. low number of foods

2. Which chronic disease is not associated with malnutrition?
   a. glaucoma
   b. end-stage renal disease
   c. chronic pancreatitis
   d. alcoholic cirrhosis
   e. cancer

3. Deficiency diseases in the elderly are usually multifactorial but one causative factor predominates. Pair the following types of malnutrition with the predominant cause.
   a. avitaminoses   i. drugs
   b. mineral deficiencies   ii. feeder neglect
   c. protein-energy malnutrition   iii. diseases

4. Protein-energy malnutrition can be acute or chronic. Which of the following are signs of acute, which of chronic malnutrition?
   a. wound edema   g. lymphocytopenia
   b. emaciation   h. impaired cellular immune
   c. apathy   function
   d. ridged nails   i. loss of subcutaneous fat
   e. delayed wound healing   j. hair brittleness
   f. crazy pavement dermatosis

5. Following are the medical terms denoting specific vitamin deficiencies. Identify the vitamin deficiency producing each of the diseases listed below:
   a. Wernicke-Korsakoff psychosis
   b. scurvy
   c. osteomalacia
   d. pellagra
   e. pernicious anemia

REFERENCES

BOARDMAN, P. L., and E. D. HART, "Side effects of indomethacin," *Ann. Rheum. Dis.*, 26 (1967), 127.

BOWERING, J., A. M. SANCHEZ, and M. I. IRWIN, "A conspectus of research on iron requirements of man," *J. Nutr.*, 106 (1976), 987–1074.

BUTTERWORTH, C. E., JR., and R. L. WEINSIER, "Malnutrition in hospitalized patients: assessment and treatment," in *Modern Nutrition in Health and Disease*, 6th Ed., eds. R. S. Goodhart and M. E. Shils, Philadelphia: Lea & Febiger, 1980, pp. 667–84.

CHANARIN, I., "Dietary deficiency of vitamin B$_{12}$ and folic acid," in *Nutritional Deficiencies in Modern Society*, eds. A. N. Howard and I. McLean Baird. London: Newman Books, Ltd., 1973, pp. 17–26.

CHANDRA, R. K., "Nutritional regulation of immune function at the extremes of life in infants and in the elderly," in *Malnutrition: Determinants and Consequences*, ed. P. White. New York: Alan R. Liss, 1984, pp. 245–51.

COFFEY, G., and C. W. M. WILSON, "Ascorbic acid deficiency and aspirin induced haematemesis," *Brit. Med. J.,* 1 (1975), 208.

DOUGLAS TALBOTT, G., "Primary alcoholic heart disease in medical consequences of alcoholism," *Ann. N. Y. Acad. Sci.,* 252 (1975), 237–42.

DRIEZEN, S., "Clinical manifestations of malnutrition," *Gerontology,* 29 (1974), 97–103.

EXTON-SMITH, A. N., "Nutritional deficiencies in the elderly," in *Nutritional Deficiencies in Modern Society,* eds. A. N. Howard and I. MacLean Baird. London: Newman Books, Ltd., 1973.

EXTON-SMITH, A. N., and P. W. OVERSTALL, *Geriatrics,* Lancaster, England: M.T.P. Press, Ltd., 1979.

FITZGERALD, F., "Clinical hypophosphatemia," *Ann. Rev. Med.,* 29 (1978), 177–89.

GARRY, P. T., "Vitamin A," *Clin. Lab Med.,* 1 (1981), 699–711.

GREGER, J. L., and B. S. SCISCOE, "Zinc nutriture of elderly participants in an urban feeding program," *Amer. J. Clin. Nutr.,* 32 (1979), 1859.

HAMPTON, D. J., B. M. CHRISLEY, and J. A. DRISKELL, "Vitamin B_6 status of the elderly in Montgomery County, VA," *Nutr. Rep. Int.,* 16 (1977), 743–50.

HODGES, R. E., et al., "Experimental scurvy in man," *Amer. J. Clin. Nutr.,* 22 (1969), 535–48.

HODKINSON, H. M., *Common Symptons of Disease in the Elderly,* 2nd Ed. Oxford: Blackwell Scientific Publications, Ltd., 1980.

HOFFBRAND, A. V., "The Megaloblastic Anaemias," in *Recent Advances in Hematology,* eds. A. Goldberg and M. C. Brain, Edinburgh: Churchill Livingston, 1971, pp. 1–76.

HURDLE, A. D. F., and P. WILLIAMS, "Folic acid deficiency in elderly patients admitted to hospital," *Brit. Med. J.,* 2 (1966), 202–5.

JACOB, R. A., "Zinc and copper," *Clin. Lab. Med.,* 1 (1981), 743–66.

JUDGE, T. G., F. I. CAIRD, R. G. S. LEASK, and C. C. MACLEOD, "Dietary intake and urinary excretion of potassium in the elderly," *Age and Aging,* 3 (1974), 167–73.

LAWSON, D. E. M., et al., "Relative contributions of diet and sunlight to vitamin D state in the elderly," *Brit. Med. J.,* 2 (1979), 303–5.

LEONARDS, J. R., and G. LEVY, "Gastrointestinal blood loss during prolonged aspirin administration," *New Eng. J. Med.,* 289 (1973), 1020.

LOTZ, M., E. ZISMAN, and F. C. BARTTER, "Evidence for a phosphorus depletion syndrome in man," *New Engl. J. Med.,* 278 (1968), 409–15.

LUMENG, L., and T-K. LI, "Vitamin B_6 metabolism in chronic alcohol abuse: pyridoxal phosphate levels in plasma, and the effects of acetaldehyde on pyridoxal phosphate synthesis and degradation in human erythrocytes," *J. Clin. Invest.,* 53 (1974), 693–704.

NARDONE, D. A., W. J. MCDONALD, and D. E. GIRARD, "Mechanisms of hypokalemia: clinical correlation," *Medicine,* 57 (1978), 435–46.

NICHOALDS, G. A., "Riboflavin," *Clin. Lab. Med.,* 1 (1981), 685–98.

PINCHOFSKY-DEVIN, G. D., and M. V. KAMINSKI, "Incidence of protein-energy malnutrition in the nursing home population." *J. Amer. Coll. Nutr.,* 6 (1987) 109–112.

PULMISSARO, D. J., "Nutrient deficiencies after intensive parenteral alimentation," *New Engl. J. Med.,* 291 (1974), 188.

RIGGS, H. E., and R. S. BOLES, "Wernicke's disease: a clinical and pathological study of 42 cases," *Q. J. Stud. Alc.,* 5 (1944), 361–370.

ROE, D. A., *Drug-Induced Nutritional Deficiencies.* Westport, CT: AVI Publishing Co., 1976, pp. 36–38.

ROE, D. A., *Alcohol and the Diet.* Westport, CT: AVI Publishing Co., 1979.

ROE, D. A.,   *Clinical Nutrition for the Health Scientist.* Boca Raton, FL: CRC Press, Inc., 1979, pp. 71–84.

ROE, D. A.,   "Interactions between drugs and nutrients," *Med. Clin. N. Amer.,* 63 (1979), 985–1007.

ROE, D. A.,   "Drug interference with the assessment of nutritional status," *Clin. Lab. Med.,* 1 (1981), 647–64.

ROE, D. A.,   "Drug-nutrient interrelationships," *Newer Knowledge Practical Gastroenterol.,* 6 (1982), 32–38.

RUDE, R. K., and F. R. SINGER,   "Magnesium deficiency and excess," *Ann. Rev. Med.,* 32 (1981), 245–59.

SAYERS, M. A.,   "Iron," *Clin. Lab. Med.,* 1 (1981), 729–41.

UNDERWOOD, E. J.,   *Trace Elements in Animal and Human Nutrition,* 4th Ed. New York: Academic Press, Inc., 1977, p. 545.

VICTOR, M., R. D. ADAMS, and G. H. COLLINS,   *The Wernicke-Korsakoff Syndrome: A Clinical and Pathological Study of 245 Patients, 82 with Post Mortem Examination.* Philadelphia: F. A. Davis Co., 1971.

VIR, S. C., and A. H. G. LOVE,   "Vitamin B_6 status of institutionalized and non-institutionalized aged," *Int. J. Vitam. Nutr. Res.,* 47 (1977), 364–72.

VIR, S. C., and A. H. G. LOVE,   "Vitamin C status of institutionalized and non-institutionalized aged," *Int. J. Vitam. Nutr. Res.,* 48 (1978), 274–80.

chapter 8

Diseases Responding to Diet Modification

Diseases responding to diet modification include both acute conditions that impair the eating ability of the elderly individual, and chronic conditions, which may cause discomfort and disability if appropriate diet restriction is not imposed. In addition, there are potentially life-threatening conditions that are preventable or modifiable by long-term modifications in the diet.

OBESITY

Obesity is common in persons 65 years or older. Common causes are failure to reduce food-energy intake in response to diminished energy expenditure in physical activity, overeating because of boredom, large meals and snacks, and institutional provision of and intake of drugs which increase appetite.

A diet higher in calories than is required for energy needs leads to energy storage and fat deposition. Excess calories (food-energy) from fat, carbohydrate, and protein food lead to obesity. Intake of calories from alcoholic beverages, consumed in addition to a diet providing sufficient food-energy to meet caloric needs, can also lead to obesity, although alcohol calories are not utilized by the body as efficiently as food calories. In the elderly, drugs which promote appetite (hyperphagic drugs) lead to obesity because of increased food intake. These drugs include tranquilizers and lithium carbonate, used in the treatment of mental disease.

The efficiency with which dietary energy sources are utilized to maintain body weight varies from person to person and is influenced by age, sex, exercise, disease, and drugs. Moderately overweight individuals require slightly excessive calories to maintain their body weight, whereas massively obese persons have to keep up a very large intake of food to keep their body weight constant but require maintenance of low-intake to semi-starvation diets over a long period of time to reduce their body weight to reach the normal range. Reduction in body weight in massively or morbidly obese persons is commonly retarded or impeded by disinclination for exercise. Exercise may also be restricted because of secondary effects of obesity leading to physical disabilities. Variables related to obesity in the elderly are shown in Table 8-1.

Obesity is the most common nutritional problem of public health concern in the United States. Although gross obesity is uncommon in the very old because persons who are morbidly obese are more likely to die

TABLE 8-1   Demographic and Medical Variables Related to Obesity in Elderly Persons

VARIABLE	RISK FACTOR
Age	Less than 75 years
Sex	Females > males
Socioeconomic status (SES)	Low SES > high SES in females
	High SES > low SES in males
Education	Less than 12th grade
History	Past obesity
	Past repeated attempts to diet
	Lack of physical exercise
Diseases	Maturity-onset diabetes
	Hypertension
	Osteoarthritis (with symptoms related to weight-bearing joints)
	Abdominal hernia
	Varicose veins ± stasis dermatitis and ulcers
	Gall bladder disease
	Gout
	Psychiatric, neurological, musculoskeletal and other diseases causing confinement to wheelchair or bed*

Drugs: Hyperphagic agents, including phenothiazine and benzodiazepine tranquilizers and lithium carbonate as well as sedatives such as barbiturates.

Drugs used in the treatment of obesity: including amphetamines, thyroid hormones.

Drugs used in the treatment of diseases complicating obesity: including oral hypoglycemic agents, diuretics, other antihypertensive drugs, and non-narcotic analgesics used to treat diabetes, hypertension, osteoarthritis, and gout, respectively.

*Obese wheelchair or bedfast elderly patients are those who maintain food energy intake in excess of their needs and do not have diseases which cause energy wastage.

earlier of complications of their obesity, obesity is still a serious disability in the elderly.

Medical disabilities are associated with the complication of obesity. Causal relationships have been identified between obesity and the development of maturity-onset diabetes, essential hypertension, and hypertensive heart disease. Obesity is also associated with the development of abdominal hernia. Gallbladder disease and gout are more common in obese people, although causal relationships are not adequately identified. Most important in the elderly, obesity is associated with increased symptoms of degenerative osteoarthritis (osteoarthrosis). Complications of varicose veins, including stasis dermatitis and stasis ulcers, are more frequent in the obese. Morbid (massive) obesity is associated with bacterial and yeast infections between folds and under the breasts. The Pickwickian syndrome, characterized by somnolence and respiratory failure, is a life-threatening complication of morbid obesity. Obese elderly patients are poor operative risks.

Massive obesity is a hindrance to independent living in the elderly. Such persons become breathless on mild exertion and therefore are unable to cope with stairs, with housework, and with the exertion required in getting to food markets. Physically disabled patients are the most difficult to care for and nurse both at home and in institutions. Problems include difficulties in lifting and bathing. Obesity also makes physical examinations difficult, and abnormal physical findings (more particularly abdominal traumas and infections) may be missed by the attending physicians (Van Itallie, 1979).

Measures for the control of obesity in the elderly have not met with outstanding success. Approaches include diet restriction (particularly prescribed restriction in food-energy intake), exercise, behavior modification, and drugs. The most effective programs utilize combinations of diet and exercise with a personalized behavior modification program. Behavior modification is difficult to achieve. In the elderly, requirements for modification of eating practices differ according to living circumstances. Independently living elderly persons must understand and interpret instructions, be motivated to lose weight, keep food records, and preferably eat away from the kitchen-refrigerator area and the TV set.

When behavior modification is proposed in a situation where the elderly person is living with a spouse, other family members, or companion, this person can be most supportive and undertake the responsibility of acting as a guide to the patient to promote compliance with the recommended change in eating activities. It is assumed that the obese, independently living elderly person would be advised to eat only when hungry, to eat in a constant place (which should be the dining area), to eat at similar times every day, and not to eat except when he or she has full awareness of the amount eaten. Snacking in front of the TV set would therefore be forbidden.

Successful modification of eating behavior in the elderly is more likely in those persons who have full preservation of mental functions and also a strong motivation to lose weight. Newly diagnosed elderly diabetics and cardiac patients with potentially life-threatening disease will often follow behavior modification programs. Compliance is facilitated by the presence of an eating partner who will follow the same regimen, by responsibility for cooking being in the hands of someone other than the patient, and by a living situation which includes a defined dining area. Specific types of behavior modification can be used in domiciliary care facilities for the elderly, in intermediate care homes, and in skilled nursing homes. When cooperation of the patient is possible, social activities at which no food is available can be provided between scheduled mealtimes. Visitors can be discouraged from bringing in snack foods. Snack carts and refrigerators in the institution to which patients have access can be stocked only with fruits or fruit juices. Obese patients can also be given nonfood token rewards for dietary compliance and weight loss (Stuart, 1974).

The use of anorectic drugs, including unsubstituted and substituted amphetamines, is never justified in the elderly, because hunger does not dictate excessive food consumption in the obese and because the side effects of these drugs, including insomnia and excitement, are serious contraindications to their use. There is also no justification for giving elderly persons thyroid hormones for the purpose of weight reduction, because these drugs may cause cardiac arrhythmias and otherwise adversely affect cardiac function. Diuretics will only produce weight loss when edema is present and should never be used in the treatment of obesity (Roe, "Interactions," 1979).

The food intake of patients receiving tranquilizers, sedative drugs, and lithium carbonate, as well as their body weight, should be monitored. If their food intakes and body weights are clearly increasing, caloric restriction is necessary. In many patients, however, weight can be controlled by decreasing intake of the prescribed hyperphagic drug.

CARDIOVASCULAR DISEASE

Common forms of cardiovascular disease in the elderly are congestive heart failure, atherosclerotic heart disease, hypertensive heart disease, and peripheral vascular disease caused by diabetes or atherosclerosis.

Salt Restriction

Indications for sodium restriction in the elderly are (1) prevention and treatment of congestive heart failure and (2) management of essential hypertension (Wintrobe et al., 1970).

High intake of sodium chloride and other sodium sources in the diet (including sodium nitrate and nitrite and monosodium glutamate), drugs such as sodium bicarbonate, and other sodium compounds mitigates against control of congestive heart failure and hypertension. Hypertension in the elderly is multifactorial and never solely attributable to high-sodium intake. Reduction in sodium intake does, however, reduce blood pressure. Weight reduction in obese, elderly patients promotes a drop in blood pressure, but the effect of weight reduction on blood pressure in these patients is enhanced by concurrent sodium restriction.

Mild, moderate, and severe hypertension should be treated by prescription of antihypertensive drugs and by sodium restriction and weight reduction if the patient is obese.

Commonly prescribed antihypertensive drugs are listed in Table 8-2, which also shows the indication for each antihypertensive drug or drug combination. Diuretics which are used in the drug management of hypertension may cause potassium, calcium, magnesium, and zinc depletion (Nickerson and Ruedy, 1975). For reference to diuretics which can cause mineral depletion, see Table 7-9.

Dietary sodium restriction has to be tailored to the needs of individual patients. Mild sodium restriction requires that the patient lower his or her intake of high-sodium foods, and high-sodium drugs should be discontinued. Moderate sodium restriction requires also that no salt be added to foods in the kitchen or at the table. Severe sodium restriction requires the use of low-sodium foods. Patients who must adhere to a very low-sodium diet should have their drinking water tested for sodium content, which should not exceed 20 mg/l (Safe Drinking Water Committee, 1980). On the assumption that the average daily intake of water is 2 l/day, the goal is to maintain an intake of sodium from drinking water and beverages made from this water at less than 50 mg/day. With a low to moderate intake of sodium from drinking water, it is possible for elderly patients with congestive heart failure to adhere to a strict low-sodium diet (500 mg/day). When

TABLE 8-2   Commonly Prescribed Antihypertensive Drugs with Indications for Their Specific Usage*

DRUG	INDICATION
Thiazide diuretics, e.g., hydrochlorothiazide triamterene resperine	Mild hypertension
Propranolol	Moderate hypertension
Methyldopa	Severe hypertension
Hydralazine	
Captopril	
Diazoxide	Hypertensive emergencies
Clonidine	
Calcium channel blockers, e.g., Diltiazem	Mild hypertension
ACE-inhibitors, e.g., Enalapril	Moderate hypertension
ACE-inhibitors + calcium channel blockers	Severe hypertension

*Combination therapy is used in moderate to severe hypertension. Use of other antihypertensive agents in the elderly imposes special hazards which must be considered. Thiazides impose the risk of elevation of blood glucose and cholesterol. Beta adrenergic blocking agents impose a risk of depression. Hydralazine imposes risk of neuropathy and of lupus nephritis (Opie, 1984).

for any reason, the sodium content of the domestic water supply is high, patients on a severely restricted sodium diet should be advised to drink from an alternate water source, e.g., bottled spring water.

Dietary guidelines to be followed by elderly patients who are on sodium-restricted diets are given in Table 8-3. Patients on moderate to strict low-sodium diets should be encouraged to avoid high-sodium foods and over-the-counter drugs. They should be also encouraged to eat nutrient-rich, low-sodium foods, including oranges and bananas.

Lipid Restriction

Epidemiological associations have been demonstrated between high intake of dietary fats, high serum cholesterol, and coronary heart disease (CHD) incidence (Glueck, 1979). The risk factors in this multifactorial disease include a high-cholesterol diet, high intake of saturated fat, hypercholesterolemia, high serum levels of low-density lipoproteins, hypertension, and cigarette smoking (Dwyer and Hetzel, 1980). A decrease in CHD mortality in European countries in the immediate post–World War II period was associated with diminished intake of total calories, fewer total calories from fat (mostly saturated fat), and a reduction in dietary cholesterol. Dietary restriction of total fat, saturated fat, and cholesterol have not, however, been shown to influence CHD mortality in older adults. This could be because atherosclerosis, causing CHD, has been so advanced that it is irreversible by the time that the lipid-restricted diet has been instituted. Regression of disease has been demonstrated in patients with atherosclerosis of the femoral arteries, but only when a lipid-restricted diet has been combined with hypolipidemic drugs (Leren, 1966; Barndt, 1977).

Elderly individuals who have adhered to a prudent diet over a lifetime or for most of their lives, with food-energy intakes in keeping with their needs and a low intake of dietary fat and cholesterol, may have a lower risk of dying from CHD, especially if they are nonsmokers. Although

---

TABLE 8-3   Dietary Guidelines for Elderly Patients on Sodium-Restricted Diets

1. Patients (or responsible household member) should be given instructions on the total amount of sodium intake permitted daily.

2. Use of Table 4 in the *Appendix* to determine the sodium content of foods is recommended to plan a mildly restricted, moderately restricted, or severely restricted low sodium diet.

3. Potassium values are also given in these tables to enable patients on diuretics to choose low sodium, high potassium foods which will offset the potassium-losing effects of the diuretics.

4. Severely restricted sodium diets must be carefully planned to ensure that the diet is nutritionally adequate, i.e., meets RDA 1980. (See *Appendix*, Table 1)

5. Patients on severely restricted, low sodium diets should be told which nondietary sodium sources to avoid, including high sodium over-the-counter and prescription drugs and water treated with domestic water softeners.

restriction of total fat, as well as of total food intake, is most advisable in the elderly to avoid obesity and the complications of obesity, sudden, stringent restriction of cholesterol in the diet of the elderly for the express purpose of reducing the risk of mortality from CHD is not presently advocated. Cessation of smoking is highly recommended. As previously mentioned, restricted cholesterol intake is also advisable in the management of diabetes in the elderly.

Alcohol Consumption

Moderate consumption of alcoholic beverages has been shown to have a protective influence against CHD mortality (Spritz, 1979). When alcohol is consumed, serum levels of high-density lipoproteins are increased, which lowers CHD risks. Although elderly people who are used to drinking a glass of wine a day should not be discouraged from doing so, both because the drink may provide a sense of well-being and because of the protective effect against CHD, we would caution against encouragement of higher alcohol intake by the elderly. Risks of heavy drinking in the elderly include not only alcoholic liver disease but also alcoholic bone disease, psychosis (Korsakoff's psychosis), alcoholic heart disease, and falls, resulting in injury (Roe, "Alcohol," 1979).

DIABETES

Diabetes in the elderly is most commonly of the maturity-onset type. Etiological factors in the development of maturity-onset diabetes include obesity and declining glucose tolerance associated with aging (Ireland, Thomson, and Williamson, 1980). Most patients with maturity-onset diabetes do not require insulin. Indeed, pancreatic insulin production is high in the early phase of the disease and may remain high throughout. In these patients, diabetes is related to peripheral insulin resistance. Maturity-onset diabetes may convert to the insulin-requiring type late in the disease because of "exhaustion" of pancreatic endocrine functions, whereby insulin is no longer produced in sufficient amounts to meet body needs. Maturity-onset diabetes may be associated with hyperlipoproteinemia.

Complications of Diabetes

Elderly insulin-requiring diabetics, however, can be juvenile diabetics who have grown older. Nutritional and dietary management of diabetes in the elderly requires full appreciation by the nutritionist that goals may be (1) weight reduction to improve glucose tolerance, (2) control of hyperlipemia in insulin-requiring diabetics, and (3) maintenance of blood sugar within an appropriate range to avert both hyperglycemia and hypoglycemia. It has been shown that persistent hyperglycemia is associated with the development of serious complications of diabetes, including renal, retinal, and degenerative vascular disease (Nutall, 1980). Complications of diabetes are shown in Table 8-4.

TABLE 8-4   Complications of Diabetes

CLASSIFICATION	COMPLICATION
Metabolic	Diabetic ketoacidosis, insulin-induced hypoglycemia
Gastrointestinal	Dysphagia, gastric distension and stasis, malabsorption
Dermatological	Cutaneous infections (e.g., pyodermas, candidiasis, dermatophytosis [fungus infections]), xanthomata, diabetic dermopathy, necrobiosis diabeticorum, gangrene
Neuropathic	Sensory loss because of mononeuropathies, polyneuropathies, or autonomic neuropathies
Cardiovascular	Peripheral vascular disease, coronary heart disease
Renal	Diabetic nephropathy
Ophthalmic	Diabetic retinopathy, cataract

Maturity-onset diabetes in the elderly can usually be controlled by diet only. Oral hypoglycemic drugs may be prescribed particularly for elderly patients for whom dietary compliance is a major problem. However, it must be understood that unwanted outcomes of oral hypoglycemic drug therapy in the elderly include increased mortality from cardiovascular disease and adverse drug reactions, usually caused by interaction of oral hypoglycemic agents with other drugs (University Group, 1970).

In the dietary treatment of maturity-onset diabetes the primary objective is weight reduction and, through weight reduction, improvement in glucose tolerance. Dietary modifications which are presently advocated to produce overall energy restriction include:

1. *Reduced intake of simple carbohydrates,* with exclusion of sucrose and sucrose-containing foods as well as exclusion of foods containing lactose, glucose, and fructose as intentional food additives. The aim is to reduce body weight to the average weight for the height and age of that individual. When reduced intake of simple sugars is inadequate to meet this goal, further advice on dietary restriction includes defined intake of fat and of animal protein foods. The desirable distribution of food-energy would have carbohydrate supplying 42 percent, protein, 20 percent, and fat, 38 percent. The approach is didactic. Complicated protein exchange lists are not discussed. Although patients are encouraged to eat vegetables with main meals, no specific instructions are given on intake of dietary fiber. Levels of complex carbohydrate are defined for each patient to meet the food-energy distribution between carbohydrates, protein, and fat.

   The simple dietary approach has been advocated in the United Kingdom as a means of meeting therapeutic goals in patients with maturity-onset

diabetes who have ingrained dietary habits and who may have difficulty in
understanding more complicated dietary instructions (Wilson et al., 1980).

2. *Reduced intake of simple carbohydrates and fats.* Guidelines to be followed are
close to the U.S. Dietary Goals, except that intake of refined sugar is minimized to avoid postprandial increases in blood glucose. Total carbohydrate
provides 55 to 60 percent of energy intake. Fat consumption is reduced or
held at not more than 30 percent of energy intake. Fats should include 10
percent saturated fat, 10 percent polyunsaturated fat, and 10 percent mono-
saturated fat. Cholesterol intake is reduced to 250 mg/day. These general
dietary guidelines are best adopted by the mildly obese diabetic. Caloric
restriction is essential. Sample menus should be provided. Foods to be included in the diet to achieve nutritional adequacy (to meet the RDA) must be
discussed with the patient. Dietary compliance is usually best achieved by use
of the exchange system.

Dietitians, clinical nutritionists, and physicians must be cautious in
advising persons of advanced age to markedly change dietary patterns
established over a lifetime, because it is unlikely that the new diet will be
followed and because if the changes are made the patients may be worried
and unhappy.

Elderly diabetics are better able to comply with prescribed diets if the
health risks of noncompliance are explained, especially risks of heart disease and other vascular complications (Roberts, Taft, and Wahlqvist, 1985).
Also, the diet instructions should be simple and the diet should contain
familiar foods. Dietitians working in nursing homes and in the community
are advised to base diet recommendations on the dietary guidelines of the
American Diabetes Association. Diets that only limit intake of sugars ("no
concentrated sweets") are not acceptable for the management of elderly
diabetics.

Improved glucose tolerance and better long-term control of the diabetic state may also be achieved by changing the carbohydrate content of
the diet, with or without energy restriction, as follows:

1. *A high-carbohydrate, high-fiber diet may be prescribed.* Complex carbohydrates
from commercially available and acceptable cereal foods and tuberous vegetables should account for about 60 percent of the total daily energy requirements. Simple sugars are restricted.

It has been suggested that the higher carbohydrate content of the diet
decreases fasting blood glucose concentrations and that diets high in fiber
reduce postprandial blood glucose concentrations. Follow-up of patients
treated by this diet has demonstrated a drop in glycosylated hemoglobin,
which indicates a long-term improvement in diabetes control (Anderson and
Ward, 1978). Whereas this diet has been successfully used in highly motivated
elderly patients with maturity-onset diabetes, doubt has been cast on any
special role for the fiber content of this diet which is derived both from cereal
grains and from vegetable sources. An alternate explanation of the good
effects of the high-carbohydrate, high-fiber diet is that benefits accrue from
the restriction in sugar intake. This is a modified fat diet in that the ratio of
polyunsaturated fatty acid to saturated fatty acid is 1:1.

The high-carbohydrate, high-fiber, modified-fat diet has also been advocated for use in the management of insulin-requiring diabetics (Simpson et

al., 1979). In these patients, diabetic control requires completion of pre-scribed meals. A problem, however, which is not inconsiderable in elderly patients, is that with a change from a low-carbohydrate to a high-car-bohydrate, high-fiber diet, the bulkier characteristics of the food make total consumption difficult. It is our experience that dietary adherence in those of advanced age is poor and that any advantage to be gained from the high-carbohydrate, high-fiber diet through small reduction in insulin require-ments may be outweighed by the discomfort imposed on the patient.

2. *Guar gum* has been used to treat patients with maturity-onset diabetes and patients with minimal insulin requirement (Jenkins, Wolevar, and Nineham, 1978). Certain unabsorbable plant polysaccharides such as guar gum, a galac-tomannan from the cluster bean, reduces postprandial hyperglycemia. The gum is used by the food industry as a thickener and emulsion stabilizer. It has been suggested that the guar gum, by increasing the viscosity of gastrointesti-nal contents, slows gastric emptying and thereby slows absorption of dietary sugar. No malabsorption of carbohydrate has been reported, but stool losses of fat are increased. Nutritionists should use caution concerning use of guar gum in any form for the treatment of elderly diabetics, in whom the risk of malabsorption of micronutrients may be greater than the advantages to be gained by this unusual pharmacological approach to the treatment of dia-betes.

It should be emphasized that the dietary management of elderly diabetics has to be tailored to the needs, the understanding, and the situation of the individual. Management requires that:

1. All elderly diabetics should be given a calorically restricted diet.
2. Elderly diabetics, irrespective of body weight, should be advised to reduce intake of fat and cholesterol.
3. Elderly diabetics should be told that there is no need to restrict intake of carbohydrate foods, provided these consist of whole grain cereals (not sweet-ened breakfast cereals) and vegetables.
4. All elderly diabetics should be given diets that will meet their nutrient re-quirements after food selection.
5. Elderly diabetics receiving insulin or long-acting oral antidiabetic agents (e.g., chlorpropamide) should be instructed to eat three small meals per day, and also a bedtime snack, to avoid nocturnal hypoglycemia and hyperglycemia.

Diabetic exchange lists should only be used in diet prescription when it is clear that the senior has an understanding of the exchange concept. Com-parison of diet essentials for diabetics not requiring insulin and for insulin-requiring diabetics is given in Tables 8-5 and 8-6. For further information on the dietary management of elderly diabetics, readers are advised to

TABLE 8-5   Guidelines on Diets for Elderly Diabetic Patients Not Requiring Insulin

Caloric restriction (use diabetic exchange list)
Total fat restriction
Cholesterol restriction
Dietary fiber increase

TABLE 8-6   Guidelines on Diets for Insulin-Requiring Elderly Diabetics

Caloric restriction (use diabetic exchange list)
Increased frequency of feeding
Consistent intake of carbohydrate, fat, and protein
Meals at the same time every day
Use food or sugar to prevent early signs of hypoglycemia
Restrict total fat and cholesterol intake

consult a handbook on diabetes (Ireland, Thomson, and Williamson, 1980) and recent position papers on diabetes management.

ORAL DISEASES

In the elderly, oral and pharyngeal diseases limit the type and consistency of food that can be consumed. Pathological conditions of the mouth and pharynx that impose the risk of diet inadequacy can be classified into the following groups (Greenberg, 1984):

1. Conditions causing extreme dryness of the buccal mucosa: These include Sjogren's disease and the late effects of radiation of the head and neck
2. Conditions causing stomatitis and glossitis: These include the following subgroups:
    a. Traumatic lesions, including those induced by ill-fitting dentures and oral prostheses
    b. Infections including candidiasis
    c. Acute radiation stomatitis induced by X-ray therapy for cancer of the head or neck
    d. Oral manifestations of dermatoses, including erosive lichen planus, pemphigus vulgaris, and cicatricial pemphigoid
    e. Oral manifestations of nutritional deficiencies, including pellagra, ariboflavinosis, scurvy, and zinc deficiency
    f. Drug-induced stomatitis, including mucositis occurring as a manifestation of the acute toxicity of cancer chemotherapeutic agents, including methotrexate
    g. Uremic stomatitis
3. Conditions causing ulceration: These include cancer of the oral cavity and pharynx
4. Conditions causing dental loss: These include periodontal disease and coronal dental caries with secondary infection (Wycoff and Epstein, 1984)
5. Conditions causing swallowing difficulties: These include Plummer-Vinson syndrome, amyotrophic lateral sclerosis, Alzheimer's disease, the late effects of stroke, systemic sclerosis, and pharyngectomy

The eating disabilities that develop in elderly with oral and/or pharyngeal problems include difficulty in chewing meats and raw vegetables, pain on chewing or swallowing, choking episodes, and regurgitation.

Oral diseases of the elderly are seen and treated by geriatric dentists, dermatologists, oncologists, and surgeons. It is however, the responsibility of nutritionists to advise health care professionals with regard to the appropriate food modifications and the nutritional support of elderly with these conditions.

Food modification that is suitable for elderly with chewing difficulties includes the use of homemade purees, baby foods, or commercially produced freeze dried purees, specifically designed and packaged to meet the needs of frail elderly men and women who experience difficulty with package opening.

For those who have extensive stomatitis, the use of formula foods is desirable, with careful prescription so that the brand selected and the volume given meet the caloric and nutrient needs of the patient (Bernard and Rombeau, 1986). However, for demented patients who push food out of their mouths, as well as for those who have chewing difficulties, the puree consistency needed for optimal intake must also be considered (Suski and Nielsen, 1989).

CONSTIPATION

In the elderly, constipation is complex in etiology (Bouchier, 1977). Contributing causes are:

1. *Low-fiber diet.* The intestinal transit time is prolonged in persons habitually consuming a diet low in dietary fiber, which contributes to fecal bulk. When low-fiber diets are eaten, stool weight and volume are reduced. The water content of the stool is diminished, and the frequency of defecation is usually reduced. Diet-related constipation can occur when dietary fiber consists of lignin (e.g., in tomato pips or fruit seeds), which does not contribute significantly to stool bulk.

2. *Irregular bowel habits.* The urge to defecate is promoted by physiological stimuli which cause mass movement of the large intestine. The gastrocolic reflex which occurs in response to food or fluid intake initiates mass movement of colon contents. When the urge to defecate is neglected or ignored, or when food or warm drinks are not taken regularly as a stimulus to the gastrocolic reflex, simple constipation results. Neglect of the urge to defecate is most likely when defecation induces pain, e.g., with hemorrhoids or anal fissure, or when the patient is confused.

3. *Debility.* Weakness and poor abdominal musculature make defecation difficult in the elderly. It is particularly difficult and may be painful for an elderly debilitated person to expel small, hard stools which occur when a low-fiber diet is consumed.

4. *Constipating drugs.* Narcotic analgesics, notably opioids such as morphine, are constipating. These drugs increase tone in the colon, and churning activity is induced in the large intestine, which together cause resistance to liminal transit. Opioids are administered to elderly patients for relief of severe pain such as may occur in cancer.

5. *Obstruction.* Change in a bowel habit in the elderly with sudden or relatively rapid development of constipation should cause suspicion that there is an

obstruction to the passage of bowel contents. Obstructive constipation in the elderly is most commonly caused by cancer of the colon or rectum.

Treatment of constipation in the elderly must be preceded by identification of the cause or causes. The physician must exclude obstruction as the cause of constipation before any dietary or drug measures are adopted. Obstructive constipation usually requires surgical intervention. Constipation occurring in patients who are receiving opioids can seldom be ameliorated by dietary management alone. Laxatives are usually also required. Debility in the elderly may be relieved by treatment of underlying disease, by nutritional rehabilitation, and by mild exercise according to the causal mechanism. When total food intake is increased and dietary quality is improved, the effect may be twofold in that stool size is increased and abdominal muscles can be stronger so that it is easier for the person to defecate.

Regularity of bowel movements in the elderly may be achieved when a hot breakfast or a hot morning beverage is supplied at the same time each morning and a visit to the toilet is encouraged soon thereafter.

Increase in dietary fiber should be achieved by inclusion of whole grain cereal breads or muffins and by giving a bowl of bran-containing breakfast cereal each morning. Other measures for increasing intake of dietary fiber include increasing the frequency of intake of vegetables, which may be cooked or raw (Mendeloff, 1976). Usually the former are preferred by the elderly.

It should be stressed that sudden increases in the fiber content of the diet of elderly people are not easily tolerated. Patients may complain of gas pain, abdominal bloating, and loose bowel movements. Further, if the "new" high-fiber diet is bulky, the elderly individual may not be able to consume that amount of food.

A moderately high-fiber diet suitable for management of constipation of dietary origin in the elderly is given in Table 2 in the Appendix.

DIVERTICULAR DISEASE

Diverticulosis and diverticulitis are disorders of later life (Bouchier, 1977). Diverticulosis denotes a condition in which pouches arise in the wall of the colon. Diverticulitis is a complication of diverticulosis in which a pouch becomes inflamed. Diverticulitis requires active treatment with hospitalization. When a diverticulum is inflamed, hemorrhage and/or perforation of the diverticulum may ensue. Elderly patients with diverticulosis should be given moderately high-fiber diets from which lignin sources are excluded. With this diet, conditions causing symptomatic diverticular disease are avoided, including constipation, diarrhea, and irregular defecation.

GLUTEN-SENSITIVE ENTEROPATHY

Gluten-sensitive enteropathy (celiac-sprue syndrome) may present for the first time in the elderly (Hovdenak, 1980). Younger "celiacs" who developed the disease in middle-life may now have lived on to become elderly, since the life-saving, gluten-free diet has been in use for more than 30 years.

Among persons who develop gluten-sensitive enteropathy in later years, most are women. Typical symptoms are loss of weight, diarrhea, steatorrhea, and evidence of multiple nutritional deficiencies. However, often the presenting clinical features are atypical. Symptoms and signs may include gurgling abdominal noises, flatulence, abdominal pain, diarrhea or constipation, aphthous stomatitis, anemia, skeletal pain (because of osteomalacia and/or osteoporosis), and confusional psychosis. Patients may present with intensely pruritic (itching), blistering, symmetrical skin lesions which, on biopsy, are shown to be dermatitis herpetiforms. Low whole-blood folacin and low fasting serum calcium levels are common.

Patients show remarkable improvement with a relief of symptoms when they are kept on a gluten-free diet. Elderly patients must be carefully instructed on cereal foods to be avoided. No foods or beverages containing wheat, oats, or rye should be taken, and patients should be told particularly to avoid high-gluten health breads and gluten-enriched pasta. During the period when disease is active, lactose intolerance may be severe and patients may be unable to take milk or other lactose-containing foods without developing fermentative diarrhea. As recovery proceeds with the patient in the gluten-free diet, tolerance for lactose gradually returns to normal.

Nutritional rehabilitation must be undertaken in accordance with findings of nutritional deficiencies. Most commonly, patients are folacin and vitamin D deficient.

QUESTIONS

Circle all correct answers (there may be more than one correct answer to each question).

1. Causes of constipation in the elderly are:
   a. debility
   b. opioids (narcotic analgesics)
   c. cheese
   d. low-fiber diet
   e. rectal cancer

2. In the dietary management of maturity-onset diabetes, which of the following guidelines should be followed?
   a. restriction of food-energy intake
   b. restriction of total carbohydrate to less than 40 percent food-energy
   c. restriction of soluble carbohydrate
   d. maintenance of dietary carbohydrate as 50 to 60 percent of food-energy
   e. restriction of dietary fat and cholesterol

3. Complications of obesity are:
   a. hypertension
   b. cirrhosis
   c. intertrigo
   d. Pickwickian syndrome
   e. diabetes

4. Justification of sodium restriction of the elderly is based on which of the following statements?
   a. High sodium intake precipitates congestive heart failure.
   b. Sodium restrictions in the elderly can prevent development of hypertension.
   c. Sodium restriction is important in the management of hypertension.
   d. Sodium restriction may induce weight reduction when edema is present.
   e. Sodium restriction will induce weight reduction when edema is absent.

5. Whole wheat bread should be avoided in patients with which of the following health problem(s)?
   a. diabetes
   b. diverticulosis
   c. gluten-sensitive enteropathy
   d. coronary heart disease
   e. obesity

REFERENCES

ANDERSON, J. W., and K. WARD, "Long term effects of high carbohydrate, high fiber diets on glucose and lipid metabolism; a preliminary report on patients with diabetes," *Diabetes Care*, 1 (1978), 77–82.

BARNDT, R. JR., D. H. BLANKENHORN, D. W. CRAWFORD, and S. H. BROOKS, "Regression and progression of early femoral atherosclerosis in treated hyperlipoproteinemia patients," *Ann. Intern. Med.*, 86 (1977), 139.

BERNARD, M. A., and J. L. ROMBEAU, "Nutritional support for the elderly patient," in *Nutrition, Aging, and Health*, ed. E. A. Young, ed. New York: Alan R. Liss, 1986, pp. 229–58.

BOUCHIER, I. A. D., *Gastroenterology*, 2nd Ed. London: Bailliere Tindall, 1977, pp. 192–93.

DWYER, T., and B. S. HETZEL, "A comparsion of trends of coronary heart disease mortality in Australia, USA and England and Wales with reference to three major risk factors—hypertension, cigarette smoking, and diet," *Int. J. Epidemiol.*, 9 (1980), 65–71.

GLUECK, C. J., "Dietary fat and atherosclerosis," *Amer. J. Clin. Nutr.*, 32 (1979), 2703–11.

GREENBERG, M. S., "Ulcerative, vesicular and bullous lesions," in *Drugs for the Heart*, 2nd Ed. Philadelphia: W. B. Saunders Co., 1984, pp. 163–208.

Hovdenak, N.,   "Prevalence and clinical picture of adult gluten induced enteropathy in a Norwegian population," *Scand. J. Gastroenterol.*, 15 (1980), 401–4.

Ireland, J. T., W. S. T. Thomson, and J. Williamson, *Diabetes Today: A Handbook for the Clinical Team.* Aylesbury, England: HM & M Publishers, 1980.

Jenkins, D. J. A., T. M. S. Wolever, and R. Nineham,   "Guar crispbread in the diabetic diet," *Brit. Med. J.*, 2 (1978), 1744–46.

Leren, P.,   "The effect of plasma cholesterol lowering diet in male survivors of myocardial infarction: a controlled trial," *Acta Med. Scand.*: Suppl. 5 (1966).

Mendeloff, A. I.,   "Dietary fiber," in *Present Knowledge in Nutrition*, 4th Ed., ed. D. M. Hegsted, New York: Nutrition Foundation, Inc., 1976.

Nickerson, M., and O. Ruedy,   "Antihypertensive agents and the drug therapy of hypertension," in *The Pharmacological Basis of Therapeutics*, 5th Ed., eds. L. S. Goodman and A. Gilman. New York: Macmillan, Inc., 1975, pp. 705–14.

Nuttall, F. Q.,   "Dietary recommendations for individuals with diabetics mellitus: summary of report from the Food and Nutrition Committee of the American Diabetes Association," *Amer. J. Clin. Nutr.*, 33 (1980), 1311–12.

Opie, L. H.   *Drugs for the Heart*, 2nd Ed. Philadelphia: W. B. Saunders Co., 1984, pp. 193–216.

Roberts, C., P. Taft, and M. Wahlqvist,   "Diet in Diabetes," in *Diabetes Mellitus: A Guide to Treatment*, ed. P. Taft. Sydney: ADIS Health Sciences Press, 1985, pp. 54–76.

Roe, D. A.,   *Alcohol and the Diet.* Westport, CT: AVI Publishing Co., 1979.

Roe, D. A.,   "Interactions between drugs and nutrients," *Med. Clin. N. Amer.*, 63 (1979), 985–1007.

Safe Drinking Water Committee,   *The Contribution of Drinking Water to Mineral Nutrition in Humans*, Vol. 3. Washington, DC: National Academy of Sciences, 1980, pp. 283–293.

Simpson, R. W., J. I. Mann, and J. Eaton,   "High carbohydrate diets and insulin-dependent diabetics," *Brit. Med. J.*, 2 (1979), 523–25.

Simpson, R. W., J. I. Mann, J. Eaton, R. A. Moore, R. Carter, and T. D. R. Hockaday,   "Improved glucose control in maturity onset diabetes treated with high carbohydrate-modified fat diet," *Brit. Med. J.*, 1 (1979), 1753–56.

Spritz, N.,   "Appraisal of alcohol consumption as a causative factor in liver disease and atherosclerosis," *Amer. J. Clin. Nutr.*, 32 (1979), 2654–58.

Stuart, R. B.,   "Behavioral control of overeating," in *Obesity in Perspective*, ed. G. A. Bray, DHEW Publ. No. (NIH) 75-708, 1974, pp. 367–85.

Suski, N. S., and C. C. Nielsen,   "Factors affecting food intake of women with Alzheimer's type dementia in long-term care," *J. Amer. Dietet. Assoc.*, 89 (1989), 1770–71.

The University Group Diabetes Program,   "A study of hypoglycemia agents on vascular complications in patients with adult-onset diabetes, II." *Diabetes*, 19, Suppl. 2 (1970), 789–830.

Van Itallie, T. B.,   "Obesity: adverse effects on health and longevity," *Amer. J. Clin. Nutr.*, 32 (1979), 2723–33.

Wilson, E. A., D. R. Hadden, J. D. Merrett, D. A. D. Montgomery, and J. A. Weaver,   "Dietary management of maturity-onset diabetes," *Brit. Med. J.*, 1 (1980), 1367–69.

Wintrobe, M. M., G. W. Thorn, R. D. Adams, I. L. Bennett, E. Braunwald, K. J. Isselbacher, and R. G. Petersdorf, eds.   *Harrison's Principles of Internal Medicine.* New York: McGraw-Hill Book Co., 1970, p. 2016.

Wycoff, S. J., and S. Epstein,   "Geriatric dentistry," in *Burket's Oral Medicine*, 8th Ed. eds. M. A. Lynch, V. J. Brightman, and M. S. Greenberg. Philadelphia: J. B. Lippincott Co., 1984, pp. 561–75.

chapter 9

Drugs
and Nutrition
in the Elderly

DRUG USE AND ABUSE

Although people 65 years and over make up only about 11 percent of the population in the United States, they consume 25 percent of the country's prescription drugs (U.S. Task Force on Prescription Drugs, 1968). Chronic diseases, for which single- or multiple-drug therapies are commonly prescribed, are more common in the elderly. Management by physicians of hypertension, ischemic heart disease, congestive heart failure, peripheral vascular disease, chronic bronchitis and emphysema, Parkinson's disease, dementias and cerebrovascular disease, diabetes, arthritis,and cancer is by prescription of drugs which confer the risk of nutritional or diet-related side effects. In any one patient, one or more drugs may be prescribed which can affect nutritional status.

The elderly also take prescription and nonprescription drugs for relief of health complaints such as weakness, headache, nervousness, forgetfulness, vertigo (dizziness), flatulence, constipation and diarrhea, and pain. They are also easily persuaded to take nutrient supplements and tonics to improve appetite, to gain in strength and well-being, and to prevent acute infections.

Excessive use or misuse of medications is common (Hulka et al., 1975; Guttman, 1977; Raffoul, Copper, and Love, 1981). Reasons for this include:

1. Prescriptions from several physicians
2. Belief that a low drug dose is ineffective in relieving symptoms and a higher dose will produce the desired effect
3. Hyochondriasis
4. Health-related obsessions (e.g., preoccupation with bowel function leading to laxative abuse)
5. Inadequate review of patient care plans
6. Failure to relate drugs in use to actual health problems present
7. Inappropriate use of drugs, including sedatives and tranquilizers, to make the patient "more manageable"
8. Forgetfulness or mismanagement, leading to increased frequency of drug intake or overdose
9. Difficulty in following medication regimens
10. Use of drugs prescribed for others (spouse, other household member, or friend)
11. Drug dose unrelated to current body weight
12. Advice from the mass media

DRUG USE AND THE QUALITY OF LIFE

Careful review has been made in recent years on the question of whether or not it is justifiable to give long-term drug therapies to elderly if the selected drug or drug combination imposes a high risk of inducing unpleasant side effects. This subject has aroused heated debate in the past, particularly when the condition for which the drug is prescribed is symptom free at the time of drug initiation. However, the knowledge that the risks of stroke and the cardiac complications of hypertension can be markedly reduced in the elderly has justified the use of antihypertensive drugs as well as diet therapy in symptom-free elderly whose blood pressure is significantly elevated. In the case of hypertension, the long-term advantages of antihypertensive drugs, relative to the prevention of stroke-related disabilities, has outweighed the short-term problems resulting from drug side effects. Also, it is now possible to select antihypertensive medications, including calcium channel blocking agents, that are well tolerated by the elderly.

Similarly it is quite unjustifiable for physicians to take a *laissez faire* approach to the drug management of other common chronic diseases of the elderly, such as diabetes, since prevention of the drug side effects may require supervision. Indeed, the advantages to be gained from maintaining long-term glycemic control, and thus preventing the devastating complications of diabetes, including blindness, signify a large gain in terms of an improved quality of life for the elderly person (Bullpitt and Fletcher, 1990).

AGING AND DRUG DISPOSITION
Drug Absorption

With aging, physiological changes occur in the GI tract which could affect drug absorption. The pH of the stomach is increased, reflecting a decrease in production of hydrochloric acid in the stomach. Splanchnic (GI) blood flow is decreased. Intestinal motility is decreased. There is a decrease in the number of cells lining the intestine which are capable of absorption of nutrients and drugs. Although there are these several aging changes in the structure and function of the GI tract which could diminish the rate or quantity of drug absorbed, no significant reduction in drug absorption attributable to aging has been identified. It is presumed that the very large capacity of the GI tract for absorption of small molecular weight compounds, such as drugs, outweighs aging effects which could reduce absorption (Vestal, 1980).

Drug Distribution

Several changes in body composition occur with aging which can affect the distribution of drugs (Novak, 1972). There is a reduction in lean body mass and a reduction in body water. Body fat is increased, and plasma albumin concentrations are decreased, even in the absence of protein malnutrition. Because of these physiological changes, the volume of distribution of drugs is reduced. Fat-soluble drugs may be retained to a greater extent because of deposition in body fat stores. Protein binding of drugs (binding to plasma albumin) is decreased. With less plasma protein binding of drugs, more free drug is available to diffuse to receptor sites, which can potentiate drug action.

Drug Metabolism

Rates of drug metabolism have been shown to be slower in the old than in the young (O'Malley, et al., 1971). Change in the rate of drug metabolism may be related to aging, to change in nutritional status or diet which may occur in the elderly, and to a decline in liver function caused by alcohol consumption or hepatic diseases. Evaluation of observed changes in the rate of metabolism in the elderly are further complicated by the interactive effects of smoking. In younger people, smoking increases the rate of drug metabolism, whereas in the elderly the effect of smoking on drug metabolism is diminished (Vestal et al., 1979).

Drug Elimination

Major routes of drug elimination are via the biliary system and via the renal tract into the urine. Decreased liver size and decreased hepatic blood flow occur with aging and could contribute to less efficient hepatobiliary excretion of drugs. However, no definitive evidence has been obtained that slowed elimination of drugs by the elderly results from these causes.

Glomerular filtration rate declines with age. Slowed elimination of certain drugs in the elderly may be caused by age-related decline in renal function, even in the absence of renal disease. The renal excretion of digitalis glycosides (e.g., Digoxin), lithium carbonate, and aminoglycoside antibiotics is reduced with decreased renal function.

Drug Disposition and Geriatric Disease

In many geriatric patients, disposition of drugs is impaired by the presence of chronic disease, including malabsorption syndromes, hepatic dysfunction associated with alcoholic cirrhosis, congestive heart failure, and chronic renal disease. Multiple-organ dysfunctions may occur in one patient. Adverse outcomes include less efficient drug absorption, metabolism, and elimination of drugs (Ouslander, 1981).

Drug Disposition in Malnourished Patients

Malnutrition also affects the transport, metabolism, and elimination of drugs (Hurwitz, 1969). Protein malnutrition leads to reduction in plasma albumin so that the protein binding of drugs is reduced. As previously stated, reduction in protein binding allows more of a drug to diffuse out of the vascular compartment (through capillaries) and across interstitial spaces and tissues to reach the drug receptor sites. Protein malnutrition also impairs drug metabolism in the liver. Other nutritional deficiency states which may impair drug metabolism include ascorbic acid, niacin, and riboflavin deficiency. Starvation or semistarvation also slows drug metabolism. Renal excretion of drugs is diminished by the presence of edema which may be associated with both protein malnutrition and congestive heart failure.

DEFINITION OF ADVERSE DRUG REACTIONS

Adverse drug reactions include (1) lack of desired therapeutic effects and (2) toxic side effects (Caranasos, Stewart, and Cluff, 1974). The elderly are at high risk for the development of adverse drug reactions caused by:

1. The chronicity of their disease processes and the multiplicity of their diseases, which increase the chances that they will take drugs over a long period of time and will take a number of drugs
2. Drug misuse because of:
   a. Sensory impairment (drug instructions are not heard or read)
   b. Lack of instruction (The physician, nurse, or pharmacist does not explain how the drug should be taken or the label is unclear.)
   c. Mental confusion
   d. Misplaced lay advice
   e. Personal decision

     f. Economic problem (It is cheaper to take old medications than to see a new physician.)
3. Delayed drug metabolism and elimination
4. Hazards of over-the-counter drugs
5. Taking medication intended for others
6. Alcohol intake while on drugs
7. Drug-food incompatibilities
8. Drug-nutrient interactions
9. Use of folk medicines
10. Circumstances which impose risks of adverse drug reactions not recognized by the physician

Adverse Drug Reactions in the Elderly

Adverse drug reactions in the elderly are most commonly caused by (1) impaired renal function and (2) conditioning factors which may be related to aging, to disease complications, or to change in nutritional status.

It has been found that whenever the glomerular filtration rate is reduced, whether this is caused by congestive heart failure or dehydration, digoxin clearance is reduced and the risk of digoxin toxicity is increased. The age-related risk of hypothermia increases the risk of severe hypothermia which may follow administration of phenothiazine tranquilizers. Age-related change in the hepatic synthesis of vitamin K–dependent clotting factors increases the risk of hemorrhage when the anticoagulant warfarin is administered. Postural hypotension is more likely to occur in elderly patients who are given the antihypertensive agent guanethidine because of an age-related impairment in baroreceptor function. Chronic renal disease increases the risk of impaired glomerular filtration from drugs such as cimetidine and procainamide and from those that are mainly eliminated by renal tubular secretion, such as aminoglycoside antibiotics. Further, because frail elderly men and women commonly reduce their intakes of potassium, they are more at risk from intake of drugs such as diuretics, which cause hypokalemia (Caird, 1985).

EFFECT OF DIET ON THERAPEUTIC EFFICACY

Food components affect drug absorption and bioavailability (Toothaker and Welling, 1980). Absorption of drugs may be increased or decreased by physiological changes which occur in the GI tract in the fed versus the fasting state. Nutrients in foods can promote drug absorption. Non-nutrient components of the diet, including specific forms of dietary fiber, may adsorb drugs, producing a transient or net reduction in drug absorption. Delayed absorption of common drugs can occur when the drug is taken at the same time as food or within 1 to 2 hours after food has been eaten. When drug absorption is delayed by food, this does not mean that less drug is totally absorbed but rather that the time for a drug to reach peak blood levels after a single dose is lengthened. Delaying effects of food on drug absorption may be caused by specific food components, e.g., pectin, or by physiological changes in the tract and its blood supply associated with food intake. Splanchnic blood flow increases after food is consumed. Stomach emptying time influences the rate of drug absorption. In the fasting state or when there is little food in the stomach, the drug leaves the stomach rapidly so that it will very soon reach the small intestine, where drugs are optimally absorbed. However, if the drug formulation is such that disintegration of drug particles, as well as dissolution of the drugs, in stomach fluid must precede absorption, then rapid stomach emptying mitigates against efficient drug absorption. Drug tablets, particularly those containing certain fillers, require more prolonged residence in the stomach for their disintegration and dissolution.

Drugs that can be absorbed from the stomach, which are either lipid soluble or non-ionized at the acid pH of the gastric environment, are more slowly absorbed when the stomach is full. Slower diffusion of the drug increases the time it takes for the drug to reach the mucosal lining of the stomach, where absorption takes place.

Slower gastric emptying times may, however, promote absorption of drugs. Reasons are either that delayed stomach emptying will permit more drug to be dissolved in the stomach before it passes into the small intestine to be absorbed or that more drug may be absorbed when it reaches the absorption site of the small intestine slowly (Welling, 1977). Slow stomach emptying occurs particularly after heavy meals or meals containing fat and, to a lesser extent, with intake of foods which are mainly sources of carbohydrate. It is now known that different dietary components may leave the stomach at different rates. Retention of dietary fiber sources in the stomach is longer than retention of fluid or semifluid components. The rate at which a drug leaves the stomach depends on whether it is adsorbed to dietary fiber or suspended or dissolved in the fluid contents of the stomach. Dietary and GI physiological factors influence the speed and efficiency of absorption of drugs which are formulated for sustained release.

The volume of beverage taken with a drug and the characteristics of the beverage also influence drug absorption. Drugs are more efficiently absorbed when they are in dilute solution and hence when the drug is taken with water or other liquids which have no specific pharmacological function (Borowitz et al., 1971).

When drugs are taken with food or beverages containing caffeine or theobromine, such as coffee, tea, chocolate, and cola drinks, metabolism of the related drug, theophylline, may be slowed. Abstention from methylxanthines promotes clearance of theophylline and related drugs (Monks, Caldwell, and Smith, 1979).

Within drug groups (groups of drugs which are used for similar therapeutic purposes), effects of food on drug absorption differ. For example, food affects the absorption of different non-narcotic anti-inflammatory drugs differently. The absorption of indomethacin is reduced by food, but the absorption of diftalone is enhanced by food and the absorption of prednisone is unaffected by food (Welling and Tse, 1983).

The effects of food or formula on drug absorption may vary with the composition of the diet or the formulation of the drug. Plasma levels of the retinoid, etretinate, which is used for the treatment of severe psoriasis, are higher when the drug is given with a high-fat meal than when given with a carbohydrate meal or under fasting conditions. Plasma levels of the active metabolite of the drug are not increased by the high-fat meal in young subjects after single doses, but it has been suggested that with chronic use of the drug higher metabolite concentrations may occur (Colburn et al., 1985).

A high-fat breakfast has also been shown to increase the rate and extent of absorption of a theophylline preparation which was formulated for once-a-day administration with the intent that absorption would be very slow (Karim et al., "Meal Composition," 1985). On the other hand, food-induced changes in the absorption of two different controlled-release formulations of theophylline have been shown to differ such that food enhanced the absorption of one product and reduced the absorption of the other (Karim et al., "Tablets," 1985).

Tables 9-1 and 9-2 show the effects of food on drug absorption. Table 9-3 shows dietary factors which influence drug metabolism.

TABLE 9-1   Drugs Whose Absorption May Be Reduced or Delayed by Food

DRUG	DOSAGE FORM	FOOD	EFFECT
ASA	Tablets	Carbohydrate, fat, and protein meals	Reduced absorption
	Enteric coated tablets	Standard breakfast	Reduced absorption
Cefaclor	Capsules	Standard breakfast	Delayed absorption
Cephalexin	Capsules	Standard hospital meal?	Delayed absorption
	Suspension	Standard hospital meal?	Delayed absorption
	Suspension	Milk, liquid formula	Reduced absorption
Cimetidine	—	Standard breakfast	Delayed absorption
Digoxin	Tablets	Standard breakfast	Delayed absorption
Erythromycin	Film-coated tablets	Carbohydrate, fat, and protein meals	Reduced absorption
	Film-coated tablets	Standard breakfast	Reduced absorption
Ibuprofen	Capsules	Standard breakfast	Delayed absorption
Isoniazid	Tablets	Standard breakfast	Reduced absorption
Nafcillin	Tablets	Breakfast?	Reduced absorption
Penicillin V	Suspension	Milk, liquid formula	Reduced absorption
Penicillin G	Suspension	Milk, liquid formula	Reduced absorption
Phenytoin	Capsules	Formula	Reduced absorption
Sotalol	Tablets	Breakfast, milk	Reduced absorption
Tetracycline	Capsules	Milk	Reduced absorption

Adapted from R. D. Toothaker and P. G. Welling, "The effect of food on drug bioavailability," *Ann. Rev. Pharmacol. Toxicol.*, 20 (1980), 173–99, by Annual Reviews, Inc.

TABLE 9-2   Drugs Whose Absorption May Be Promoted by Food

DRUG	DOSAGE FORM	FOOD
Diazepam	Tablets	Standard breakfast
Dicoumarol	Tablets	Standard breakfast
Diftalone	Capsules	"Standard Italian lunch"
Erythromycin ethylsuccinate	Suspension	Milk, children's formula
Erythromycin estolate[a]	Capsules	Standard breakfast
Erythromycin stearate[a]	Film-coated tablets	Standard breakfast?
Hydralazine	Tablets	Standard breakfast
Hydrochlorothiazide	Tablets	Standard breakfast
Lithium citrate	Tablets	Standard breakfast
Metoprolol	—	Standard breakfast
Nitrofurantoin	Tablets	Standard low-lipid meal
Propranolol	—	Standard breakfast
Riboflavin	Tablets	Standard breakfast or carbonated beverage

[a]Single and repeated dose study.

Adapted from R. D. Toothaker and P. G. Welling, "The effect of food on drug bioavailability," *Ann. Res. Pharmacol. Toxicol.,* 20 (1980), 173–99, by Annual Reviews, Inc.

TABLE 9-3   Dietary Factors Which Influence Drug Metabolism

Protein level

Alcohol content

Charcoal broiling

Vegetables eaten
(cabbage, brussels sprouts)

Coffee, tea, cocoa
(methylxanthine-containing foods)

Dietary fiber
(or other factors influencing intestinal microflora)

Eating times (in relation to drug intake)

Adapted from A. H. Conney, E. J. Pantuck, C. B. Pantuck, J. G. Forbner, A. P. Alvares, K. E. Anderson, and A. Kappas, "Variability in human drug metabolism," in *Proc. First World Conf. Clin. Pharmacol. Therap.* London, Aug. 3–9, 1980 (London and Basingstoke: Macmillan Publishers, 1980).

Absorption of levo-dopa is diminished when this drug is taken with a high-protein meal or with an amino acid mixture. Competitive inhibition of L-dopa absorption occurs when other amino acids, absorbed from the same intestinal absorptive site, are present (Goldin and Goldman, 1973). Similarly, a high-protein meal taken with methyl dopa may diminish absorption of the drug because absorption of amino acids derived from protein foods in the meal is competitive with the drug, which, like levo-dopa, is an amino acid (Sved, Goldberg, and Fersham, 1980).

Important diet-related factors which promote drug metabolism include:

1. The protein content of the diet (A high-protein diet increases the rate of drug metabolism. Low-protein, high-carbohydrate diets slow drug metabolism. Change in the rate of drug metabolism may be caused by changes in the protein content of the diet, which is likely to occur with hospitalization or on discharge of a patient from hospital.)
2. Eating of vegetables of the *Brassica* family, including cabbage and brussels sprouts
3. Eating charcoal-broiled meats

Changes in the diet which increase drug metabolism will shorten or modify the duration of effective blood levels. Higher blood levels of drugs will be sustained longer when the diet is changed so that drug metabolism is retarded (Anderson et al., 1979). There is a critical need to monitor blood levels of drugs with change in diet to improve drug efficacy and prevent toxicity, which can occur when the drug is retained at high levels in the body for an excessive time. Particular consideration must be given to the frequency of drug administration, which must be related to the rate of metabolism and clearance of drugs.

ALCOHOL USE AND ABUSE IN THE ELDERLY

Although the elderly may metabolize alcohol as efficiently as younger individuals, it has been shown that in the elderly higher peak levels of alcohol may occur when similar amounts of alcohol are ingested as are consumed by younger people. This is due to the changes in the distribution of the alcohol in the body, which are explained by age-related differences in body composition. The practical risks of high blood levels of alcohol after relatively low levels of intake include the risk of accidents in the home and accidents while driving, as well as the risk of falls and hip fractures during periods of inebriation.

Problems in assessing whether or not health problems in the elderly are alcohol related include those problems caused by faulty memory, confabulation, and the inappropriateness of tests that are available. Also many symptoms of alcohol abuse, including depression, cognitive impairment, and loss of libido, may be mistaken for changes due to aging.

Premature disability occurring in the 50s and 60s, and leading to the homebound condition or necessitating institutionalization, is frequently linked to alcoholic psychoses, alcoholic liver disease, and alcoholic nutritional deficiencies. Further, in the elderly the risk of adverse drug reactions and drug-nutrient interactions is higher in alcohol abusers (Roe, 1989a; Stinson et al., 1989).

In diabetics taking antidiabetic drugs, alcohol abuse imposes a serious risk of hypoglycemic episodes.

It should also be remembered that alcohol abuse is frequently associated with smoking, which not only contributes to poor appetite but also over time to the risk of emphysema and lung cancer, which both lead to protein-energy malnutrition and premature death.

EFFECT OF ENTERAL FORMULA FEEDING AND TPN ON DRUG DISPOSITION AND ADVERSE REACTIONS

Nutritional support of the elderly in hospitals and in nursing homes is frequently carried out by means of tube feeding. Before a decision is made to start tube feeding, there is a special need to decide whether the failure to eat reflects drug-induced anorexia in elderly patients. Such a loss of appetite, which results from drug toxicity, is particularly common when digoxin is being given in higher dosage than that required by an elderly patient with impaired renal function (Roe, 1989).

Medical indications for tube feeding include an inability to ingest sufficient food to meet nutritional needs because of anorexia, swallowing difficulties, or impaired consciousness, as well as maldigestion and malabsorption. However, in those elderly who have grossly impaired intestinal absorptive function due to surgical resection of the gut or due to disease, total parenteral alimentation (TPN) may be the only feasible method to prevent death due to malnutrition. While these special feeding methods are desirable, both tube feeding and TPN produce major effects on drug disposition and efficacy. If drugs are added to feeding solutions, this can reduce drug as well as nutrient stability. Further, drugs passed down enteral feeding tubes can cause tube blockage. Liquid formulations of drugs that are acidic are particularly likely to be incompatible with enteral formula solutions because drug formula mixture may form a gel or precipitate in the tube. This is likely to cause tube blockage, and it also reduces the availability of the drug being given as well as the nutrients in the formula which is being administered. Examples of drug formulations that are incompatible with enteral formulas include oral preparations of digoxin and thioridazine, which is a commonly used phenothiazine drug given to disturbed elderly patients (Cutie et al., 1983). Because of these problems, which arise from physico-chemical interactions between drug and formula constituents, it is recommended that when liquid formulations of drugs are to be given via enteral feeding tubes, the formula infusion first be stopped. After the flow of formula is stopped, the tube should be washed thoroughly with water; then the medication should be given via the tube. Finally, after a 45-minute period, the tube should be irrigated again before the formula infusion is restarted (Roe, 1989).

Nutrients in parenteral formulas may be unstable and may undergo chemical breakdown if the solution is exposed to ultraviolet light. Also, certain nutrient constituents of parenteral formulas (e.g., thiamin), as well as drugs like insulin, which may be added to the formula, can also cause allergic reactions in elderly, as well as in younger patients (Niemec and Vanderveen, 1984).

NUTRITIONAL PROBLEMS RELATED TO SELF-MEDICATION

Laxative Use and Abuse

Laxative use increases with age. Surveys have shown that approximately 50 percent of people in the United States who are 60 years or older take occasional or regular doses of laxatives. It is reported that only a quarter of these people consider themselves constipated (Fingl and Freston, 1979).

Reasons for laxative use and abuse are:

1. Simple constipation caused by low-fiber diet
2. Medical disorders mitigating against easy defecation or defecation unattended by physical distress
3. Long-term use of laxatives
4. Intake of drugs which are constipating
5. Bowel obsessions

Laxatives are classified into six groups as follows:

1. *Bulk-forming agents.* These include natural and semisynthetic disaccharides or polysaccharides. Laxative properties are related to the hydrophilic, bulk-forming properties of these compounds. An additional laxative effect is caused by intestinal bacterial fermentation of these compounds with release of osmotically active substances. Bulk-forming agents include methyl cellulose, food fiber source (particularly cereal brans), psyllium seeds, and lactulose. Lactulose is a semisynthetic disaccharide which is not hydrolyzed by intestinal enzymes. Its laxative properties are similar to those of lactose in people with lactase deficiency. This unabsorbed disaccharide is metabolized by intestinal bacteria, with formation of acetic, lactic, and other organic acids. The pH in the colon is reduced by this fermentation. Water and electrolytes are kept in the intestinal lumen by the intact disaccharide. The organic acid derivatives increase GI motility. Large doses of lactulose can induce fermentative diarrhea.

2. *Osmotic agents.* Magnesium and sodium sulfate are osmotic, saline laxatives. After administration these salts are incompletely absorbed. By osmosis, more fluid is drawn into the intestine. The stool passed is admixed with liquid. Osmotic diarrhea occurs when larger doses of osmotic or saline laxatives are

taken. It has been suggested that both magnesium and sodium sulfate may release intestinal hormones, including cholecystokinin, which can increase both secretion and motility in the small intestine.

3. *Agents that alter electrolyte transport.* Surface-active agents that are used as laxatives include bile salts, which normally contribute to "bowel evacuation," and dioctylsulfosuccinate.

4. *Agents that alter intestinal motility.* Intestinal motility may be increased by dietary fiber. Fiber sources which increase intestinal motility include hemicellulose from cereal brans and fruits and vegetables containing pectin and lignin. Lignin from fruit and vegetable seeds is not employed as a laxative because of its irritant effect on the intestine. Although natural fiber sources affect intestinal motility and may also act as bulk-forming agents, other substances that promote intestinal motility also alter transport of electrolytes in the intestine.

5. *Agents that alter both electrolyte transport and intestinal motility.* Examples of laxatives which have these dual effects are castor oil, anthraquinone drugs, including senna and cascara, and diphenylmethane derivatives, including phenolphthalein and bisacodyl. These drugs induce net intestinal losses of sodium and water. Glucose and amino acid absorption may be inhibited. Mucosal permeability may be increased, particularly with high and prolonged intake of these drugs. Ricinoleic acid, the active metabolite of castor oil, not only inhibits absorption of sodium and glucose but also increases the intestinal permeability to macromolecules. Plasma protein losses into the intestine may thereby be increased. Dietary fiber sources which have some effect on intestinal transport do not exert significant effects on intestinal absorption except by adsorption of micronutrients such as trace elements in the intestinal lumen (Reinhold et al., 1976).

6. *Stool softeners.* Drugs function as stool softeners if they increase stool bulk or if they prevent absorption of water from the feces in the large intestine by providing a physical barrier to water loss. Mineral oil provides an inert physical barrier to water loss from the feces in the large intestine. It also lubricates the stool thereby facilitating defecation.

Side Effects of Laxatives

In the elderly, bulk-forming agents taken before food can reduce appetite because the individual feels full. Although intake of bulk-forming laxatives seldom has a major anorectic effect, it may be a contributing cause of early satiety. Animal studies, presently unconfirmed in elderly people, indicate that bulk-forming laxatives such as psyllium seed reduce absorption of dietary minerals, including calcium, magnesium, and zinc (Smith et al., 1980).

Laxative abuse can cause potassium deficiency (Schwartz and Relman, 1953). Hypokalemia with or without clinical evidence of potassium deficiency is most likely to develop in elderly people taking laxatives to excess who are also on a marginal potassium intake and take potassium-losing diuretics (Roe, "Interactions," 1979). Types of laxatives most commonly associated with potassium deficiency are agents that affect electrolyte transport.

Malabsorption with steatorrhea can occur in laxative abusers when the laxative taken has a primary effect on the small as well as on the large intestine. Severe malabsorption has been reported in abusers of phenolphthalein and bisacodyl in steatorrhea and decreased calcium absorption. Decreased calcium absorption is a contributory cause of osteomalacia, which may develop in elderly laxative abusers. Protein-losing enteropathy with massive plasma protein loss via the GI tract is another complication of laxative abuse, which occurs in persons taking phenolphthalein, bisacodyl, or castor oil. Protein-losing enteropathy causes hypoalbuminemia and edema (Heizer et al., 1968; Levine, Goode, and Wingate, 1981).

Mineral oil, if taken at mealtimes or in the postprandial absorptive period, will prevent or reduce absorption of beta carotene and the fat-soluble vitamins. The most common vitamin deficiency reported in the elderly mineral oil abusers is osteomalacia. Osteomalacia in these patients is usually multifactorial, being determined not only by intake of mineral oil but also by very low consumption of vitamin D and little or no exposure to sunlight so that vitamin D synthesis in the skin is minimized (Curtis and Ballmer, 1939; Fitzgerald, 1978).

Antacid Abuse

Antacid abuse is of frequent occurrence in elderly people for the following reasons:

1. Upper GI tract symptoms, including flatulence and belching, are common complaints.
2. Antacids may be taken to counteract gastric side effects of other drugs, e.g., corticosteroids and non-narcotic analgesics such as aspirin and indomethacin.
3. Antacids may be taken to relieve acute alcoholic gastritis.
4. Antacids are taken to relieve pain or acute indigestion associated with organic disease of the stomach, e.g., cancer of the stomach.
5. Media advertising strongly suggests that antacids have a positive effect on health.
6. Antacids are taken by cardiac patients with angina or with postprandial dyspnea.

Antacids may contain aluminum or magnesium hydroxide or mixtures of these substances. A phosphate depletion syndrome is known to occur in elderly people on heavy doses of these antacids. Dietary phosphate combines with aluminum and magnesium hydroxide to form insoluble aluminum and magnesium phosphate which are excreted by the GI tract. The risk of phosphate depletion is greatest when there is an interactive effect with a low-phosphate diet. Symptoms of phosphate depletion are profound muscle weakness, which may be limited to proximal limb muscles; malaise; paresthesias (pins and needles); anorexia; and convulsions. In some patients phosphate depletion leads to low-phosphate osteomalacia or hemolytic anemia.

Sodium overload with development of congestive heart failure can result from intake of antacids containing sodium bicarbonate (Yokel, 1977).

Analgesic Abuse

Elderly people commonly have arthritis or other painful musculo-skeletal disorders for which they take aspirin or non-steroidal anti-inflammatory drugs (NSAIDs). Long-term use of high doses of aspirin causes erosion of the GI mucosa, leading to multiple small hemorrhages and chronic blood loss via the GI tract. Aspirin overuse is a prominent cause of iron deficiency anemia in the elderly. It should be pointed out that although aspirin has the potential for causing these nutritional side effects, it is a most useful drug and is a safer drug than other analgesics. However, if iron deficiency anemia is discovered in an elderly person, questions should be asked about aspirin usage, and dosage should be modified to avoid GI bleeding. NSAIDs, commonly used to treat degenerative arthritis in the elderly, can also cause GI bleeding and iron deficiency anemia.

Aspirin overuse is also a contributory cause of folacin deficiency, although the causal mechanism is not well identified (Weiss, 1974). The risk of folacin deficiency leading to macrocytic anemia in aspirin users is greater in those whose folacin intake is low (Gough, 1964).

Another non-narcotic analgesic which can cause toxicity, having nutritional implications, is acetaminophen. Acetaminophen is the active ingredient of Tylenol and is also present in over-the-counter sedatives and cold mixtures. High doses cause hepatic and renal damage. Massive doses of acetaminophen cause liver necrosis, which can be prevented or diminished by administration of sulfur-containing amino acids and related compounds, such as methionine or cysteamine. The nephrotoxic effects of acetaminophen develop with prolonged intake. Manifestations include a progressive loss of renal function and hypoalbuminemia (Rumack and Peterson, 1980).

Use and Abuse of Over-the-Counter Stimulants

Over-the-counter stimulants that contain ephedrine or ephedrine-like drugs that may be used by the elderly as nasal decongestants or to reduce appetite can increase blood pressure and the risk of stroke. The stimulants which may have these effects in these drugs include phenylpropanolamine, pseudoephedrine, and ephedrine (Pentel, 1984). These same drugs can increase blood glucose levels in diabetics (Hansten, 1985).

Abuse of Alcohol-Containing Mixtures

Numerous over-the-counter drugs in liquid formulation contain alcohol. The alcohol may be present in up to 25 percent of the total volume. Over-the-counter drugs which contain alcohol include cough syrups (elixirs), cold medicines, geriatric tonics, and sleep medicines (Roe, "Alcohol," 1979).

Reasons why elderly people take alcohol-containing mixtures are as follows:

1. Alcohol has a sedative effect.
2. Elderly alcoholics want a socially acceptable form of alcohol.
3. Alcohol-containing mixtures are promoted as palliative treatment for common health problems which disable the elderly, e.g., coughs, insomnia, poor appetite, and loss of memory. Certain geriatric tonics which contain nicotinic acid (niacin) in an alcohol-containing vehicle are claimed to induce dilatation of cerebral blood vessels and thus improve memory. There is no scientific basis for these claims. Vitamin mixtures in an alcohol base are to be avoided, both because of the risks of alcohol intake in the elderly, e.g., risk of falls because of alcohol-related confusion, and because the vitamins present in these mixtures, e.g., thiamin, may not be stable or optimally available for absorption.

Alcohol-based tonics may contain methionine. Methionine supplements taken by elderly alcoholics with liver disease can precipitate liver failure (hepatic encephalopathy).

Abuse of Nutrient Supplements—Vitamins

Hypervitaminoses in the elderly are likely to result from self-medication. Elderly people should be warned against self-medication with potent vitamin preparations. Whereas in the United States, availability of the fat-soluble vitamins A and D has been reduced by legislation which controls over-the-counter sale of individual capsules or tablets containing high doses of these vitamins, it is still possible for elderly people to obtain an unlimited supply of these vitamins by buying more of the lower dose tablets or capsules. Elderly people may be encouraged to take vitamin A to improve their eyesight and vitamin D to prevent or control fragile bones. Hypervitaminosis A causes bone pain, headache, and alopecia and may also cause jaundice. Hypervitaminosis D causes hypercalcemia, hypertension, and progressive renal failure (Roe, 1966).

Other vitamins commonly taken in excess by the elderly are vitamins E and C and niacin (Herbert, 1979). High doses of vitamin E can be dangerous in patients receiving anticoagulants, because the vitamin E enhances the antivitamin K effects of the drug. Megadoses of vitamin C are not dangerous but can cause GI disturbances, including "gas" and diarrhea. Claims that megadoses of vitamin C prevent or cure colds or prevent or cure cancer are unfounded. High doses of nicotinic acid may produce unpleasant flushes and may also cause impairment of liver function.

Abuse of Mineral Supplements

Claims have been made that elderly people have special mineral needs which are not supplied in the diet. Calcium, particularly calcium from "natural" sources such as bone meal, is advocated for persons with osteoporosis to harden bones. Zinc is advised to promote healing of ulcers and to improve taste sensation. Iodine, especially from kelp, is supposed to be health-giving and to improve thyroid function. Risks are that bone meal may contain lead, and therefore cause lead poisoning, that high intake of zinc causes zinc toxicity, and that kelp, because of the high iodine content, can cause iodide goiter and, in people with pre-existing thyroid enlargement, hypo- or hyperthyroidism, depending on previous thyroid status and cancer of the thyroid. Cancer of the thyroid is a rare complication of prolonged iodide overdose. Life-threatening hypersensitivity reactions can occur when iodide is taken in cough medicines by elderly people who are allergic to iodine (Roe, "Interactions," 1979).

Other Nutrient Supplements

Elderly people may be persuaded that massive intake of fructose or of amino acids such as lysine confers protection against metabolic or infectious disease. There is no scientific basis for these claims.

Elderly people with health complaints are advised to seek advice, diagnosis, and treatment from their physicians and not to self-medicate. Pharmacists can provide guidance to the elderly on the advisability of taking over-the-counter drugs.

ADVERSE NUTRITIONAL EFFECTS OF DRUGS

The two principal adverse effects of drugs on the elderly's nutritional health are obesity and malnutrition (Roe, "Interactions," 1979; Roe, 1980). Drugs which enhance the risk of obesity are hyperphagic drugs or drugs that increase appetite. Psychotropic drugs, including phenothiazine and benzodiazepine tranquilizers, and antidepressant drugs, including the monoamine oxidase inhibitors and tricyclics as well as lithium carbonate, may cause marked increases in appetite which, if food is available, lead to excessively large food intake and development of obesity. Change in appetite with these drugs is related to relief from anxiety, depression, and phobias. Conversely, when phenothiazine or benzodiazepine tranquilizers are given to elderly, underweight, bedridden patients, they may eat less because the tranquilizing and sedative effects of these drugs detract from interest in food. Because drug metabolism and elimination are slowed in the elderly, "sleep time" after sedative or tranquilizing drugs may be prolonged so that patients may not be awake at meal times.

Drugs which induce protein-energy malnutrition are most commonly those which induce nausea, vomiting, or other adverse reactions to food. Cancer chemotherapeutic drugs commonly cause nausea and vomiting immediately after drug administration, but with certain cancer chemotherapy regimens nausea is prolonged after the drugs are given (Carter, 1981). Combined chemotherapy and radiation therapy produce profound anorexia and, unless nutritional support is given, severe weight loss will follow. Elderly patients who have repeated courses of cancer chemotherapeutic drugs may develop aversion to foods which are offered in the immediate postdrug period, and subsequently they may refuse to eat these foods.

Digoxin in high dosages (high dose for body weight) causes serious anorexia with or without nausea and vomiting. "Digitalis cachexia" is a severe type of chronic protein-energy malnutrition which may stimulate cancer cachexia. Loss of weight in elderly people on digitalis glycosides may also be caused by loss of edema fluid and therefore may be desirable (Banks and Nayab, 1974).

Protein-energy malnutrition may occur in the elderly, as in younger people, as a consequence of drug-induced maldigestion or malabsorption. Drugs causing maldigestion and malabsorption are listed in Table 9-4, which also shows fecal nutrient losses.

Vitamin deficiencies may be caused by inadequate intake because of drug-induced anorexia, maldigestion, malabsorption, hyperexcretion, or impaired vitamin utilization.

TABLE 9-4 Drug-Induced Malabsorption

DRUG	USAGE	NUTRIENTS LOST	MECHANISM
Aluminum & magnesium hydroxide	Antacid	Phosphate	Formation of insoluble phosphate
Cholestyramine	Hypocholesterolemic agent	Fat soluble vitamin and folate	Binding of bile acid and absorption of nutrients (e.g., folacin)
Cimetidine	H$_2$ receptor antagonist (used in peptic ulcer patients)	Vitamin B$_{12}$	Hypochlorhydria
Colchicine	Anti-inflammatory agent in gout		Mitotic arrest; structural defect in intestinal mucosa
Colestipol	Hypocholesterolemic agent	Fat soluble vitamin and folacin	Binding of bile acid and absorption of nutrients (e.g. folacin)
Methotrexate	Cancer chemo-therapeutic agent	Calcium	Acute folacin deficiency
Mineral oil	Laxative	Fat soluble vitamins	Physical barrier to absorption; nutrient dissolved (beta-carotene); micelle formation ↓
Neomycin	Antibiotic	Fat; nitrogen; K; Fe; calcium; lactose; vitamin B$_{12}$	Mucosal "injury" pancreatic lipase ↓ Maldigestion
Phenytoin	Laxative	Calcium; fat	Intestinal hurry; K depletion; loss of structural integrity

TABLE 9-5   Vitamin Antagonists

	DRUG	USAGE
Folacin antagonists	Methotrexate	Cancer chemotherapy
	Pyrimethamine	Antimalarial
	Triamterene	Diuretic
	Trimethoprim	Antibacterial
Vitamin B₆ antagonists	Isoniazid	Antituberculosis agent
	Hydralazine	Antihypertensive agent
	Cycloserine	Antituberculosis agent
Vitamin K antagonists	Warfarin	Anticoagulants

Taken from D. A. Roe, "Interactions between drugs and nutrients," *Med. Clin. N. Amer.*, 63, 5 (1979), 1001. © W. B. Saunders Co. Reprinted by permission.

Acute vitamin deficiencies occur when vitamin antagonists are administered. Vitamin antagonists commonly used in the elderly are coumarin anticoagulants (vitamin K antagonists) and methotrexate, a folacin antagonist used in the treatment of cancer (Carter, 1981). Although the desired pharmacologic effects of these drugs are related to their antivitamin properties, high drug doses can cause life-threatening situations, e.g., hemorrhage with the anticoagulant drugs because of inability to use vitamin K and failure of hemopoiesis when methotrexate is given because of inability of the body to form folacin coenzymes because of methotrexate-induced enzyme block (block of the dihydrofolate reductase enzyme). The antidote for methotrexate toxicity is folinic acid. Table 9-5 lists vitamin antagonist drugs and their usage.

TABLE 9-6   Mineral Depletion Induced by Drugs

Diuretics	Calcium (not thiazides)
	Potassium
	Magnesium
	Zinc
Laxatives (Laxative abuse)	Potassium
	Calcium
Glucocorticoids	Calcium
	Potassium
Chelating agents (penicillamine)	Zinc
	Copper
Ethanol	Potassium
	Magnesium
	Zinc
Antacids	Phosphates
Non-narcotic analgesics (aspirin, indomethacin)	Iron (by GI blood loss)

Taken from D. A. Roe, "Interactions between drugs and nutrients," *Med. Clin. N. Amer.*, 63, 5 (1979), 998. © W. B. Saunders Co. Reprinted by permission.

Mineral depletion is often caused by drugs in the elderly. As described earlier, severe forms of mineral depletion may result from abuse of over-the-counter drugs. Other drugs causing mineral depletion are oral diuretics (Morgan and Davidson, 1980). However, although a fall in serum potassium levels is a well-known effect of the thiazide and "loop" diuretics (furosemide and ethacrynic acid), chronic intake of these diuretics does not commonly result in severe hypokalemia in patients taking these drugs for hypertension or congestive heart failure unless intake of potassium from the diet is marginal or patients are laxative abusers. Drugs causing mineral depletion are shown in Table 9-6 on page 199.

Other folacin (folate) antagonists commonly taken by the elderly are the antibacterial drug trimethoprim and the potassium-sparing diuretic triamterene. These two drugs are mild folacin antagonists.

DRUGS ADVERSELY AFFECTING THE CONTROL OF DIET-RELATED DISEASE

Diabetes

Drugs which increase blood glucose and may account for short-term or persistent hyperglycemia in diabetic patients include corticosteroids, thiazide diuretics, loop diuretics, and stimulants containing ephedrine or ephedrine-like drugs. Alcohol and beta-adrenergic blocking agents such as propranolol as well as high doses of aspirin can induce hypoglycemia, particularly in patients receiving oral antidiabetic drugs (Dargaville, 1985).

Hypertension

The control of hypertension may be reduced by intake of prescription or over-the-counter drugs which are high in sodium, including antacids containing sodium bicarbonate (Roe, 1984). Hypertensive drugs include alcohol, corticosteroids, disulfiram, the monamine oxidase inhibitors, and drugs containing ephedrine or related stimulants (Roe, 1982).

ACUTE INCOMPATIBILITY REACTIONS CAUSED BY INTERACTION OF DRUGS WITH BEVERAGE AND FOOD COMPONENTS

Adverse reactions to drugs can be precipitated by intake with certain foods or alcoholic beverages. Reactions vary greatly in intensity, some being sufficiently unpleasant to make the person want to avoid going through the experience again, whereas other reactions are life-threatening (Roe, "Interactions," 1979). The major types of drug-food and drug-alcohol incompatibilities are summarized in Table 9-7.

TABLE 9-7 Drug-Food and Drug-Alcohol Incompatibilities

CLASSIFICATION	REACTANTS		EFFECT
	1	2	
1. Tyramine reactions	*MAO Inhibitors*	*High tyramine/ dopamine foods*	
	Antidepressants, e.g., phenelzine	Cheese	Flushing
		Red wines	Hypertension
	Procarbazine	Chicken liver	Cerebrovascular
	Isoniazid (INH, Isonicotinic acid hydrazide)	Broad beans Yeast extracts	accidents
2. Disulfiram reactions	*Aldehyde dehydrogenase inhibitors*	*Ethanol*	
	Disulfiram	Beer	Flushing, headache
	(Antabuse)	Wine	Nausea, vomiting
	Calcium carbimide	Liquor	Chest and
	Metronidazole	Foods containing	abdominal pain
	Nitrofurantoin	alcohol	
	C. atramentarius*		
	Sulfonylureas		
3. Hypoglycemic reactions	*Insulin releasers*	*Ethanol*	Weakness
	Oral hypoglycemic agents		Mental confusion
	Sugar (as in sweet mixers)		Irrational behavior
			Loss of consciousness
4. Flush reactions	*Miscellaneous*	*Ethanol*	Flush
	Chlorpropamide [in diabetes]		Dyspnea
	Griseofulvin		Headache

*Coprinus atramentarius = Inky cap mushroom.

Taken from D. A. Roe, "Interactions between drugs and nutrients," *Med. Clin. N. Amer.*, 63, 5 (1979), 985. © W. B. Saunders Co. Reprinted by permission.

Major risk factors related to adverse nutritional effects of drugs and drug-food incompatibilities occur when:

1. The drug is an antinutrient.
2. The drug, which has adverse nutritional effects, is taken for a long time.
3. The patient is on a multidrug regimen.
4. The diet is nutritionally inadequate.
5. There is excessive drug use or abuse of prescription or over-the-counter drugs.
6. Disease-related malabsorption is present.
7. The patient is malnourished.
8. The patient is not given special diet instructions.
9. Physicians and nutritionists are unaware of the risks.

PREVENTION OF ADVERSE DRUG REACTIONS
IN THE ELDERLY

Guidelines to physicians and physicians' assistants on means to decrease the incidence of adverse drug reactions include the following strategies proposed by Oppeneer and Vervoren (1983):

1. Obtaining a careful drug history from patients on their use of prescription and over-the-counter drugs
2. Avoiding multiple-drug therapies whenever possible
3. When multiple-drug therapies are required, minimizing interactions by pre-prescription consideration of need to use the safest drugs which will provide the desired therapeutic effect
4. Adjusting dose in accordance with the patient's renal function
5. Avoiding unnecessary changes in the drug regimen
6. Carefully monitoring patients who are receiving drugs which are known to cause interactions
7. Instructing the patient about the possible risks of drug interactions with the medications they are taking

When considering dose adjustment for patients with renal impairment, Santoro and Kaye (1984) have emphasized the need for substantial reduction in the dose of specific groups of antibiotics, including the aminoglycosides such as amikacin, kanamycin, gentamicin, and tobramycin. It has also been stressed by these authors that to avoid renal toxicity, cephalosporin antibiotics should not be given with aminoglycosides, since the risk of renal failure is enhanced by this drug combination.

To avoid unwanted or adverse outcomes of drug-nutrient interactions in the elderly, the following is also recommended:

1. The times that the patient's drugs are given should be set so that there is no conflict with mealtimes and so that drug absorption is optimized.
2. Diet changes should not be made without prior review by the physician so that changes in the rate of drug metabolism, and hence changes in the duration of drug effect, are avoided.
3. Drugs should not be given via enteral feeding tubes when the liquid formula is being infused, and drugs should never be given by this route if they have been demonstrated to be incompatible with the contents of the formula that is being administered.
4. To avoid diarrhea, use of oral broad-spectrum antibiotics should be avoided in patients who are being tube fed.
5. Drug dosage should be modified in accordance with the patient's body weight.
6. Patients receiving drugs which can induce nutritional deficiencies should be monitored by biochemical assessment of their vitamin and mineral status.
7. Patients receiving drugs which can alter appetite and food intake should be weighed weekly.

8. Patients receiving drugs which can cause hypertensive crises through interaction with amines in foods (e.g., monamine oxidase inhibitors such as the antidepressant phenelzine, isoniazid, and procarbazine) should be given instructions on which foods to avoid, e.g., aged cheese, pickled herring, chicken livers, and wine.

9. Elderly patients on drug regimens which include sedative or other drugs incompatible with alcohol should be instructed not to drink alcoholic beverages.

10. Patients on prescription drugs whose action is altered by concurrent intake of vitamins should be instructed not to take such nutrient supplements.

QUESTIONS

Circle all correct answers (there may be more than one correct answer to each question).

1. Over-the-counter drug abuse in the elderly is related to:
   a. chronic allergies
   b. chronic constipation
   c. chronic aches and pains
   d. promotional advertising
   e. alcohol content of drug mixtures

2. Potassium deficiency is associated with:
   a. high sodium intake
   b. low-cholesterol diet
   c. intake of oral diuretics
   d. heavy use of laxatives
   e. diet of bread, cold cuts, and sodas

3. Tranquilizing drugs may lead to gain in weight. Reasons are:
   a. increased appetite and food intake
   b. fluid retention
   c. decreased physical activity
   d. gain in muscle mass
   e. gain in bone mass

4. Adverse drug reactions occur more frequently in the elderly because:
   a. more drugs are taken
   b. patients do not understand medication instructions
   c. drug metabolism is slowed with aging
   d. over-the-counter drugs are abused
   e. drugs are taken which are intended for others

5. Acute adverse reactions (drug-food and drug-beverage incompatibilities) occur under one or more of the following circumstances:
   a. Aspirin is taken with eggs.
   b. Milk is taken with antihistamines.
   c. Aged cheese is taken with antidepressants (MAOI).
   d. Alcohol is taken with metronidazole (Flagyl).
   e. Cookies are taken with propranolol (Inderal).

6. Risks of alcohol abuse in those over 50 include:
   a. Greater risk of falls and hip fractures
   b. Disability from alcoholic psychoses
   c. Poorer glycemic control in those who are diabetics
   d. More laxative abuse
   e. More adverse drug reactions

REFERENCES

ANDERSON, K. E., A. H. CONNEY, and A. KAPPAS, "Nutrition and oxidative drug metabolism in man: relative influence of dietary lipids, carbohydrate and protein," *Clin. Pharmacol. Ther.*, 26 (1979), 483–501.

BANKS, T., and A. NAYAB, "Digitalis cachexia" (letter), *New Eng. J. Med.*, 290 (1974), 746.

BAUER, L. A., "Interference of oral phenytoin absorption by continuous nasogastric feedings," *Neurology*, 32 (1982), 570–72.

BOROWITZ, J. L., P. F. MOORE, G. K. W. YIM, and T. S. MIYA, "Mechanisms of enhanced drug effects produced by dilution of the oral dose," *Toxicol. Appl. Pharmacol.*, 19 (1971), 164–68.

BULLPITT, C. J., and A. E. FLETCHER, "Drug treatment and quality of life in the elderly," in *Clinics in Geriatric Medicine: Clinical Pharmacology*, Vol. 6, ed., P. P. Lamy. Philadelphia: W. B. Saunders, 1990, pp. 309–17.

CAIRD, F. I., "Towards rational drug therapy in old age," *J. Roy. Coll. Physicians Lond.*, 19 (1985), 235–39.

CARANASOS, C. J., R. B. STEWART, and L. E. CLUFF, "Drug-induced illness leading to hospitalization," *J. Amer. Med. Assoc.*, 228 (1974), 713–17.

CARTER, S. K., "Nutritional problems associated with cancer chemotherapy," in *Nutrition and Cancer, Etiology and Treatment*, eds. G. R. Newell and N. M. Ellison. New York: Raven Press, 1981, pp. 303–17.

COLBURN, W. A., D. M. GIBSON, L. G. RODRIGUEZ, C. J. L. BUGGE, and H. P. BLUMENTHAL, "Effect of meals on the kinetics of etretinate," *J. Clin. Pharmacol.*, 25 (1985), 583–89.

CONNEY, A. H., et al., "Variability in human drug metabolism," in *Proceedings of the First World Conference in Clinical Pharmacologic Therapy*, London, Aug. 3–9, 1980. London: Macmillan Publishers, Ltd., 1980.

CURTIS, A. C., and R. S. BALLMER, "The prevention of carotene absorption by liquid petrolatum," *J. Amer. Med. Assoc.*, 113 (1939), 1785–88.

CUTIE, A. J., E. ALTMAN, and L. LENKEL, "Compatibility of enteral products with commonly employed drug additives," *J. Parent. Ent. Nutr.*, 7 (1983), 186–91.

DARGAVILLE, R., "Drug interactions in treatment," in *Diabetes Mellitus: A Guide to Treatment*, ed. P. Taft. Sydney: ADIS Health Science Press, 1985, pp. 77–83.

FINGL, E., and J. W. FRESTON, "Antidiarrhoeal agents and laxatives: changing concepts," *Clin. Gastroenterol.*, 8 (1979), 161–86.

FITZGERALD, F., "Clinical hypophosphatemia," *Ann. Rev. Med.*, 29 (1978), 177–89.

GOLDIN, B. R., and P. GOLDMAN, "The metabolism of L-dopa: the role of the intestinal microflora," *Fed. Proc.*, 32 (1973), 798.

GOUGH, K. R., et al., "Folic acid deficiency in rheumatoid arthritis," *Brit. Med. J.*, 1 (1964), 212–17.

GUTTMAN, D. V., "A study of legal drug use by older Americans," *Services Research Report* (NIDA), 1977.

HANSTEN, P. D., *Drug Interactions*, 5th Ed. Philadelphia: Lea & Febiger, 1985, p. 155.

HEIZER, W. D., A. L. WARSHAW, T. A. WALDMAN, and L. LASTER, "Protein losing gastroenteropathy and malabsorption associated with factitious diarrhea," *Ann. Intern. Med.*, 68 (1968), 839–52.

HERBERT, V. D., "Megavitamin therapy," in *Contemporary Nutrition Controversies*, eds., T. P. Labuza and E. A. Sloan. St. Paul, MN: West Publishers, 1979, pp. 223–27.

HULKA, B. S., L. L. KUPPER, J. C. CASSEL, R. L. ERD, and J. A. BURDETTE, "Medication use and misuse: physician-patient discrepancies," *J. Chronic Dis.*, 28 (1975), 7–21.

HURWITZ, N., "Predisposing factors in adverse reactions to drugs," *Brit. Med. J.*, 1 (1969), 536–39.

KARIM, A., T. BURNS, L. WEARLY, J. STREICHER, and M. PALMER, "Food induced changes in theophylline absorption from controlled-release formulations. I. Substantial increased and decreased absorption with Uniphyl tablets and Theo-Dur Sprinkle," *Clin. Pharmacol. Ther.*, 38 (1985), 77–83.

KARIM, A., T. BURNS, D. JANKY, and A. HURWITZ, "Food induced changes in theophylline absorption from controlled-release formulations. II. Importance of meal composition and dosing time relative to meal intake in assessing changes in absorption," *Clin. Pharmacol. Ther.* 38 (1985), 642–47.

LEVINE, D., A. W. GOODE, and D. L. WINGATE, "Purgative abuse associated with reversible cachexia hypogamma globulinaemia and finger clubbing," *Lancet*, 1 (1981), 919–20.

MONKS, T. J., J. CALDWELL, and R. L. SMITH, "Influence of methylxanthine-containing foods on theophylline metabolism and kinetics," *Clin. Pharmacol. Ther.*, 26 (1979), 513–24.

MORGAN, D. B., and C. DAVIDSON, "Hypokalaemia and diuretics: an analysis of publications,"*Brit. Med. J.*, 1 (1980), 905–8.

NIEMEC, P. W., JR., and T. W. VANDERVEEN, "Compatability considerations in parenteral nutrient solutions," *Amer. J. Hosp. Pharm.*, 41 (1984), 893–95.

NOVAK, L. P., "Aging, total body potassium, fat-free mass and cell mass in males and females between ages 18 and 85 years," *J. Gerontol.*, 27 (1972), 438–43.

O'MALLEY, K., J. CROOKS, E. DUKE, and I. H. STEVENSON, "Effect of age and sex on human drug metabolism," *Brit. Med. J.*, 3 (1971), 607–9.

OPPENEER, J. E., and T. M. VERVOREN, *Gerontological Pharmacology: A Resource for Health Practitioners*. St. Louis: The C. V. Mosby Co., 1983, p. 40.

OUSLANDER, J. G., "Drug therapy in the elderly," *Ann. Intern. Med.*, 95 (1981), 711–22.

PENTEL, P., "Toxicity of over-the-counter stimulants," *J. Amer. Med. Assoc.*, 252 (1984), 1898–1903.

RAFFOUL, P. R., J. K. COPPER, and D. W. LOVE, "Drug misuse in older people," *Gerontologist*, 21 (1981), 146–50.

REINHOLD, J. G., B. FARADJI, P. ABADI, and F. ISMAEL-BEIGI, "Decreased absorption of calcium, magnesium, zinc and phosphorus by humans due to increased fiber and phosphorus consumption as wheat bread," *J. Nutr.*, 106 (1976), 493–503.

ROE, D. A., "Nutrient toxicity with excessive intake. 1. Vitamins," *New York State J. Med.*, 66 (1966), 869–71.

ROE, D. A., *Alcohol and the Diet*. Westport, CT: AVI Publishing Co., 1979.

ROE, D. A., "Interactions between drugs and nutrients," *Med. Clin. N. Amer.*, 63 (1979), 985–1007.

ROE, D. A., *Nutrition and the Health Scientist*. Boca Raton, FL: CRC Press, Inc., 1979, pp. 67–69.

ROE, D. A., "Nutrition and chronic drug administration: effects on the geriatric patient," *American Pharmacy*, NS20 (1980), 33–35.

ROE, D. A., *Handbook: Interactions of Selected Drugs and Nutrients in Patients*. Chicago: American Dietetic Association Publications Department, 1982, pp. 32, 19, 100, 109.

ROE, D. A., "Adverse nutritional effects of OTC drug use in the elderly," in *Drugs and Nutrition in the Geriatric Patient*, ed. D. A. Roe. New York: Churchill Livingstone, 1984, pp. 121–33.

ROE, D. A., "Drug-nutrient interactions in the elderly," in *Nutrition, Aging and the Elderly*, eds. H. N. Munro and D. E. Danford. New York: Plenum Press, 1989, pp. 363–84.

ROE, D. A., *Drug and Nutrient Interactions: A Problem-Oriented Reference Guide*, 4th Ed. Chicago: American Dietetic Association, 1989, pp. xiii–xv.

ROE, D. A., *Diet and Drug Interactions*. New York: Van Nostrand Reinhold, 1989, pp. 29–58.

RUMACK, B. H., and R. G. PETERSON, "Clincial toxicology," in *Casarett and Dou-ll's Toxicology, The Basic Science of Poisons*, 2nd Ed., eds. J. Doull, C. D. Klaassen, and M. O. Amdur. New York: Macmillan, Inc., 1980, pp. 682–83.

SANTORO, J., and D. KAYE, "Antimetabolites and antifungal agents," in *CRC Handbook on Pharmacology of Aging*, eds. P. B. Goldberg, J. Roberts, R. C. Adelman and G. S. Roth. Boca Raton, FL: CRC Press, Inc., 1984, p. 228.

SCHWARTZ, W. B., and A. S. RELMAN, "Metabolic and renal studies in chronic potassium depletion resulting from overuse of laxatives," *J. Clin. Invest.*, 32 (1953), 258–71.

SMITH, R. G., M. J. ROWE, A. N. SMITH, M. A. EASTWOOD, E. DRUMMOND, and W. G. BRYDON, "A study of bulking agents in elderly patients," *Age and Aging*, 9 (1980), 267–71.

STINSON, F. S., M. C. DUFOUR, and D. BERTOLUCCI, "Alcohol-related morbidity in the aging population," *Alc. Health Res. Wld.*, 13 (1989), 80–86.

SVED, A. F., I. M. GOLDBERG, and J. D. FERNSHAM, "Dietary protein intake influences the antihypertensive potency of methyl dopa in spontaneously hypertensive rats," *J. Pharm. Exp. Therapeut.*, 214 (1980), 147–51.

U. S. TASK FORCE ON PRESCRIPTION DRUGS, *The Drug Users*. Washington, DC: U.S. Department of Health, Education, and Welfare, 1968, pp. 126–29.

VESTAL, R. E., "Methodological problems associated with studies of drug metabolism in the elderly," ed. P. Turner, *First World Conf. on Clin. Pharmacol. and Therapeut., London, Aug. 3–9, 1980*. London: Macmillan Publishers, 1980, pp. 110–16.

VESTAL, R. E., A. J. J. WOOD, R. A. BRANCH, D. J. SHAND, and G. R. WILKIN-

SON, "Effects of age and cigarette smoking on propranolol disposition," *Clin. Pharmac. Therap.*, 26 (1979), 8–15.

WEISS, H. J., "Aspirin—a dangerous drug?" *J. Amer. Med. Assoc.*, 229 (1974), 1221–22.

WELLING, P. G., "Influence of food and diet on gastrointestinal absorption: a review," *J. Pharmacokinet. Biopharmaceut.*, 5 (1977), 291–331.

WELLING, P. G., and F. L. S. TSE, "Food interactions affecting the absorption of analgesic and anti-inflammatory agents," *Drug-Nutrient Interact.*, 2 (1983), 153–68.

YOKEL, R. A., "Sodium and potassium levels in antacids," *Amer. J. Hosp. Pharm.*, 34 (1977), 200–202.

chapter 10

Nutrition Services

Nutrition services for the elderly comprise those available to the healthy elderly, those designed for the sick and disabled elderly in the community, those used in acute care hospitals, and those used in nursing homes. The services have been established with the following goals:

1. To provide nutrition education to:
    a. seniors in the classroom, clinic, or other formal setting
    b. seniors in the informal setting of the home
    c. community-based health and personal care providers
    d. nursing home staffs
2. To give food-shopping assistance for:
    a. seniors who need assistance in selecting foods for special diets
    b. homebound seniors who cannot get to the food markets
3. To provide meals services for:
    a. healthy or moderately disabled seniors who prefer to eat their main meal with others in a community setting.
    b. homebound elderly who cannot cook at all, or who cannot prepare dinner-type meals.
4. To combat food emergencies associated with:
    a. homelessness
    b. food insecurity
    c. terminal illness

5. To prevent or combat diet-related disease through:
   a. changes in the regular food supply
   b. providing special diet foods
   c. nutrition research
6. To provide quality assurance by using:
   a. state and local auditing of food services in nursing homes
   b. surveys of community meals programs
7. To contribute to the overall care of the elderly by:
   a. referral of seniors to other community agencies
   b. planning for future needs

NUTRITION EDUCATION PROGRAMS

Nutrition education programs for the elderly are quite frequently initiated by nutritionists or by nutrition students, not only for the purpose of dietary counseling but also with the aim of imparting nutrition knowledge which is unrelated or only indirectly related to diets. Such nutrition education programs may be provided at senior citizens centers, at congregate meal sites supplying Title IIIC meals to the elderly, in churches, in domiciliary care facilities, and even in nursing homes. One or more lectures are usually given. The topics are likely to be chosen by the speaker, although sometimes choice of subject matter is decided by college teachers or by social program directors in community organizations. The elderly target groups are assumed to be eager to have the latest information on advances in nutritional science and may retain this information. Whereas this assumption may be correct when the talk or talks are being given to socially and intellectually active elderly, it is naive to believe that nutritional science or even tips on good nutrition are of concern to elderly people who are either intellectually impaired or whose diet and nutrition are the responsibility of others (Templeton, 1978).

Realistic goals of nutrition education programs for the elderly are:

1. To provide reliable nutrition information to active older people on topics of current interest or dispute
2. To provide basic nutrition education to such groups when this is requested by group members
3. To explain recent policy changes at the federal or local level on food assistance programs to the elderly
4. To teach interested elderly how to cook special or fun dishes of high-nutrient content
5. To provide structured and reliable instruction to groups of elderly with specific chronic diseases requiring dietary management (e.g., diabetics, cardiac patients)
6. To provide recreational activity to groups of aged people inside and outside institutions
7. To provide nutrition education experience to students in training

Studies of nutrition education as part of group feeding programs have been conducted, and it has been reported that both improved eating habits and a greater knowledge of nutrition for the participants has come about as a result of the educational program. Kim, Schriver, and Campbell (1981), commenting on these results of nutrition education for the elderly, noted that these changes could have been brought about from the social contact of the group-meal situation and not just from the nutrition education program.

Constraints on nutrition education programs for the elderly have been identified by these authors as follows:

1. The normal aging process may cause physical changes which interfere with the learning process, such as reduced hearing capacity or an inability to follow rapid speech.
2. Impaired vision can make it impossible for elderly audiences either to see slides on a screen or to read instructional materials.
3. Elderly people whose dietary practices have been shaped by an extended lifetime are not easily persuaded by talks or lectures to change their dietary practices.

In spite of these reservations about nutrition programs for the elderly, Kim, Schriver, and Campbell (1981) decided to set up a nutrition education program in a nursing home to try to improve the eating habits of nursing home residents. At the same time they established a means to evaluate the effectiveness of their program on the dietary intakes of the residents. Nutrient intakes were measured before, during, and after presentation of the nutrition education in a small nursing home. The nutrition education presentations were given to small groups of residents during the noon meal weekly for a period of 4 weeks. The weekly talks were videotaped and played back to the residents toward the end of the noontime meal in a room which was next to the dining room.

Changes in nutrient intake were observed in the experimental group, i.e., in the residents of the nursing home receiving the nutrition education (while the program was in progress), but these improvements in nutrient intake were not maintained after the program was over. It was pointed out by the investigators that whereas it is possible that the nutrition education program was responsible for the temporary changes in nutrient intake, it could also be that the focus of attention on the nursing home residents could have altered their intakes.

Attempts have also been made to improve the food and the actual dietary intake of nursing home residents by education of the facility staff. Holme and Kim (1981) developed nutrition education lessons for weekly presentation to nursing home staffs. These sessions were conducted in one nursing home. Sessions were voluntary and considered as in-service workshops. Each presentation was for a period of one-half hour, and these sessions were conducted at weekly intervals. Pretest and post-test questionnaires were developed to assess the nutrition knowledge of the nursing home staff before the lesson and thereafter. Questionnaires also investigated the staff attitudes before the presentation and after as to the importance to the residents of a nutritionally adequate diet. Material presented included food plan (the nutritional basis of a sound diet), a videotape-illustrated lecture which showed eating patterns of the elderly, changes in these eating patterns which could occur and why they occur when these people enter the nursing home, and lastly, a lecture on interpersonal relationships between the food service staff and the residents.

As a result of this program it was found that the staff increased their nutrition knowledge. The staff rated the presentations according to quality and responded positively to a videotape entitled "Meals: Then and Now." They also responded well to the opportunity to use role-playing in the last lesson. Another positive outcome of this program was that, at its completion, 78 percent of the staff members felt that they could now talk to residents about their feelings about meals that were served in the nursing home and that they could further encourage the residents to make better food choices.

NEW FINDINGS AND IDEAS ON NUTRITION EDUCATION FOR THE ELDERLY

One environmental factor that fosters good nutrition in the elderly is access to nutrition education (Austin, 1989). "Written materials, including books, magazines, pamphlets, posters, and food labels, have been found to be the most frequent source of nutrition information both for urban and rural elderly. Elderly also obtain information from TV and radio programs. Among the elderly, females use food labels, books, and magazines more than men (Briley et al., 1990). Wellness programs in which nutrition and exercise are combined are popular among the better-educated groups of retirees.

It has been proposed that retirees should be a prime target for multiple types of nutrition education aimed to improve their ability to follow dietary guidelines, since it has been demonstrated that those who have been retired for approximately one year make significant changes in their patterns of food budgeting, food shopping, and eating. Proposed methods of nutrition education for retirees include dramatic presentations, group discussions, food-tasting groups, cooking demonstrations, the use of nutrition and recipe books, and reminders to take home (Davies, 1990). The types of nutrition education that should be developed and made available to the elderly should vary with the specific aims of the educational process as well as with the educational level of the audience, their familiar language, and depending on whether or not they are visually impaired or deaf.

In addition, while formal nutrition education in college settings is presently more often provided to health care professionals charged with the care of the elderly than to the elderly themselves, it is proposed that elder hostels, community colleges, and university summer schools develop nutrition courses for older men and women.

NUTRITIONAL COUNSELING FOR THE ELDERLY

In recent years, target groups for nutrition education have included the elderly. The overall aim has been to influence older people to consume an adequate diet (U.S. Select Committee, 1974; Harper et al., 1978; Wurtman, 1979). Recognition that certain elderly people need nutrition counseling is due in part to a growing awareness of the difficulties these people may have in buying and preparing food and, more especially, in choosing and obtaining foods required for special diets (Clarke and Wakefield, 1975). Other special needs of the elderly, coming under the umbrella of nutrition education, include strategies to modify eating times and content of meals to avoid symptoms generated by food and adverse drug reactions, combatting nutrition misinformation, and instruction on the risks of food and alcohol abuse (Roe, 1979; Roe, 1980). Nutrition counseling for the elderly may be direct education in a classroom or a community setting but more commonly is by counseling of elderly individuals or groups or by giving information to those with responsibility for the direct care of the elderly.

Goals of nutritional counseling are:

1. To explain personal food-energy and nutrient needs
2. To show how nutritional requirements can be met using available foods
3. To offer simple and feasible menu and exercise plans for weight control or reduction
4. To develop skills in food procurement and preparation which are related to situational factors and disabilities present
5. To give information on locally available nutrition-support services, food-delivery services, and congregate meal centers.
6. To interpret prescribed diets intended for the control of chronic disease and to ensure that restrictive diets are nutritionally adequate.
7. To give practical advice on foods which are desirable to prevent GI complaints, including flatulence and constipation.
8. To establish eating times which allow optimal absorption, utilization, and tolerance of prescribed medications.
9. To combat use of fad diets
10. To encourage socialization at meal times
11. To obtain information on alcohol abuse, to make referrals on alcoholism counseling, and to counsel alcoholics on dietary needs
12. To promote the best use of a limited food budget

The following should receive counseling:

1. The elderly individual if he or she is living independently and is responsible for food procurement and preparation
2. The homemaker who purchases and/or prepares food for the elderly person
3. The food service manager at a domiciliary care facility or nursing home
4. The nurse or personal care attendant who is responsible for feeding and assisting in feeding the individual

Guidelines on Implementation
of Counseling Goals

Meeting energy and nutrient needs. The food-energy needs of the individual should be explained, with emphasis on adjustment of calorie intake downwards in accordance with age, lower metabolic rate, decreased muscle mass, and most important, physical exercise. Using oral presentation and charts as shown in Figure 10-1, it should be emphasized that if the person's weight is within the desirable range for his or her height, usual food-energy intake meets requirements.

Food sources of key nutrients should be explained. Special emphasis should be placed on food sources rich in calcium, vitamin D, riboflavin, and folacin, which are frequently deficient in the diets of the elderly (Lawson et al., 1979). It should also be stressed that if a variety of foods rich in essential nutrients are consumed this will markedly increase the chance that the diet will be nutritionally adequate.

Weight reduction. When weight reduction is required, it is necessary to determine the person's current and/or usual food-energy intake. For an individual who is living independently, this requires repeated 24-hour

FIGURE 10-1
Food sources of key nutrients
(to be consumed daily).

Food/beverage	Nutrient
Enriched bread, pasta, and flour	Carbohydrate, B vitamins
Milk	Protein, Vitamin A, Vitamin D, Calcium
Margarine	Fat, Vitamin A
Fruit juices (citrus)	Vitamin C, Potassium
Fortified breakfast cereals	Carbohydrate, Vitamin A, Vitamin D, Vitamin C, B vitamins, Iron
Green leafy vegetable	Folic acid, Potassium

dietary recalls (a minimum of three so that the average daily intake can be calculated) or a diet record. It is seldom feasible to obtain a diet record for more than 3 days, one of which should be a weekend day. Instruction should be given either to the elderly individual or to a responsible spouse, home companion, or domestic worker on how the diet record should be kept. It is very important that the 24-hour recalls or diet records indicate eating times, all foods and beverages consumed, and portion sizes. Then the individual's weight and height should be measured. An ideal body weight for a man or woman of that height can be determined using Table 10-1. By subtracting the ideal weight from the patient's weight, a desirable weight loss can be calculated. It is only justifiable, however, to calculate the desired weight loss by this means if edema and ascites are absent. When a diuretic is prescribed to treat edema but has not yet been taken, then measurement of body weight and calculation of desirable weight loss should be delayed until a "dry" weight can be obtained, i.e., the patient should be weighed again when the edema fluid has been lost. When the patient has ascites, prescription of weight-reducing diets is seldom justifiable.

The feasibility of attaining the desired weight loss has to be evaluated by the nutritionist in consultation with the patient's physician and preferably following discussion with another family member or a close companion of the patient, who can assess motivation and ability of the patient to change or modify his or her eating habits.

The food-energy content of the weight-reducing diet has to be selected. Severe food restriction and semifasting regimens are inappropriate in elderly persons.

Predicted rate of weight loss of sedentary elderly people on diets of

TABLE 10-1   Suggested Desirable Weights for Heights and Ranges for Adult Males and Females

HEIGHT[a]		WEIGHT[b]							
		MEN				WOMEN			
in.	cm	lb		kg		lb		kg	
58	147	—		—		102	(92–119)	46	(42–54)
60	152	—		—		107	(96–125)	49	(44–57)
62	158	123	(112–141)	56	(51–64)	113	(102–131)	51	(46–59)
64	163	130	(118–148)	59	(54–67)	120	(108–138)	55	(49–63)
66	168	136	(124–156)	62	(56–71)	128	(114–146)	58	(52–66)
68	173	145	(132–166)	66	(60–75)	136	(122–154)	62	(55–70)
70	178	154	(140–174)	70	(64–79)	144	(130–163)	65	(59–74)
72	183	162	(148–184)	74	(67–84)	152	(138–173)	69	(63–79)
74	188	171	(156–194)	78	(71–88)	—		—	
76	193	181	(164–204)	82	(74–93)	—		—	

[a]Without shoes.
[b]Without clothes. Average weight ranges in parentheses.

TABLE 10-2   Defining Goal of Weight Loss, Rate of Weight Loss, and Kilocalorie Level of Diets for Sedentary Obese Elderly

1. Obtain measurements of weight and height of patient.
2. Determine, by use of Table 10-1, the "ideal" weight for a person of the individual's sex, height, and age. We will assume the goal of weight reduction is attainment of "ideal" weight.
3. Obtain a 3-day diet record and, from this record, determine the person's current food-energy intake in kcal.
4. Estimate on the basis of the individual's medical needs and food-related behavior whether it is better to recommend loss of 1 or 2 lbs per week.
5. a. To lose 1 lb per week, subtract 500 kcal daily from current intake in kcal.*
   b. To lose 2 lbs per week, subtract 1000 kcal daily from current intake in kcal.
6. Explain to individual or responsible household member or health professional how long it will take for the individual to reach the "ideal" weight without change in activity pattern.

---

*Estimation of kcal reduction is from the following calculation:

1 lb of body fat = 454 gm

1 gm of body fat yields 7.7 kcal

454 gm of body fat yields 454 × 7.7 = 3,496 kcal/lb body fat (3500 kcal)

If 3500 kcal is divided into 7 days, then to reduce 1 lb in body fat per week requires reduction of $\frac{3500}{7}$ = 500 kcal/day.

defined caloric content can be calculated using the information shown in Table 10-2.

Simple menus for use in weight reduction which are planned to provide an adequate intake of nutrients are illustrated in Figures 10-2 and 10-3. By using exchange lists, these menus can be varied.

Further increase in the rate of weight loss could be obtained by increasing energy expenditure through exercise. Appropriate forms of physical activity in a person over 65, who does not have severe cardiac or respiratory disease or other severe physical handicaps, are walking, bicycling, gardening, golf, bowling, and daily exercises. Gradual acclimation to increased physical activity is essential. Individuals using a walker can exercise under supervision.

Individuals who are confined to a wheelchair may also be able to increase their energy expenditure by performing simple exercises which involve arm and head movements. However, the extent to which such exercise can contribute to weight loss in a wheelchair patient is very limited. Exercise plans for the disabled elderly person need to be worked out by a physiatrist or physical therapist who has extensive experience in working with geriatric patients.

Food procurement and food preparation for special diets. Skills in food procurement and preparation in which independently living elderly persons can be instructed include:

Breakfast
  Prune juice, 1/4 cup
  Cereal, fortified, 3/4 cup
  Skim milk, 8 oz.
  Tea

Lunch
  Lean roast beef, 3 oz.
  Carrots, 1/2 cup
  Rice, 1/2 cup
  Fruit (fresh orange), 1 small
  Margarine, 1 tsp.
  Coffee

Dinner
  Cottage cheese, 1/2 cup
  Tomato
  Lettuce
  Whole wheat enriched bread, 1 slice
  Margarine, 1 tsp.

Snack
  Cantaloupe, 1/4 medium
  Skim milk, 8 oz.

For 1200 kcal, add 1 meat, 1 bread, and 1 fat.

FIGURE 10-2
Simple menu for weight reduction (1000 kcal).

FIGURE 10-3
Alternate menu for weight reduction (1000 kcal).

Breakfast
  Orange juice, 1/2 cup
  Cereal, fortified, 3/4 cup
  Skim milk, 8 oz.
  Coffee

Lunch
  Whole wheat enriched bread, 1 slice
  Cottage cheese, 1/2 cup
  Fruit, unsweetened, 1/2 cup
  Margarine, 1 tsp.
  Tea

Dinner
  Tomato juice, 1/2 cup
  Chicken (baked), 3 oz.
  Spinach, 1/2 cup
  Potato, baked, 1 small
  Margarine, 1 tsp.

Snack
  Skim milk, 8 oz.
  Banana, 1/2 small

For 1200 kcal, add 1 meat, 1 bread, and 1 fat.

1. How to obtain transportation to the market
2. How to obtain local information on food stores where assistance may be obtained in carrying bagged groceries to the car
3. How to buy foods that have a high nutrient-to-calorie ratio (Appendix Table 3)
4. How to understand food labeling (It is advised that if the elderly person has a visual impairment, use of a magnifying lens in the market may be helpful.)
5. How and where to procure foods to follow a therapeutic diet, e.g., low-sodium products, and how to determine which foods are appropriate (Appendix Table 4)

Unless sodium restriction is severe (<1000 mg/day), it is rarely necessary to deliberately shop for special low-sodium products, but rather it is necessary to explain high-sodium foods which should be avoided, including instant, dried, and canned soups (unless bearing the label "low sodium"), canned, smoked, and dried fish, sea food (especially if canned), ham, bacon, hot dogs, cold cuts, meat spreads, cheeses unless of the low-sodium varieties, salted snack foods (including nuts), potato chips, crackers, and canned vegetables unless packed in water. For the sodium content of foods, Table 4 in the Appendix should be consulted, and a list of high-sodium foods should be given to the elderly individual. It must be stressed that sodium restriction requires that salt not be added to foods either in cooking or at the table.

When the need is to seek low-sodium staples, then markets supplying low-sodium bread, margarine, and canned goods should be identified.

When elderly people are receiving diuretics, they should usually increase potassium intake. Instructions in food sources rich in potassium should be given, and preconceived notions about bananas or oranges being the only good sources of potassium should be dispelled. Rich food sources of potassium which are also low in sodium are given in Table 4 in the Appendix.

Guidelines on obtaining and preparing low-fat and low-cholesterol diets should be given through explanation of foods to be avoided and through instruction on foods to be selected. Verbal instruction should be supplemented by distribution of short lists of low-fat and low-cholesterol foods as in Table 5 in the Appendix. It must be emphasized that compliance with low-fat diets requires that foods should not be fried or cooked with addition of fat other than that approved by the prescribed diet.

For guidelines on foods and cooking methods which are appropriate to elderly diabetic patients, see section on diabetes in Chapter 8.

It is often important to instruct elderly men and women on good food sources of dietary fiber. In recommending high-fiber foods, it is important to remember that elderly people will often be unable to consume bulky foods or foods that require a lot of chewing.

Kitchens and cooking for the disabled. When elderly persons are physically disabled, special instruction is necessary for modification to be made in the kitchen and in kitchen appliances to make it possible for the person to function alone. Utensils, dishes, glassware, and silverware should be within reach of a person using a walker or wheelchair. Redesign or change in the installation or modification of kitchen cabinets, stovetops, and ovens may be necessary. When the nutritionist is inexperienced in these matters, consultation should be held with the persons or societies having expertise in the rehabilitation of elderly persons following stroke or other chronic diseases associated with long-term and/or permanent handicaps.

Information on meal and food distribution programs. Elderly individuals need also to be given information on locally available meal and food distribution systems, including meal facilities under Title IIIC, Meals-on-Wheels, or local agencies providing low-cost meals. Program eligibility has to be determined on the basis of income, domicile, and age (Pelcovitch, 1972). Elderly persons who are found to be eligible to receive Food Stamps may need assistance in obtaining the Food Stamps from the Department of Social Services. It may be important for the individual to be accompanied to the market, particularly if the food layout in the market is unfamiliar, if assistance is required in food selection, or if guidance is needed on obtaining special foods necessitated by therapeutic diets. Community resources which may provide for the needs of the elderly include Home Help Service, commonly made available through the Public Health Department, as well as home health aides and homemakers working under local agencies.

Explaining prescribed diets. The interpretation of prescribed diets must include:

1. Dietary guidance which imposes the least change in the individual's pattern or food preference
2. Menu planning such that each daily menu includes permitted food and intake of essential nutrients

When dietary history and/or clinical anthropometric, hematological, or biochemical assessment of nutritional status indicates that prior to implementation of the special diet the patient's nutritional status is unsatisfactory, the physician should be consulted about the need for a nutrient supplement.

If a nutrient supplement is prescribed, its composition must be such as to conform with the restriction of the diet. For example, elderly persons who have developed chronic radiation enteritis following x-ray or other radiation treatment of the abdomen for cancer usually need to adhere to a low-lactose diet. In these persons liquid nutrient supplements must also be of the low-lactose type.

Instructions on prevention of gastrointestinal systems. Practical advice on foods which are desirable to prevent GI complaints in the elderly usually has to be combined with gentle but firm dissipation of old wives' tales (e.g., the idea that cheese constipates or that orange juice, and sometimes a wide variety of foods, are "too acid" and therefore to be avoided by the elderly for fear of digestive disorders). It should be taught that common beverages likely to cause heartburn and upper abdominal pain or discomfort are coffee and alcohol. Coffee and alcohol can also potentiate signs of rosacea with flushing of the face and particularly of the nose, which is most marked at certain times of the day and week (i.e., when these beverages are taken in greatest amount or volume). More acute upper right-sided abdominal pain, in a patient with a history of gallbladder disease, is usually caused by intake of fatty foods. Lower abdominal pain with discomfort and gassy diarrhea can be caused by lactose intolerance following radiation therapy to the abdomen or is associated with alcohol abuse. Constipation with attendant abdominal discomfort can be caused by:

1. Intake of a low-fiber (lower residue) diet
2. Failure to consume breakfast or to take a warm early morning beverage which will initiate the gastrocolic reflex
3. Inactivity leading to weakness of the abdominal muscles so that expelling feces from the rectum is difficult

Constipation or self-diagnosed constipation associated with intermittent diarrhea is associated with the irritable bowel syndrome but also with laxative abuse. Constipation per se is also associated with intake of therapeutic drugs which are constipating, particular examples being the narcotic analgesics used to relieve intractable pain such as that associated with metastasis and inoperable cancer which have not responded to chemotherapy or radiation therapy.

Intermittent constipation and diarrhea in the elderly may occur in diverticular disease as well as with mismanagement of the diet, e.g., sudden or irregular change from a low-fiber to a high-fiber diet (hemicellular rich foods) or intake of foods high in lignin, i.e., foods which contain seeds and pips such as strawberries and tomatoes. Diarrhea can be caused by gluten-sensitive enteropathy and inflammatory bowel disease and by lactose intolerance and laxative abuse.

It cannot be overemphasized that in the elderly abdominal symptoms are frequently associated with underlying serious abdominal disease or intake of therapeutic drugs which are necessitated for the control of systemic disease.

Other common causes of abdominal symptoms are abuse of food substances, including coffee and alcohol; abuse of drugs such as laxatives and cathartics; and dietary mismanagement.

Abdominal symptoms, particularly constipation, may be caused by debility and muscle weakness, particularly if the individual has been confined to bed for long periods of time or if wheelchair confinement or obesity give little opportunity or inclination for physical exercise.

The elderly may complain excessively of abdominal symptoms or may relate abdominal symptoms to the types of food consumed or to the methods of cooking (particularly institutional cooking) when in fact no such relationships exist. The nutritionist from whom advice is sought by an elderly person or by another person taking care of the elderly individual should not offer dietary advice unless the cause of the abdominal symptoms has been established by a physician, nurse, or clinician and causes other than diet have been eliminated. Dietary guidelines appropriate to elderly persons with commonly encountered abdominal symptoms are indicated in Table 10-3.

Meals and medication usage. Elderly persons or their attendants need information which can be given by the nutritionist, but the nutritionist must always first consult with the patient's physician and the pharmacist on eating times which will allow optimal absorption of prescribed drugs. For lists of drugs which are better absorbed in the fasting or fed state, the nutritionist should consult Tables 9-1 and 9-2 in Chapter 9.

Modification of eating schedules to promote compliance with therapeutic drug instructions may require a change in mealtimes or advising the individual to take milk and iron-containing foods away from times of drug (e.g., tetracycline) intake. It may also be necessary to discuss with the patient appropriate small snacks to take with drugs to lessen gastric distress. A cracker or rusk may be taken with antibiotics such as tetracycline without impairment of drug absorption.

Combatting fad diets. Elderly persons are attracted by fad diets because of advertisements in magazines and claims made in fad diet books which suggest that adherence to a particular diet will protect the individual from acute or chronic illness, will increase vitality, or will relieve health complaints which are commonly associated with aging. Writers of fad diet

TABLE 10-3   Dietary Guidelines for Elderly Patients with Gastrointestinal Symptoms

All elderly persons with gastrointestinal symptoms or change in bowel function should be examined by a physician to exclude upper GI, colon, and rectal cancer. Dietary guidelines given here are for elderly persons with GI symptoms which are not due to cancer or accompanied by other gastrointestinal pathology requiring surgical or drug therapy.

Indigestion or flatulence. Avoid fruit and fatty food, alcohol, coffee.

Bloating or "Gas." Avoid large meals, boiled or baked beans, and very large volumes of citrus fruit juice.

Constipation. Establish cause. Increase intake of high fiber foods including foods containing cereal brans such as bran breakfast cereals, breads and muffins. Increase intake of carrots, squash, celery, and leafy green vegetables as well as fruits including apples and apple sauce. Drink one (4 oz.) glass of prune juice per day. Drink warm beverages on arising each morning at breakfast and make a regular visit to the toilet thereafter.

Diarrhea. Establish cause. If due to chronic radiation enteritis with nonreversible malabsorption and lactose intolerance, omit milk and substitute other high-calcium foods. Decrease fat intake. If due to gluten-sensitive enteropathy, omit breads and other foods containing gluten.

books may also advocate intake of "health foods" or megadoses of nutrients, including amino acids such as lysine, sugars such as fructose, vitamins, minerals, and trace elements. Nutritionists working with the elderly should be familiar with current fad diet literature and should be able to point out to their elderly clients the fallacies and dangers of the fad diet regimen which has attracted interest or is being followed. High-protein, high-fat diets impose special health risks in elderly persons whose hepatic, pancreatic, or renal function is impaired. Complications arising from intake of these diets include liver failure (high protein), acute pancreatitis (high fat), and renal failure (high protein). Weight-reducing diets which suggest an intake of soups and bouillon high in sodium can precipitate congestive heart failure.

Counseling on avoidance of fad diets requires that the nutritionist gain the complete confidence of the elderly client and that a rational alternative diet be provided which will ameliorate or modify health problems from which the person is seeking relief. In the event that a fad diet is being followed as an alternative measure to proper medical care, the elderly person should be assisted in obtaining primary health care from a family physician or, if appropriate, from a medical specialist.

Need for socialization at mealtime. Loneliness is a very common problem among elderly persons. Contributory causes are loss by death, institutionalization of or separation from spouse or long-term companion, breakdown of family ties, lack of participation in social organizations such as senior citizens or church groups, lack of transportation, eccentricity, physical disability, depression, and insensitivity of younger persons (including care givers) to the special needs of older people.

The nutritionist can help to relieve loneliness in elderly clients or patients by giving advice on congregate meal sites for independently living persons. Home-delivered meals' clients have the special opportunity for conversation with the delivery persons for these frail elderly. Elderly patients in nursing homes should be encouraged to eat their meals with other patients in a communal dining room, in a group in the recreation area, or around the nursing station. When elderly persons have organic brain syndromes and are likely to disturb other patients having their meals by making noise or by unattractive eating habits, it is often possible to find patients with similar problems to eat together. Socialization at mealtimes for patients in nursing homes requires establishment of specific, stepwise goals in the patient care plan, whereby the withdrawn individual is encouraged both by the nutritionist and/or the dietitian, by the nurse, and by the social worker to gradually accept the presence of other patients during eating times, to take pride in his or her personal appearance when at meals with others, to learn to enjoy interchange of conversation or words with other patients, and to make friends.

Combating alcohol abuse. Alcohol abuse is a problem in the elderly as in younger age groups. Nutritionists have special opportunities to identify the problem, to counsel clients on temperance, and to initiate referral to alcoholism counseling services. Alcohol abuse is indicated by observation of liquor, beer, or wine bottle in the home, particularly in unusual places such as in arm chairs, at the back of the sofa, or at the bedside; by dietary history indicating a high level of daily intake or binge drinking; by admitted intake of single or multiple medications containing alcohol; by history of alcoholism or hospitalization for alcohol-related diseases; by erratic or unusual behavior suggesting inebriation during visits by the nutritionist or nutrition aide; by a history of blackouts or frequent falls; or by impairment of nutritional status which fails to respond to changing diet or administration of nutrient supplements.

Nutrition counseling for elderly alcoholics cannot be successful unless the patient becomes abstinent through medical supervision, alcoholism counseling, or use of an alcohol-aversive drug. Use of an alcohol-aversive drug (disulfiram [Antabuse]) may be hazardous for elderly persons who have severe impairment of liver function or who are receiving interactive drugs. When abstinence is achieved, alcoholics will often crave sweet foods and may eat a diet low in essential nutrients although adequate in calories. The nutritionist counseling such a patient should develop menu plans which encourage use of foods that are high in essential nutrients. Milk may not be tolerated by newly abstinent elderly alcoholics who are lactose intolerant. Restricted protein intake is necessary for elderly alcoholics with liver disease, and fat restriction is necessary for patients with alcoholic pancreatitis. Restriction of sodium intake is necessary for cirrhotic patients with ascites (Roe, 1979).

Nutrition counseling for the alcoholic must be preceded by consultation between the nutritionist and the patient's physician. Diets must be prescribed by a physician, and it is the nutritionist's responsibility to promote dietary compliance.

Advice on nutrient supplements. The administration of specific vitamin and/or mineral supplements should be based on need defined by clinical and biochemical assessment of nutritional status. However, all nutritionists should be fully aware that alcohol excess produces damage to the liver, bone marrow, and brain which increases the requirements for B vitamins, including riboflavin, folacin, vitamins B_6 and B_{12}, and thiamin. Although diets high in these vitamins should be recommended to all elderly patients who have had a recent or long-term history of alcohol abuse, therapeutic doses of folic acid should *not* be recommended until pernicious anemia has been excluded, and thiamin needs to avoid alcoholic brain damage (Korsakoff's psychosis) must be either determined on the basis of biochemical tests (erythrocyte transketolase assay) or may be derived form standard recommendations for amount of the vitamin required. The experienced clinical nutritionist will often be the member of the health care team who can best emphasize to the physician the urgent need for high doses of parenteral thiamin for the elderly alcoholic who has been subsisting on a semistarvation diet. Pharmacological doses of thiamin given intravenously by the physician to these patients is prophylaxis against development of the permanent brain damage associated with Korsakoff's psychosis.

Food budgeting. Intake of an inadequate diet by elderly people may be related to the high prices of foods which are thought to be most nutritious. Elderly people who are conservative in their food habits need encouragement by a nutritionist to use cheaper foods which are alternate sources of essential nutrients but are seldom used because of unfamiliarity or prejudice. Food likes and dislikes must be carefully assessed before meal planning to increase the chance of dietary compliance.

FOOD-SHOPPING ASSISTANCE

Shopping assistance programs have been developed in many communities to assist the homebound elderly, as well as elderly without adequate means of transportation and without family or friends, to obtain their groceries. Staffing of these programs may be by volunteers, including retirees, or by paid shopping aides. For these programs to be useful in improving food access to seniors, and to avoid financial dishonesty on the part of the aides, it is necessary that these programs be under the management of the local office for aging.

COMMUNITY FEEDING PROGRAMS FOR THE ELDERLY IN THE UNITED STATES; TITLE IIIC PROGRAMS

In 1973 the Congress of the United States first appropriated monies to establish a feeding program for the elderly on a national basis. The Nutrition Program for Older Americans (NPOA) was mandated by the 1972 Title VII Amendment to the Older Americans Act of 1965. The Director of the Commission on Aging of the Administration on Aging (AoA) within the Department of Health, Education, and Welfare was empowered to administer the Title VII program through AoA in consultation with other departments of the federal government. AoA is divided into ten regional offices, each containing three to eight states. The regional offices must review and approve the annual operating plans of states and territories in their regions and carry the responsibility for providing assistance to state offices on aging for development of their Title VII plans. The State Agencies on Aging are responsible for producing operating plans to carry out the Title VII program in accordance with federal goals and guidelines. The State Agencies award funds to local projects.

From the annual appropriation, Title VII funds were made available to 50 states and to the District of Columbia, Guam, American Samoa, the Virgin Islands, and the Trust Territories of the Pacific Islands. The funds that were made available supported up to 90 percent of the cost of development and implementation of the Title VII program.

State Agencies were responsible for:

1. Identifying eligible target groups among the elderly in the state and approving projects serving these individuals

2. Establishing a minimal project size for effective program implementation
3. Approving local project plans and awarding of Title VII grants
4. Monitoring and evaluating the program
5. Reviewing project menus

Community-based meals are now provided under the Title IIIC program, whereas formerly community-based meals were under Title VII. Meals are served to people over 60 years of age. Congregate meals, which constitute most of the meals served, are made available at Title IIIC sites, which may be senior citizens centers, religious facilities, schools, public housing, restaurants, or community centers. Local nutrition projects under the County Offices of the Aging are responsible, under the State Agency or Area Agency, for delivery of services. Local community projects have some professional administrative staff and direct providers of services, including dietitians, nurses, and social workers, and nonprofessional paid staff and volunteers. Paid staff are assisted by volunteers in the provision and delivery of congregate and home-delivered meals.

Local goals of the Title IIIC program administrative staffs are:

1. To establish nutrition projects that serve at least one hot meal a day for the elderly in congregate meal settings and by home delivery
2. To assure that the meal provided includes a minimum of one third of the RDA
3. To serve individuals 60 years of age or older who may not eat adequately either because they cannot afford to do so, because they do not have the requisite skills to purchase and prepare nourishing meals, because they have limited mobility, or because they do not have the motivation to prepare meals. (Persons having these characteristics, as well as minority individuals, are "target" groups.)
4. To set up feeding sites as close to the eligible individuals as possible and to furnish transportation to the sites
5. To encourage participation of target groups
6. To provide special menus to meet special dietary needs which may be related to health problems, religious beliefs, or ethnic preference
7. To provide health and welfare counseling and nutrition education
8. To provide training to paid staff and volunteers who are purchasing, preparing, transporting, and serving meals
9. To give staffing preferences to persons 60 years of age or older
10. To undertake program evaluation

There is no cost for meals, but individuals may make a voluntary contribution. There is no test of eligibility by income. Main meals that are delivered to homes are the same or similar to those served at the congregate sites.* An additional light meal consisting of a sandwich, a piece of fruit, and milk may be packed with the hot meal and delivered to provide food for supper.

*Meals-on-Wheels is a separate program under the auspices of local volunteer groups.

In most Title IIIC programs the aim is to provide five hot meals per week. Weekend meals may be delivered to the home in some sites.

Local, state, and federal goals in program evaluation are to examine program inputs and outputs in relation to effects and benefits of the Title IIIC program. Program inputs include food, funds, staff, equipment, program consultants, and technical equipment. Program outputs include meals, transportation, outreach, referral services, nutrition education, counseling, and escort services. Effects which may be examined include program satisfaction, availability of services, target group of elderly persons served, and financial savings for participants. Long-term benefits which may be evaluated are the improved health and nutritional status of those served, an improvement in mental and social well-being, and maintenance of an independent lifestyle.

Program evaluations have shown that the major positive effects are increased socialization and improved life satisfaction of participants. Participants have also found that their food bills have been reduced. Diet, nutrition, and health benefits have varied. In several studies it has been shown that the diet of participants has a higher nutrient content than the diet of nonparticipants. Criticism of the program by participants has included dissatisfaction with Title IIIC meals. Elderly persons expressing satisfaction with the programs have also reported the most benefits (Posner, 1979).

Nonparticipation in the Title IIIC program by eligible persons may reflect an ability to cope with food purchase and preparation, the provision of meals by family members or others, or a disinterest in eating and health.

Several experimental programs have been undertaken by Area Agencies on Aging. These have been designed to cover unmet nutritional needs of the elderly or to assist those who have not been reached by the regular Title IIIC program (Watkin, 1977).

In 1984 the Supplemental Nutrition Assistance Program was initiated in New York State. Funded through the New York State Department of Health and administered by the State Office for Aging, this program provides home-delivered meals to homebound elderly who are deemed eligible but are not provided for by the Title IIIC program. Goals of this program, in addition to provision of meals, are to employ nutritional surveillance methods to estimate the unmet need of the frail elderly for access to food, for nutrition-related services, and for health services necessary to the prevention of diet-related diseases and their complications (Roe, 1985).

EMERGENCY FOOD SERVICES

Emergency food services include soup kitchens, food pantries (food banks), and the distribution of free foods derived from food surplus stores. In general these programs are not targeted to meet the needs of the elderly but rather to provide for indigent and homeless people irrespective of their age. No attempt is made by these services to provide diets that would be appropriate for seniors with diet-related diseases (Chan et al., 1990).

COMBATING DIET-RELATED DISEASE

In order to combat diet-related disease, screening programs are available, including hypertension and cholesterol screening. Pamphlets provide information on ways to reduce the risk of hypertension and coronary heart disease, and are usually available in the screening clinics.

Ingredient and nutrition labeling of foods, as well as health messages on food packages, can assist elderly in making wise food purchases. However, misleading health messages can be harmful, especially if unreasonable claims are made about the ability of special foods to prevent or cure geriatric diseases. The Food and Drug Administration plays an important role in controlling food manufacturers' claims about their products (Pennington, 1989).

DIETETIC SERVICES IN NURSING HOMES IN THE UNITED STATES

The Social Security Amendments of 1972 (P. L. 92-603) require the development of uniform dietetic standards of all skilled nursing facilities. Standards are mandated for facilities certified under Medicare and Medicaid (Social Security Administration, 1974). These standards pertain to (1) staffing, (2) menus and nutritional adequacy, (3) therapeutic diets, (4) preparation and service of foods, (5) hygiene of staff, and (6) sanitary conditions.

Staffing

A full-time dietetic service supervisor must be employed. This person must either be a qualified dietitian, a graduate of a dietetic technicians program or a dietetic assistant training program approved by The American Dietetic Association, or a graduate of a state-approved course of instruction in food service management and have had experience as a supervisor in a health care or military facility. If the dietetic service supervisor is a food service manager, then consultation must be provided by a qualified dietitian. If the supervisor of dietetic services is not a dietitian, then consultant visits are supposed to be of sufficient duration and frequency to meet the dietetic needs of the facility.

Menus and Nutritional Adequacy

Menus need to be planned and followed based on physicians' orders to meet the nutritional needs of patients. The RDA are to be followed to the extent that it is medically possible. All menus are to be approved by the full-time or consultant dietitian.

Therapeutic Diets

Therapeutic diets are to be prescribed by the physician. Special therapeutic menus must be planned in writing and prepared and served as ordered with supervision by the dietitian or in consultation with the dietitian. An up-to-date diet manual, approved by the dietitian, must be available to the attending physician, nursing staff, and dietetic personnel in the facility.

Preparation and Service of Food

At least three meals or their equivalent must be served daily, at regular hours, with not more than 14 hours between a substantial evening meal and breakfast.

To the extent that it is medically possible, bedtime nourishments are to be offered to all patients.

Foods are to be prepared by methods that conserve nutritive value, flavor, and appearance and be attractively served at the proper temperatures and in a form to meet individual needs. If a patient refuses food served, appropriate substitutes of similar nutritive value are to be served.

Hygiene of Staff

Dietetic service personnel are to be free of communicable disease. They must practice hygienic food-handling techniques.

In the event that food service employees are assigned duties outside the dietetic service, these duties must not interfere with the sanitation, safety, or time required for dietetic work assignments.

Sanitary Conditions

Food must be procured from sources approved or considered satisfactory by federal, state, or local authorities. Food must also be stored, prepared, distributed, and served under sanitary conditions. Waste must be disposed of properly.

Written reports of inspections by state and local health authorities must be kept on file at the facility, with notations made of action taken by the facility to comply with any recommendations.

Conditions for participation of skilled nursing homes under Medicare and Medicaid which apply to physicians' and nurses' services also pertain to the nutritional care of patients. Each patient's total program of care must be reviewed by the attending physician and/or medical director of the facility at least once every 30 days or more often as required for the first 90 days. The total program of care includes dietary orders which must be reviewed by the physician and decisions made as to whether the orders should be continued, changed, or discontinued according to the patient's needs. Dietary needs of each patient are to be identified with the assistance of the dietitian.

Nursing personnel are required to gain awareness of the nutritional needs of the patients. Nurses must also monitor and record the food and fluid intake of patients. They are further required to assist patients with their meals whenever such help is needed. It is expected that a close liaison will be established between physicians, nurses, and dietary service personnel in skilled nursing homes.

State guidelines for dietary services as well as medical and nursing services relating to the nutritional care of patients in skilled nursing homes are generally similar to federal guidelines. Intermediate care homes which may be designated "health-related" must comply with the 1974 federal standards to be certified and to participate in Medicare and Medicaid. Domiciliary care facilities (also known as personal care homes), residential care facilities for adults, and rest homes are not covered by the federal or state standards set for skilled nursing and intermediate care homes. Guidelines for the management of their food service operations are set by state departments of social services.

Responsibilities of the operator or administrator of skilled nursing homes relating to dietary services are as follows:

1. To organize and administer the dietetic service
2. To integrate the dietetic service into administrative and patient care services and assure that the dietetic service is represented on all committees whose work affects dietetic service operations and provision of nutritional services
3. To maintain records of diet orders and changes, nutritional care plans, and nutrition counseling afforded to patients
4. To develop a monitoring system that provides for "appropriate and timely review" of the nutritional care provided to all patients
5. To prepare patients for discharge by providing information and methods to the patient to manage his or her own nutritional care or by transferring appropriate information to another agency or facility for continuity of care
6. To furnish evidence that sufficient and appropriate foods have been purchased, prepared, and served to patients and to maintain such records for 1 year
7. To ensure that the dietetic service select food and drink and prepare menus with regard to the cultural background and food habits of patients and that they write and date menus and keep records of general and therapeutic diets
8. To provide a dining room area equipped and arranged for regular use by all patients who can get there unaided or come assisted for regularly scheduled meals
9. To maintain a file on specifications and maintenance for all major and fixed dietetic service equipment
10. To provide the dietary service with sufficient and suitable space and equipment to ensure efficient sanitary operation of all required functions
11. To assure that all employees, including those in the dietetic service, maintain personal cleanliness and hygiene
12. To maintain the following records for the dietary service:
    a. A plan for organization, management, and day-to-day operations
    b. A master plan and weekly work schedules for staffing
    c. The name, qualifications, and terms of agreement with the dietitian
    d. A current diet manual

The standards of the Joint Commission on Accreditation of Extended Care Facilities also require that pertinent information on each patient should be assembled and the short- and long-term goals should be established. Discharge plans must also be formulated.

Patient care and discharge plans should include nutritional components. It is the duty of the dietitian to assemble information from the physician, nurses, and social workers which may relate to the patient's nutrition. The dietitian and physician together should make a nutritional assessment of each patient and determine nutritional needs (Treadwell, 1974).

Patient care plans are the joint responsibility of the health team in long-term care facilities, including skilled nursing homes and intermediate care homes. The health team includes the medical director and/or the attending physician, the nurse directly responsible for the care of the particular patient, the social worker, and, in some instances, other health professionals such as physical therapist and an occupational therapist. At weekly meetings within the facility, at which patient care plans are developed and reviewed, the administrator of the facility is usually also present.

The nutrition component of the patient care plan is developed by the dietitian. It must be integrated into the total patient care plan. Goals must be set by each team member. These nutritional goals include:

1. Providing each patient with food of sufficient energy and nutrient content to meet his or her needs
2. Evaluating change in the nutritional and health status of the patient in response to general or therapeutic diets
3. Retraining the patient to feed himself or herself
4. Increasing socialization at eating times
5. Responding to the patient's food-related concerns

Plans must be developed which detail procedures by which these goals can be accomplished. The procedures are then implemented insofar as this is feasible in a sequential manner. Evaluation of progress in meeting the nutritional goals is a primary responsibility of the dietitian, but other members of the health team may well contribute. For example, the nurse will be able to provide records of the patient's food intake and body weight and the physician will have reports on blood counts and a biochemical profile which should include screening tests of nutritional status. If the dietitian is employed on a consultant basis, then the supervisor of the dietetic service, whether a food service manager or a dietetic technician, must evaluate progress when the dietitian is absent. Actual consumption of food and beverages by the patient should be monitored.

Modification in nutritional care plans must be undertaken to deal with the following conditions:

1. Patient refusal to eat or dislike of the diet
2. Physical signs and laboratory test results indicating unwanted change in nutritional and/or health status
3. Identification of special or newly present nutritional needs relating to poor appetite, disease, or medications
4. Special behavioral problems

When the patient is ready for discharge or is to be sent to another facility offering a higher or lower level of care, nutrition discharge plans made by the dietitian should include guidelines for the person(s) who will be undertaking the care of the patient or instructions to the patient, if the patient will be caring for himself or herself, relating to diet, food preparation, appetite, eating problems, and more recent nutritional assessment.

Problems Relating to Nutritional Care of Patients in Skilled Nursing Homes

Dietetic services are inadequate when:

1. The dietetic service supervisor is not a dietitian.
2. Standards for nutritional adequacy of menus are not followed.
3. Presented therapeutic diets are not followed.
4. Meals are badly cooked and/or served.
5. Food-borne infection occurs because nutrition staff does not follow hygienic food-handling practices.

Nursing service is inadequate when:

1. Food and beverage intake is not monitored or not monitored regularly.
2. Patients are not weighed.
3. Patients are not assisted in feeding themselves.

Physician service is inadequate when:

1. The physician is ignorant of the nutritional needs of patients.
2. The physician prescribes an inappropriate therapeutic diet.
3. The attending physician rarely sees the patient.
4. An assessment of nutritional status is not carried out.

Team problems include:

1. Inadequate concern for the patient.
2. The desire to meet standards only to pass federal or state inspection.

QUALITY ASSURANCE

The quality of home-delivered meals service programs is monitored when county health departments inspect the site of nutrition kitchens to determine if food storage and preparation meet local standards for food safety and to see if staff are following basic health guidelines to avoid food-borne disease. Monitorings and surveillances of the home-delivered meals systems to assess whether or not the most nutritionally needy elderly are being served are not routinely carried out. Surveys of federal and state congregate and home-delivered meals services have found that poorer services (such as less weekday meals, no weekend meals, and no provision of special diets) are provided in poorer areas. This may be explained by the fact that in these areas it is more difficult to raise money from private donors to supplement the budget provided to the nutrition programs from Title IIIC funds or state funds.

Other issues that degrade the coverage of the nutritional needs of the frail elderly include a local program policy to serve those who are closest or most accessible to the delivery route. State agency administrators and local program directors may explain that geographically isolated seniors may be unserved as a matter of budgetary constraint. Other reasons may include staffing problems and problems in the modification of food delivery routes in order to better reach those who are most isolated (Roe, 1990).

Maintenance of the quality of nutritional services for the elderly is a major problem both in the community and in nursing homes. Regulatory procedures are used by state health departments and federal agencies to ensure the compliance of nursing homes with state codes and national standards of nutritional care and health care.

Quality assurance methods are also used to examine whether or not nursing home services meet Medicare and Medicaid standards. Through nutritional service audits there are regular systematic screenings to uncover problems, as seen in New York State's Sentinal Events system. Care modalities of nutritional importance examined through this system include the appropriateness or otherwise of special diet prescription, the indications used for the prescription of vitamins, the documentation of nutritional assessment, the quality of food services, and patient morale. Data is collected from patient records, staff interviews, and inspections by audit teams. Reports are then sent to the nursing homes that contain the identification of specific problems and recommendations for corrective action. Follow-up studies are conducted to examine whether or not the deficiencies have been corrected (Zimmer, 1989).

THE ROLES AND TASKS OF THE DIETITIAN IN GERIATRIC PRACTICE

I. The work of the dietitian in the community.
    Dietitians working with seniors in the community may be on the staff of a federal or state nutrition program for the elderly or may be in private practice. The dietitians' responsibilities in these two different work situations differ though to some extent their roles overlap. Major activities and responsibilities of public sector and private sector dietitians need to be understood for purposes of work success and efficiency.
    A. Dietitians working with nutrition programs.
        When working with a nutrition program, the dietitian usually has three types of work responsibility. First, the dietitian may be responsible for providing group nutrition education for seniors at attending congregate meal sites. In this role, it is important for the dietitian to first gauge the audience's views and expectations about what they want to learn and what they expect from their learning opportunity. Identification of their concerns can be carried out through use of focus groups (Crockett et al., 1990).

The dietitian is more commonly responsible for assessing the need of seniors for home delivered meals and for reassessing their need for these meals at stipulated time intervals. Assessment of need for home delivered meals requires that following referral to the program by a hospital discharge worker, a family physician, a public health nurse, a family member, or after self-application, the senior is visited to find out if he or she meets the eligibility criteria of age and being confined to the home. Low socioeconomic status usually increases the priority for meals (Cass, Ryan, and Bower, 1989). Other factors which need to be considered in defining priority status for elderly to receive home delivered meals include inability to cook, lack of an informal or a formal caregiver available to assist in food preparation, and a report by the senior that he or she has less than 7 hot meals a week or goes days without food. Other purposes of this assessment are also to determine need for a special diet and also the need for nutrition counselling.

Whereas other nutrition program staff may carry out assessments of referred clients, the unique role of the dietitian, relative to homebound elderly, consists of providing in-home nutrition counseling. Skills required in order to conduct effective nutrition counseling with homebound seniors include the following:

1. Interviewing skills.

    a) To be able to elicit information on the factors which determine the usual food habits of the senior. The dietitian needs to discuss use of high salt or high fat ethnic foods, which may be preferred even if a low salt or low fat diet has been prescribed (Chau et al., 1990).

    b) To be able to obtain information on the barriers which the senior may have in assimilating new diet information. These include deafness and impaired vision if the information is in written form.

    c) To be able to assess the practical problems the senior may have in making dietary changes or indeed in the whole arena of problems with food selection, food purchase, and food preparation. These include loss of mobility and loss of manual dexterity.

2. Observational skills.

    a) To be able to observe the senior in his or her home and to note disabilities present which may make food preparation difficult or hazardous. These include upper arm disabilities which make it difficult to turn the stove on and off and prevent use of the wrists to open jars and cans. These also include lower limb disabilities which make standing at the stove difficult or impossible. The degree of visual impairment should be observed in a practical sense to check whether the senior would be able to tell when the stove is on. Further, to observe the extent of mental confusion and to see whether it fluctuates in such a way that the senior might become unaware of how to turn stove burners on and off.

    b) To be able to observe informal and formal caregivers, the extent of their assistance with food preparation, and their skills in preparing a regular or therapeutic diet.

    c) To observe the home including the state of cleanliness, the kitchen facilities, whether or not the kitchen appliances work, and the food storage arrangements. The dietitian should note whether or not food is left around at room temperature at inappropriate times. The contents of the icebox, including whether outdated and inedible foods are present should also be investigated.

The geriatric dietitian who has responsibility for seniors in the community must be prepared not only to make frequent home visits but also to observe changes in the actual ability of the senior to prepare food, to open food and beverage containers, to cut food, and to eat independently. Changes in formal caregivers, such as the appearance of a new and unskilled home attendant, must also be assessed. It is essential that this new person's limited cooking skills be determined by direct observation. Furthermore, the dietitian should be on the alert for evidence that the home attendant or even family members may be consuming food intended for a frail elder.

3. Counseling and teaching skills.
   Nutritional counseling and teaching skills include:

   a) The ability to provide new nutrition information to the senior in an understandable and acceptable manner. In a survey of the sources of nutrition information which the elderly commonly use, dietitians and health food stores were mentioned second to physicians (Probart et al., 1989). Therefore, there is a challenge for the dietitian to provide seniors with information about their real nutritional concerns rather than those who are less familiar with their nutritional requirements.

   b) The dietitian should have the ability to explain not only desirable diet changes but also to describe why these are required. An example of a desirable diet change which may have to be explained and justified to a senior includes changing from whole milk to low fat milk consumption. However, the desired change may be more complex and may require exclusion of certain favorite foods which are too high in fat or salt. Such a need for change must be explained in terms of the health benefit.

   c) The dietitian must have the ability to convert the dietary changes into the practical terms of actual foods which are usually consumed by the senior. If the senior is being advised to make dietary changes, these must not be unrealistic given the senior's culture of origin, living conditions, health status, and possible denial of the need for change.

   d) The dietitian must be able to interpret therapeutic diets. The noon meal may be supplied by the nutrition program as a special diet and in some nutrition programs, the evening meal is also prepared to meet the special diet specification. Nevertheless, the dietitian is responsible for explaining the appropriate frequency of meals and snacks on the diet, for interpreting the times medications should be taken in relation to these meals, and for describing what foods are appropriate for breakfast.

4. Follow up and evaluation.

   a) The dietitian working with the nutrition program needs to determine whether advice to the homebound seniors has been understood and is being implemented. Verbal assurance that the necessary dietary changes have been made may reflect the senior's desire to please the dietitian rather than tell the truth. Furthermore, exaggerated claims of sudden use of "health foods" suggests confabulation, i.e., that the information is fabricated. The more convincing evidence of dietary change includes actual observation of the senior eating these foods.

B. Geriatric dietitians in private practice.

Dietitians in private practice, who are working with seniors, are in the role of consultants. They are usually called upon to give diet advice by the senior or by a family member. The dietitian may be asked to assess the nutritional quality of the diet currently being consumed or may be required to answer such questions as whether or not the senior should take vitamin supplements or eat some particular food which has been extolled by the media. Additionally, the dietitian may be asked to explain or assist the senior in the selection of foods to meet a diet prescription.

In order to work effectively with their older clients, these dietitians must seek out the underlying reason for the consultation. Caution is needed by the dietitian because the senior may be seeking a magic diet which will cure a chronic disease such as cancer or which will provide assurance of health and increased longevity. The dietitian must disclaim the ability to provide cures and change of destiny.

In order to effectively fulfill the various roles of a nutrition counselor to the elderly in the community, it is important for the dietitian to understand the cultural, social, economic, and medical factors which explain the eating habits of the older adult. Dietitians may consider themselves uniquely capable of finding out why seniors have particular food patterns, why seniors avoid certain foods which they have been advised to eat, and why seniors want to take high potency vitamin pills. The dietitian should have professional training in obtaining such information, but the dietitian of today needs to understand that anthropologists are also trained to find out the factors which determine eating patterns. Indeed, dietitians should not only recognize that anthropologists have this skill but should learn how these social scientists approach the problem of eliciting diet information from seniors using both the traditional methods of the ethnographer and recently developed rapid assessment methods (Scrimshaw and Hurtado, 1987). Social scientists, skilled in ethnography, utilize direct and participatory observation as well as interviews to better understand their respondents' beliefs, attitudes, and habits (Fetterman, 1989). It is advocated that geriatric dietitians use these same approaches which decrease the risk that nutritional counselling will be ineffective. Other essential knowledge for dietitians working with minority seniors living in their own homes is the diversity of their respondents' health beliefs and cultural practices (Johnson et al., 1990). Acceptance of the dietitians' advice depends on whether or not the advice given is more compelling than the advice concurrently being given by family, friends, and the media. In order to understand the client's acceptance or refusal of dietary advice, the dietitian needs to understand that the client has a deep rooted system of beliefs about lifestyle changes. Furthermore, these beliefs may be overlaid a recent depression which decreases the ability of the senior to make the choice for a change in their diet in the desirable direction.

II. Work of the dietitian with geriatric patients in acute care hospitals.
Geriatric patients in acute care hospitals include those admitted from their
own homes and those admitted from nursing homes. The dietitian working
with these patients is required to make assessments of their nutritional needs
at the time of admission and at frequent intervals thereafter. A particular goal
of the dietitian is to prevent malnutrition due to dietary insufficiency, disease
related problems, and drugs. The dietitian will assist patients to make appropriate food choices from the hospital menu. As a member of the hospital's
nutrition team, the dietitian is also responsible for monitoring the fluid,
calorie and nutrient intake of patients whether they are eating normally or
receiving enteral or total parenteral nutritional support.

III. Work of the dietitian in long-term care facilities.
The dietitian working in a long-term care facility has to prepare menus and
supervise food preparation for patients on regular and special diets including
diets of modified consistency. The dietitian is responsible for assessing the
nutritional needs of patients on admission and thereafter at monthly or more
frequent intervals. The responsibilities also include counselling patients with
chronic diet related diseases such as diabetes about diet compliance. Further,
the dietitian usually works closely with the nursing staff in the management of
patients on tube-feeding regimens. In this task, the dietitian's particular
function is to monitor the fluid, calorie and nutrient intakes of these patients.
Additional duties of the dietitian in the nursing home include presiding over
the patients' council on which they have the opportunity to make their food
likes and dislikes known. Institutional diet changes recommended by the
patients may then be made by the dietitian given that these would not
contribute to nutritional risk for those on special diets. The dietitian has to
maintain the federal and state standards for dietary care of nursing home
patients and today is also usually required to work with physicians and with
the pharmacist to minimize the risk of drug-nutrient interactions.
The Omnibus Budget Reconciliation Act of 1987 (OBRA 87) requires that
skilled nursing facilities and intermediate care facilities maintain quality assessment and assurance committees (Herbelin, 1989). Each committee has to
meet at least quarterly to discuss quality assessment and assurance issues.
Plans must be developed by the staff to correct previous deficiencies in the
quality of care. Responsibility for the quality assessment and assurance plans
for dietary services rests on the dietitian(s) and the food service supervisor.
It is expected that the geriatric dietitian monitor patients' weight and make a
concerted effort to maintain the patients' weight within their appropriate
weight for stature range. The dietitian (or the food service supervisor) has the
responsibility of documenting nutrition interventions which are implemented
for all patients who have lost or gained weight. Furthermore, the dietitian
must make weekly evaluations of the response to the nutrition interventions
and if these interventions are not effective they must be modified and documented once again.

STUDENT GUIDE TO NUTRITION EDUCATION PROGRAMS FOR THE ELDERLY

Nutrition education programs require a definition of overall goals as well
as a specific goal. One must consider the motives of the person presenting
the program, learn about the characteristics of the audience, develop the

program, and decide on the means of evaluation of the program, program production, and results of the program.

Define Your Goals

What are you trying to do?

1. To provide nutrition information in response to the requests of elderly people in the community
2. To give dietary counseling in response to patient wishes or in response to requests by a physician or nurse
3. To expand the nutrition knowledge of public health or home health aides having responsibility for the care of the homebound elderly
4. To teach food service personnel or other staffs of the geriatric facility the nutritional value of food, the nutritional requirements of the elderly, meals which will meet nutritional needs, and skills which will facilitate interpersonal relationships with the residents
5. To give individual counseling to the elderly on special diets
6. To help elderly people spend their food dollars wisely
7. To explain food labeling
8. To talk in lay terms to elderly people who are captive audiences (e.g., in congregate meal sites) about nutrition topics which may be relevant to their health (e.g., the dangers of high-sodium foods, drug-nutrient interactions)

Consider Your Motives

Why are you concerned with the development of a nutrition education program for the elderly? Motives could be:

1. To provide nutrition information to those elderly who seek it
2. To give information on nutrition to those elderly you think would benefit
3. To change the attitudes of geriatric caregivers to nutrition
4. To improve the quality of the diet for geriatric patients
5. To change the food habits of the elderly
6. To entertain groups of elderly people
7. To fulfill a class requirement

Find Out About Your Audience

1. Who are they?
2. What are their food-related or nutrition problems?
3. Where are they going to be when you make your presentation?
4. What is their attention span likely to be?
5. Are they visually impaired?
6. How long can they stay at your presentation(s)?
7. Will the audience really come to hear you, or are they present for other primary purposes?

8. Are they likely to find a selected topic(s) relevant and interesting?
9. What is their educational level?
10. Will you be speaking to the same audience each time you give a talk?
11. Is the audience hearing impaired so that you will need a microphone?
12. What means will you have for determining your audience's immediate response to your presentation and whether you have fulfilled your goal?

Develop Your Program

Bearing in mind your goals and motives, are they justified and appropriate to your audience?

Example of a Nutrition Education Program for Senior Citizens

Stimulus. A request has come from a senior citizens group for a nutritionist (or nutrition student) to talk to them for 1 hour about their need for B vitamins and how they can get these vitamins from their food.

Goal. Your goal is to respond to this request. Your motive is to fulfill a class requirement. The projected audience will consist of approximately 50 women and men between the ages of 65 and 86. None of these persons are likely to be blind, but about 50 percent are visually impaired and 50 percent have hearing problems. All have at least a high school education.

The facility provided is a large, well-lit room which has a screen and a slide projector with a carousel. There is an overhead projector and a microphone.

Program plan. Handouts should include:

1. A pamphlet describing the functions of essential B vitamins written in lay language and produced in large print
2. Charts showing food sources rich in B vitamins, preferably multicolored bar graphs

Pretest and post-test questionnaires should be developed:

1. *Pretest.* A pretest quiz should be given to the audience to find out if they know what B vitamins there are, what foods are good sources of these vitamins, and why these vitamins are needed for good health.
2. *Post-test.* Questionnaires should be developed before the program to evaluate whether the audience has learned the nutrition information and to determine their overall responses to the program.

Lecture and time frame. A 30-minute lecture is given, illustrated with slides which show elderly people eating foods containing rich sources of B vitamins. Functions of these vitamins, their food sources, and the requirements of the elderly for the major B vitamins (thiamin, folate, riboflavin, niacin, vitamin B_6, and vitamin B_{12}) are emphasized.

The overhead projector is used to show transparencies on which there are large, clearly drawn diagrams of foods which are rich sources of these vitamins. The microphone is used throughout the presentation so that those in the audience with moderate hearing impairment can hear the presentation.

A 10-minute question period follows. Questions are requested from the audience. The speaker should repeat the question asked, using the microphone. Discussion is encouraged, and the speaker should be prepared to clear up misunderstandings.

After the lecture, a second quiz is given to find out if the audience has taken in the message and if they thought the talk was interesting, clear, and useful. For each of these ratings, a scale should be used. Rating should also be requested for the audiovisual materials used.

Program record. Record forms should be prepared and used by the speaker or by an assistant present at the lecture, on which the following information can be tabulated:

1. The number of people present at the program
2. The age structure of the class
3. The female-to-male ratio
4. The number of persons leaving the presentation
5. The number of pre- and post-test quizzes completed and returned
6. The number of persons falling asleep during the class
7. The number of questions posed at question time and after the class
8. The number in the audience who request the speaker to return for another nutrition program

The program can be evaluated by considering:

1. Process—program development
2. Product—the lesson plan, its presentation, the handout materials, and the audiovisual materials
3. Outcome—the audience evaluation of the quality of the program and the change in the nutrition knowledge of the audience

QUESTIONS

Circle all correct answers (there may be more than one correct answer to each question).

1. Which of the following community nutrition services are currently intended to meet the needs of the elderly?
   a. Soup kitchens
   b. Home-delivered meals
   c. Food pantries

   d. College nutrition courses
   e. Congregate meal centers

2. Goals of nutrition counseling for the elderly are:
   a. to explain personal food-energy and nutrient needs
   b. to interpret prescribed diets
   c. to promote best use of a limited food budget
   d. to encourage intake of nutrients which prevent aging
   e. to establish optimal eating times which allow optimal absorption, utilization, and tolerance of prescribed medications

3. The Nutrition Program for Older Americans (Title IIIC) provides meals for the elderly in which of the following locations?
   a. skilled nursing homes
   b. congregate meal centers
   c. private homes
   d. hospitals
   e. domiciliary care facilities

4. Staff of skilled nursing homes have certain responsibilities under Medicare and Medicaid in providing for the nutrition of patients. Pair the following staff members with their responsibilities:

   a. physician   i. approval of diet manual
   b. dietitian   ii. food purchase
   c. food service manager iii. Rx therapeutic diets
   d. nurses   iv. organization of dietetic service
   e. operator or administrator v. recording food intake of patients

5. Common problems relating to the nutritional care of patients in skilled nursing homes include which of the following?
   a. Patients are not weighed.
   b. Therapeutic diets are not followed.
   c. Meals are not served regularly.
   d. Assessment of nutritional status is not carried out.
   e. The dietetic service supervisor is not a dietitian.

6. In counseling elderly people on weight reduction, certain objectives should be stressed. Select the three most important and practical goals:
   a. severe food restriction
   b. moderate increase in exercise
   c. regular intake of anorectic drug
   d. development of nutritionally adequate diet
   e. menu planning to meet prescribed food-energy level

REFERENCES

AUSTIN, A. G., "Environmental assessment of the elderly," in *Practical Nutrition: A Quick Reference for the Health Care Practitioner*, eds. M. D. Simko, C. Cowell, and M. S. Hreha. Rockville, MD: Aspen Publications, 1989, pp. 245–54.

BRILEY, M E., M. S. OWENS, M. B. GILLHAM, and S. W. SHAPLIN, "Sources of nutrition information for rural and urban adults," *J. Amer. Dietet. Assoc.*, 90 (1990), 986–87.

CARRILLO, T. E., J. A. GILBRIDE, and M. M. CHAN, "Soup kitchen meals: an observation and nutrient analysis," *J. Amer. Dietet. Assoc.*, 90 (1990), 989–90.

CASS, RYAN V., and M. E. BOWER, "Relationship of socioeconomic status and living arrangements to nutritional intake of the older person." *J. Amer. Dietet. Assoc.*, 89 (1989), 1805–1807.

CHAU, P., H. LEE, R. TSENG, and N. J. DOWNES, "Dietary habits, health beliefs and food practices of elderly Chinese women," *J. Amer. Dietet. Assoc.*, 90, (1990), 579–80.

CLARKE, M., and L. M. WAKEFIELD, "Food choices of institutionalized vs. independent-living elderly," *J. Amer. Dietet. Assoc.*, 66 (1975), 600–4.

CROCKETT, S. J., K. E. HELLER, J. M. MERKEL, and J. M. PETERSON, "Assessing beliefs of older rural Americans about nutrition education: use of focus group approach," *J. Amer. Dietet. Assoc.*, 90, (1990), 563–67.

DAVIES, L., "Retirement courses: Should they include nutrition? *J. Royal Soc. Health*, 110 (1990), 20–21.

FETTERMAN, D. M., *Ethnography*, (vol. 17), Newbury Park, London, New Delhi: Sage Publications, (vol. 17), (1989), 41–64.

HARPER, A. E., "Recommended dietary allowances for the elderly," *Geriatrics*, 33 (1978), 73–80.

HARPER, J. M., G. R. JANSEN, C. T. SHIGETOMI, and A. L. FREY, "Menu planning in the nutrition program for the elderly," *J. Amer. Dietet. Assoc.*, 68 (1976), 529–34.

HERBELIN, K., "Quality assessment and assurance in a long-term care facility: meeting current federal requirements." *J. Am. Dietet. Assoc.*, 89 (1989), 1499–1500.

HOLME, D. S., and S. KIM, "Nutrition education programs for nursing home staff," *J. Amer. Dietet. Assoc.*, 78 (1981), 366–39.

JOHNSON, H. R., R. C. GIBSON, and I. LUCKEY, "Health and social characteristics: implications for service." *In Black Aged*, eds. Z. Harel, E. A. McKinney, and M. Williams, Newbury Park, London, New Delhi: Sage Publications.

KIM, S., J. E. SCHRIVER, and K. M. CAMPBELL, "Nutrition education for nursing home residents," *J. Amer. Dietet. Assoc.*, 78 (1981), 362–68.

LAWSON, D. E. M., A. A. PAUL, A. E. BLACK, T. J. COLE, A. R. MANDAL, and M. DAVIE, "Relative contributions of diet and sunlight to vitamin D state in the elderly," *Brit. Med. J.*, 4 (1979), 303–5.

"New Federal Regulations for Skilled Nursing Homes, Commentary," *J. Amer. Dietet. Assoc.*, 64 (1974), 467–69.

PELCOVITCH, S. J., "Nutrition to meet the human needs of older Americans," *J. Amer. Dietet. Assoc.*, 62 (1972), 99.

PENNINGTON, J. A. T., "The Food and Drug Administration and the dietary guidelines," *Fam. Commun. Health*, 12 (1989), 1–13.

POSNER, B. M., *Nutrition and the Elderly: Policy Development, Program Planning, and Evaluation*. Lexington, MA: Lexington Books, D.C. Heath and Co., 1979.

PROBART, C. K., L. G. DAVIS, J. H. HIBBARD, and R. E. KIME, "Factors that influence the elderly to use traditional or non-traditional nutritional information sources," *J. Amer. Dietet. Assoc.*, 89 (1989), 1758–1762.

ROE, D. A.,   *Alcohol and the Diet.* Westport, CT: AVI Publishing Co., 1979.

ROE, D. A.,   "Nutrition and chronic drug administration—effects on the geriatric patient," *Amer. Pharmacy,* NS20, 1980, 30–35.

ROE, D. A.,   "Development and current status of home-delivered meals programs in the United States," *Nutr. Rev.,* 48 (1990), 181–85.

ROE, D. A., D. F. WILLIAMS, and E. A. FRONGILLA,   1984–1985 Survey of Elderly Recipients of SNAP Home-Delivered Meals in New York State. Final Cornell Report, July, 1985 (Unpublished).

SCRIMSHAW, S. C. M., and E. HURTADO,   *Rapid Assessment Procedures for Nutrition and Primary Health Care.* Los Angeles: UCLA Latin American Publ. Univ.

SMITH, C. E.,   "Influence of standards on the nutritional care of the elderly," *J. Amer. Dietet. Assoc.,* 73 (1978), 115–19.

SOCIAL SECURITY ADMINISTRATION,   "Skilled nursing facilities: standards for certification and participation in Medicare and Medicaid programs," *Federal Register,* 39, 12 (Jan. 1974), 2237.

TEMPLETON, C. L.,   "Nutrition counseling needs in a geriatric population," *Geriatrics,* 33 (1978), 58–66.

TREADWELL, D. D.,   "Planning the nutrition component of long-term care," *J. Amer. Dietet, Assoc.,* 64 (1974), 56–60.

U. S. SENATE SELECT COMMITTEE ON NUTRITION AND HUMAN NEEDS,   "Nutrition and the Elderly," June 19, 1974.

WATKIN, D. M.,   "The nutrition program for older Americans: a successful application of current knowledge in nutrition and gerontology," *World Rev. Nutr. Dietet.,* 26 (1977), 26–40.

WURTMAN, J. J.,   *Eating Your Way Through Life.* New York: Raven Press, 1979, pp. 204–7.

ZIMMER, J. G.,   "Quality Assurance," in *Principles and Practice of Nursing Home Care,* eds., P. R. Katz and E. Calkins. New York: Springer Publications Co., 1989, pp. 91–109.

chapter 11

Geriatric Nutrition in Third World and Immigrant Populations

Until recently, Third World countries were characterized by youthful populations. Injury, infection, and malnutrition were the major causes of early death, and most people did not achieve their genetic potential for longevity. Although these problems continue to exist, improved health services and, more particularly, successful programs aimed at the eradication of infectious disease have led to longer survival of men and women in these countries. This has especially been the case in those countries that are in a condition of transition from a preindustrialized to an industrialized society. These countries may be called "Second World Countries." They include both countries which enjoy a democratic form of government, such as India, Jamaica, and Kenya, and countries where Communism is practiced or where there are dictatorships. Thus, in the People's Republic of China, in Chile, and in Cuba, many people are living longer.

What are the outcomes of change in the age structure of these populations? The major unwanted outcome of the phenomenon has been an escalating incidence of degenerative diseases. However, the prevalence of diabetes, and, in the Caribbean and African countries, of hypertension cannot be related solely to the aging of the population but also to conditions accompanying industrialization and relative prosperity, e.g., increased food-energy intake, decreased activity, and psychosocial stress.

A further social problem has arisen in many, but not all, of these countries: The traditional responsibility of the family to care for the elderly is being lost or becoming less feasible because of urban living conditions, changes in lifestyles, and, unfortunately, loss of the older generation's prestige. A major unsolved problem, resulting both from the concurrent change in population age structure and change of attitude and practice toward the elderly in these countries, is that of providing for their care. Community care for the elderly, wherever the family have relinquished their responsibilities, is commonly lacking. In particular, food distribution programs for the frail elderly do not exist, except insofar as the churches have elected to accept their traditional responsibility of providing for the needy. Further, institutional care is often of an outdated variety. Long-term care facilities that do exist are workhouses or warehouses for the indigent, or the disabled elderly may be cared for in psychiatric or medical wards in general hospitals.

Several major factors which have determined change in the prevalence of chronic diseases in the Third World are of particular importance to nutritionists. These are increased intake of food-energy, fat, and salt; decreased physical exercise; and increased stress. It is these changes in diet and lifestyle, as well as the fact that these populations may now live long enough to develop chronic disease because of excessive intake of ingested substances, that explain the newly recognized degenerative disease picture in countries that are undergoing rapid socioeconomic development.

HYPERTENSION

Elevation of blood pressure and an increased prevalence of hypertension with age have been found in certain populations, including some in Third World countries. Surveys in South Africa have shown a high prevalence of hypertension among the Zulu and Xhosa populations (Seedat, 1979; Seedat and Seedat, 1982; Seedat et al., 1982). In these populations a higher prevalence of hypertension has been found in the city than in the rural groups, females have shown slightly more hypertension than males, and there has been a marked increase in older age groups. Demographic risk factors for hypertension in these people include residence in cities and low income.

The findings in South Africa are but one example of a much wider phenomenon of the rise in the prevalence of hypertension, with both migration from rural to urban areas within Third World countries and migration from Third World countries to industrialized parts of the world by peoples of African origin (Cassel, 1975).

Acculturation, i.e., change in cultural practices occurring in societies undergoing modernization and urbanization, has been shown to be associated with increase in blood pressure with age (Marmot, 1984). However, to understand the actual elements of acculturation that explain elevation in blood pressure with age and an increased prevalence of hypertension, it is necessary to consider particular psychosocial factors, dietary changes, and drug exposures that contribute causally to the problem. Recent studies of the psychosocial factors associated with alterations in blood pressure have indicated that, among men, those with low self-confidence and less perceived control over their lives have higher systolic and diastolic pressures (Cottington et al., 1985).

A fatalistic attitude bred out of social failure has been found in under- and unemployed men and women in the United States, whether of African origin or Caucasians (Roe, 1971). The important message that these findings communicate is that perhaps it is not ambition but rather nonachievement in a competitive and often hostile society that may influence blood pressure levels.

Dietary factors and nutritional changes that have been associated with an increased prevalence of hypertension include increased sodium intake through consumption of processed foods. Observations by Joossens and Geboers (1983) offer support for the etiological role of high-salt diets in explaining regional differences in hypertension and stroke mortality. Further, Ohambo, Okanga, and Karkar (1974) have stressed the importance of increased salt intake as a major factor explaining the increased prevalence of hypertension in urbanized African populations, particularly in the African middle class. A decreased intake of high-potassium foods, associated with a decline in intake of vegetable foods, has also been suggested as playing an etiological role in the evolution of hypertension in people moving from rural to urban areas (Marmot, 1984).

An increased intake of calories, coupled with decreased activity levels and resultant obesity, has also been linked to hypertension in urbanized populations in the Third World (Pobee et al., 1977).

Excessive alcohol ingestion is foremost among drug exposures that have been related to the exacerbation of hypertension and perhaps etiologically associated with its development in urbanized populations in Third World countries. In one of the forms of cardiomyopathy, which has been described in Ghana (Ikeme, 1976) and may be found in other African countries and in other places in the Third World, high alcohol consumption is the major etiological factor. In about 10 percent of these cases, hypertension may occur as a sequel.

In conclusion, it can be seen that the changes brought about in conferring the so-called advantages of industrialized society on the Third World have, in fact, resulted in the application of multiple risk factors for hypertension. Further, since people in these countries are now likely to live longer because of the better control of infectious disease, it is necessary to address the urgent matter of intervention. An all-out effort must be made to reduce the multiple risks for hypertension that are now present and that are in great part of the responsibility of those in the high-income countries who provoked and supplied the agents of cultural change.

CORONARY ARTERY DISEASE

The incidence of coronary artery disease is increasing in some black populations in Third World countries in Africa and in the Caribbean. In these populations there are indications of an increase in coronary heart disease (CHD) mortality with age. In the Caribbean, data indicate a higher mortality for CHD in males than in females, but this male sex preponderance is not as marked as with Caucasian populations (Strong, 1972; McGlashan, 1982).

However, even in those populations of the Third World in which CHD is increasing, it is not a very common cause of death. Risk factors related significantly to CHD, including hypercholesterolemia, are less prevalent than in high-income countries, and HDL cholesterol tends to be higher both in younger and older males, which may have a protective effect. However, it is already noticeable that in urban areas of increasing affluence, lower high-density (HDL) cholesterol and higher low-density (LDL) cholesterol are found. Hypertension, which, as previously noted, is common in these communities, is not highly correlated with CHD mortality. Indeed, not only is hypertension less frequently associated with CHD in black populations in Third World countries but also hypercholesterolemia and diabetes appear to pose less risk for CHD morbidity and mortality (Watkins, 1984).

Despite a certain optimism at present concerning the risk of CHD in the countries under discussion, such optimism may only be transient, since at the present time CHD is the leading cause of death among U.S. blacks (Gillum, 1982). Moreover, data indicate that in Third World countries that are undergoing rapid development, such as Malaysia, CHD mortality is increasing. This may be attributable not only to changing lifestyle and diet but also to longer survival (Harlan, Harlan, and Oii, 1982).

With our current knowledge of the risk factors for CHD, and the prospect that these risk factors may be increasing at an alarming rate in the Third World (this includes cigarette smoking), it is recommended that national and international guidance be given on the need for a prudent diet that is limited in total calories, cholesterol, and total fat. Every effort must be made to decrease the cultivation and smoking of tobacco so that (1) an escalating prevalence of CHD morbidity and mortality can be prevented and (2) at the same time there will be a lower risk of premature death from emphysema and lung cancer.

DIABETES

Major studies of diabetes prevalence in Third World countries have been conducted in the last 20 years. In contrast to earlier reports that diabetes was uncommon in most underdeveloped areas of Asia and Africa, findings of these studies (summarized in Table 11-1) indicate that the prevalence within these continents varies widely. Indeed, specific populations have an extremely high prevalence of the disease. Further, areas of high prevalence of diabetes in Asia, in Africa, on islands of the Pacific and the Caribbean, and on the North American continent among Pima Indians have been shown to have an escalating diabetes incidence in recent years (West, 1978).

Deviant types of diabetes in Third World countries include so-called tropical diabetes, which is associated with malnutrition, and diabetes associated with pancreatic calcification, which may result from ingestion of cyan-

TABLE 11-1   Prevalence Rates Found in Epidemiological Studies of Diabetes Mellitus in Industrialized and Third World Countries

		AGE GROUPS	PREVALENCE (%) MALES	PREVALENCE (%) FEMALES
Australia (Welborn et al., 1968)		40–49	0.3	0.6
		50–59	0.5	1.2
		60–69	4.5	5.6
		≥70	8.5	9.6
England (Reid et al., 1974)		50–59	1.4	
		60–64	2.5	
Greenland (Sagild et al., 1966)		40–49	0.3	0
		50–59	1.7	0.8
		60–69	0	0
		>70	0	0
Pacific (Zimmett et al., 1977)		40–49	9.1	16.3
		50–59	12.1	25.8
		>60	4.8	47.6
USA (Kannel, Danel, and McGee, 1979)		45–54	5.4	3.5
		55–64	9.5	7.4
		>65	12.7	11.8
Papua, New Guinea (Martin et al., 1980)		18–54	15.75	
India (Gupta, Joshi, and Dave, 1982)	Urban:	41–50	4.7	4.6
		51–60	13.6	6.5
		>60	16.6	15.3
	Rural:	41–50	1.3	0.7
		51–60	1.3	1.3
		>60	5.7	4.8

	ALL AGES	BOTH SEXES
Africa (Owusu, 1984)		
Botswana		0.23
Ghana		0.2–0.4
Kenya		1.5
Malawi		0.6
Mali		1.4
Nigeria		0.43
South Africa		2.7
Uganda		0.24
Zimbabwe		0.28

ogenic glycosides in cassava (Mngola, 1982). However, the predominant form is Type I non-insulin dependent diabetes (NIDDM), which is of major public health importance and which has a high prevalence among Pima Indians; Nauru Islanders; the Hindu and Moslem populations of India; the Arab-Moslem population in Kenya and Middle Eastern countries; and people of African origin in Jamaica, Tobago, and Trinidad

(Mngola, 1974; Bennett et al., 1976; Ajgaonkar, 1982; Morrison, 1983). Ecological studies of NIDDM have shown that this form of the disease occurs more in urban than in rural populations, and that the incidence increases with age (Zimmet, 1982). In India, for example, all of the major field investigations have shown that the maximal prevalence of the disease is in people who are at least middle-aged. Whereas the increased affluence of people in these countries has been considered to be a proxy indicator of risk, etiological variables include factors contributing to obesity, including excessive food-energy intake and decreased energy expenditure caused by change from a physically active to a sedentary lifestyle (Richter, Ruderman, and Schneider, 1981).

Both in a Jamaican study (Florey et al., 1972) and in a more recent study of the Tobago population (Patrick and Boyd-Patrick, 1985), elevation of blood sugar has been significantly associated with increasing body mass index. In these populations there has also been a concurrent increase in postload blood sugar levels and in body weight with increasing age, both in men and women. A finding in the 1985 Tobago study which is of particular interest to geriatric nutrition is an apparent decrease in height with increasing age. This decrease may, as in other populations, reflect bone loss but is more probably a late consequence of early malnutrition (Bajaj, 1982). Indeed, it has been postulated that NIDDM may occur more commonly in those who become obese after early food deprivation. The extent to which genetic predisposition accounts for the high prevalence of NIDDM in specific populations and the extent to which this is determined by particular dietary characteristics have not been elucidated. Major problems exist in Third World countries having to do with diabetes management, particularly among the elderly. Patients frequently do not present themselves at health care facilities until they have major complications of their disease, including gangrene or blindness. Further, clinic attendance thereafter may be very poor because of indigence, lack of transportation, or ignorance of need. Even for those who do attend clinics, maintenance of normoglycemia is extremely difficult, because (1) management is largely at primary health care centers, (2) education is lacking on the need for drug and diet compliance, and (3) prevalence of skin infections is high.

The following are World Health Organization (WHO) recommendations on diabetes:

1. Health care for the diabetic incorporated into the community-based health care system
2. National guarantee on the availability of insulin
3. Development of centers within Third World countries for promotion of research into diabetes
4. Patient and care provider education on diabetes
5. International standardization of diabetes testing procedures, classification of types, provision of insulin and availability of educational materials
6. Intensive efforts at primary prevention including decreasing risk factors
7. Intensive efforts to reduce the burden of complications
8. Establishment of registries of diabetics

9. Investigation of traditional methods of treatment
10. WHO promotion of these recommendations

MUSCULOSKELETAL DISEASES

Musculoskeletal diseases occurring in Third World countries, which can lead to severe deformity and impairment in mobility, include many of those found elsewhere but in addition include some which are related to diseases endemic to specific areas. For example, in East Africa, degenerative musculoskeletal diseases include rheumatoid arthritis (Kanyerezi, 1969), osteoarthritis (Kanyerezi, 1976), cervical spondylosis with and without fluorosis (Makene and Lodha, 1976; Sezi, 1976), and gout (Kibukamusoke, 1968). In the Punjab in India these diseases also occur, with a marked regional preponderance of endemic skeletal fluorosis with bony changes (Jolly et al., 1968).

Whereas in the past these diseases have been major causes of disability, the extended life span of populations in the Far East, the Caribbean, and in Africa may soon produce a situation in which these diseases present as serious chronic disease problems. Furthermore, with greater affluence, it may be anticipated that gout may become more prevalent.

The nutritional implication of these predictions is twofold. First, there is a need to consider to what extent prevention of these diseases can be brought about by nutritional intervention. Examples include (1) reduction in fluoride intake by water treatment and discouragement of heavy tea drinking in high-fluoride areas and (2) diet modification to decrease intake of alcohol and high-purine foods for those with gout. Second, the more important issue to consider is the extent to which deformity and loss of mobility can be prevented so that the elderly in the Third World countries are not put at greater risk of hunger because they are unable to get food, to prepare it, or even to eat it unaided.

DIET-RELATED DISEASE IN ELDERLY IMMIGRANTS TO THE UNITED STATES

Over the last 20 years, Hispanics have been entering the United States from Mexico, Cuba, and Puerto Rico. Migration patterns show that older Mexicans go predominantly to California, Cuban migration is to Florida, and Puerto Ricans go via Florida to New York City. Independent residence is not as common for these immigrants as for other Hispanics who have been in the United States since they were young or middle aged. Poverty is a serious problem in immigrant households (Biafora and Longino, 1990), and living in extended family households may improve access to social services for elderly immigrants. However, due to poverty and linguistic barriers, the diagnosis and management of diet-related disease is poor.

A high prevalence of uncontrolled non-insulin dependent diabetes has been found in both elderly Puerto Rican immigrants and elderly

Puerto Ricans who have been in the United States since they were less than 65 years of age. Contributory factors in this problem include the inability to understand prescription labels for antidiabetic agents, a lack of blood glucose monitoring, infrequent clinic and medical office visits, and a failure to comprehend and/or to follow diet instructions (Ekoe, 1988).

The adverse effect of a lack of diabetes control has been examined in older Hispanics from Mexico and it has been shown that renal complications are particularly common (Pugh et al., 1988).

CROSS-CULTURAL STUDY OF NUTRITION AND AGING

The International Union of Nutritional Scientists (IUNS) is currently sponsoring a cross-cultural study of food habits and health in later life. The major aim of this study, which is being carried out in Australia, New Zealand, Greece, the United Kingdom, Sweden, Kenya, China, Japan, and the United States, is to define the lifestyle and eating habits associated with living to a healthy old age. Investigators are studying elderly men and women using anthropological and nutritional assessment methods incorporated into a single basic questionnaire as well as into similar measurement techniques. Data will be pooled so that the information, which is of worldwide importance, can be examined for the relevant commonalities of long-term diets and living habits as well as for lifestyle modifications with aging (Kouris et al., 1989).

QUESTIONS

Circle all correct answers (there may be more than one correct answer to each question).

1. List the three major degenerative diseases occurring in Third World countries.
2. Which of the following demographic and psychosocial factors have been associated with an increased prevalence of hypertension in the Third World?
   a. rural living
   b. high income
   c. urban living
   d. low income
   e. low self-confidence
3. Which of the following statements are true?
   a. Type I is the predominant form of diabetes in the Third World.
   b. Increased body mass index is associated with increased blood sugar levels.

   c. Diabetics in the Third World present themselves for treatment whenever they need more medication.

   d. Diabetics in the Third World often do not present themselves for treatment until they have major complications of their disease.

   e. The prevalence of diabetes increases with age.

4. Summarize the WHO recommendations on diabetes.

5. Which of the following factors is *not* related to the development of endemic skeletal fluorosis?

   a. high intake of water

   b. high intake of fluoride

   c. high intake of sugar

   d. extended life expectancy

   e. heavy tea drinking

6. Write a brief account of each of the following:

   a. Diet-related disease in elderly Hispanic migrants

   b. The cross-cultural study of nutrition and aging

REFERENCES

AJGAOKAR, S. S., "Status of diabetes in India," in *World Book of Diabetes in Practice,* ed. L. Krall. Amsterdam: Excerpta Medica, 1982, pp. 167–70.

BAJAJ, J. S., "Nutritional factors in the etiology of diabetes," in *World Book of Diabetes in Practice,* ed. L. Krall. Amsterdam: Excerpta Medica, 1982, pp. 173–75.

BENNETT, P. H., P. M. LeCOMPTE, M. MILLER, and N. B. RUSHFORTH, "Epidemiological studies of diabetes in the Pima Indians," *Recent Prog. Horm. Res.,* 32 (1976), 333.

BIAFORA, F. A., and C. F. LONGINO, JR., "Elderly Hispanic migration in the United States," *J. Gerontol.,* 45 (1990), S212–29.

CASSEL, J. C., "Studies of hypertension in migrants," in *Epidemiology and Control of Hypertension, Papers and Discussion from the Second International Symposium on the Epidemiology of Hypertension, 1974.* Stratton Intercontinental Medical Book Co., 1975, pp. 41–61.

COTTINGTON, E. M., B. M. BROCK, J. S. HOUSE, and V. M. HAWTHORNE, "Psychosocial factors and blood pressure in the Michigan statewide blood pressure survey," *Amer. J. Epidemiol.,* 121 (1985), 515–29.

EKOE, J. M. *Diabetes Mellitus: Aspects of the World Wide Epidemiology of Diabetes Mellitus and Its Long Term Complications.* New York: Elsevier, 1988, pp. 119–28.

FLOREY, C., duV., H. M. McDONALD, J. McDONALD, and W. E. MIALL, "The prevalence of diabetes in a rural population of Jamaican adults," *Int. J. Epidemiol.,* 1 (1972), 157–66.

GILLUM, R. F., "Coronary heart disease in black populations. I. Mortality and morbidity," *Amer. Heart J.,* 104 (1982), 839.

GUPTA, O. P., M. H. JOSHI, and S. K. DAVE, "Prevalence of diabetes in India," *Adv. Metab. Disord.,* 9 (1978), 147.

HARLAN, W. R., L. C. HARLAN, and W. L. OII, "The implications for cardiovascular disease when developing countries achieve 'middle income' status," *Cardiovasc. Epidemiol. Newsletter,* 31 (1982), 24.

IKEME, A. C., "The pathogenesis of idiopathic cardiomyopathy," in *Degenerative Disorders in the African Environment: Epidemiology and Consequences,* eds. F. J. Bennett, A. M. Nhonoli, and H. Nsanzumuhire. Nairobi: East Africa Literature Bureau, 1976, pp. 317–24.

JOLLY, S. S., B. M. SINGH, O. C. MATHU, and K. C. MALHOTRA, "Epidemiological, clinical, and biochemical study of endemic dental and skeletal fluorosis in Punjab," *Brit. Med. J.,* 4 (1968), 427.

JOOSENS, J. C., and J. GEBOERS, "Salt and hypertension," *Prev. Med.,* 12 (1983), 53–59.

KANNEL, W. B., L. DANIEL, and L. McGEE, "Diabetes and cardiovascular risk factors: the Framingham study," *Circulation,* 59 (1979), 8–13.

KANYEREZI, B. R., "Rheumatoid arthritis in Uganda," *East Afr. Med. J.,* 46 (1969), 71–75.

KANYEREZI, B. R., "Skeletal degenerative disorders: polyarthritis among Ugandan Africans," in *Degenerative Disorders in the African Environment: Epidemiology and Consequences,* eds. F. J. Bennett, A. M. Nhonoli, and H. Nsanzumuhire. Nairobi: East Africa Literature Bureau, 1976, pp. 21–31.

KIBUKAMUSOKE, J. W., "Gout in Africans," *East Afr. Med. J.,* 45 (1968), 378.

KOURIS, A., M. WAHLQUIST, A., TRICHOPOULOS, and E. POLYCHRONOPOULOS, *Food Habits and Health of Elderly in Sparta, Greece: Application of Survey Instrument.* Seoul, Korea: 14th Int. Cong. Nutr., August 1989.

MAKENE, W. J., and S. M. LODHA, "Cervical spondylosis and its complications: role of excessive fluorine content of water," in *Degenerative Disorders in the African Environment: Epidemiology and Consequences,* eds. F. J. Bennett, A. M. Nhonoli, and H. Nsanzumuhire. Nairobi: East Africa Literature Bureau, 1976, pp. 43–46.

MARMOT, M. G., "Geography of blood pressure and hypertension," *Brit. Med. Bull.,* 40 (1984), 380–86.

MARTIN, F. I. R., G. B. WYATT, A. R. GRIEW, M. HAURAHELIA, and L. HIGGINBOTHAM, "Diabetes mellitus in urban and rural communities in Papua New Guinea," *Diabetologia,* 18 (1980), 369–74.

McGLASHAN, N. D., "Causes of death in ten English-speaking Caribbean countries and territories," *Bull. Pan Amer. Health Organ.,* 16 (1982), 212.

MNGOLA, E. N., "Diabetes mellitus," in *Health and Disease in Kenya,* eds. L. C. Vogel, A. C. Muller, R. S. Odingo, Z., Onyango, and A. De Geus. Nairobi: Kenya Literature Bureau, 1974.

MNGOLA, E. N., "African pancreatic diabetes," in *World Book of Diabetes in Practice,* ed. L. Krall. Amsterdam: Excerpta Medica, 1982, pp. 176–79.

MORRISON, E. Y., "Diabetes mellitus in Jamaica," *West Indian Med. J.,* 32 (1983), 199–200.

OHAMBO, H. P., J. OKANGA, and A. H. T. KARKAR, "The pattern of heart disease," in *Health and Disease in Kenya,* eds. L. C. Vogel, A. S. Muller, R. S. Odingo, Z. Onyango, and A. De Geus. Nairobi: Kenya Literature Bureau, 1974, pp. 473–78.

OWUSU, S. K., "Endocrine and metabolic disease," in *Principles of Medicine in Africa,* ed. E. H. O. Perry. Oxford: Oxford University Press, 1984.

PATRICK, A. L, and H. A. BOYD-PATRICK, "Blood sugar levels, weights, and heights of Tobagonians," *West Indian Med. J.,* 34 (1985), 114–22.

POBEE, J. M., E. B. LARBI, D. W. BELCHER, F. K. WURAPA, and S. R. A. DODU,

"Blood pressure distribution in rural Ghanian population," *Trans. Roy. Soc. Trop. Med. Hyg.*, 71 (1977), 66.

PUGH, J., M. STERN, S. HAFFNER, C. EIFLER, and M. ZAPATA, "Excess incidence of treatment of end-stage renal disease in Mexican Americans." *Amer. J. Epidemiol.*, 127 (1988), 135–44.

REID, D. D., G. Z. BRETT, P. S. HAMILTON, R. J. JARRETT, H. KEEN, and G. ROSE, "Cardiorespiratory disease and diabetes among middle-aged male civil servants," *Lancet* (1974), 469–73.

RICHTER, E. A., N. B. RUDERMAN, and A. H. SCHNEIDER, "Diabetes and exercise," *Amer. J. Med.*, 70 (1981), 201.

ROE, D. A., *Health and Nutritional Status of Working and Non-working Mothers in Poverty Groups*, USDL Contract 51-36-71-02, Final Report. Ithaca, NY: Cornell University, 1971.

SAGILD, U., J. LITTAUER, C. S. JESPERSEN, and S. ANDERSEN, "Epidemiological studies in Greenland 1962–64. I. Diabetes mellitus in Eskimos," *Acta Med. Scand.*, 197 (1966), 29–39.

SEEDAT, Y. K., "The prevalence, etiology, and complications of hypertension in the South African black population," in *Prophylactic Approach to Hypertensive Diseases*, eds. Y. Yamori, W., Lovenberg, and E. D. Freis. New York: Raven Press, 1979, p. 7.

SEEDAT, Y. K., and M. A. SEEDAT, "An interracial study of the prevalence of hypertension in an urban South African population," *Trans. Roy. Soc. Trop. Med. Hyg.*, 76 (1982), 62.

SEEDAT, Y. K., M. A. SEEDAT, and D. B. T. HACKLAND, "Biosocial factors and hypertension in urban and rural Zulu," *S. Afr. Med. J.*, 61 (1982), 999.

SEZI, C. L., "Clinical presentation of cervical spondylosis at Mulago Hospital," in *Degenerative Disorders in the African Environment: Epidemiology and Consequence*, eds. F. J. Bennett, A. M. Nhonoli, and H. Nsanzumuhire. Nairobi: East Africa Literature Bureau, 1976, pp. 47–54.

STRONG, J. P., "Atherosclerosis in human populations," *Atherosclerosis*, 16 (1972), 193.

WATKINS, L. O., "Coronary heart disease risk factors in underdeveloped countries: the case for primordial prevention," *Amer. Heart J.*, 108 (1984), 850–62.

WELBORN, T. A., D. H. GURNOW, J. T. WEARNE, K. I. CULLAN, M. G. McCALL, and N. S. STENHOUSE, "Diabetes detected by blood-sugar measurement after a glucose load: report from the Busselton Survey, 1966," *Med. J. Aust.* (1968), 778–83.

WEST, K. M., *Epidemiology of Diabetes and Its Vascular Complications*. New York: Elsevier-North Holland, Inc., 1978.

ZIMMET, P., "The global epidemiology of diabetes," in *World Book of Diabetes in Practice*, ed. L. Krall. Amsterdam: Excerpta Medica, 1982, pp. 4–10.

ZIMMET, P., A. SELUKA, J. COLLINS, P. CURRIE, J. WICHING, and W. DEBOER, "Diabetes mellitus in an urbanized, isolated Polynesian population: the Funafuti survey," *Diabetes*, 26 (1977), 1101–8.

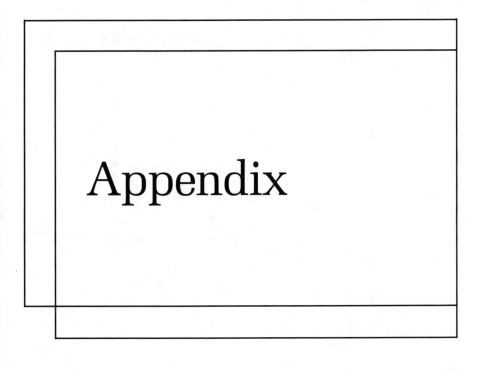

Appendix

TABLE 1 Calculation of Food Energy Intake, Nutritive Value of Common Foods[a]

	AMOUNT	CAL	PRO-TEIN (G)	FAT (G)	CARBO-HYDRATE (G)	CAL-CIUM (MG)	PHOS-PHORUS (MG)	IRON (MG)	SOD-IUM (MG)	POTAS-SIUM (MG)	VITA-MIN A (IU)	THIA-MIN (MG)	RIBO-FLAVIN (MG)	NIA-CIN (MG)	AS-CORBIC ACID (MG)	USDA HAND-BOOK NO. 456/REF. NO.
Milk																
Buttermilk	1C	88	8.8	0.2	12.5	296	233	0.1	319	343	10	0.10	0.44	0.2	2	509b
Milk, skim	1C	88	8.8	0.2	12.5	296	233	0.1	127	355	10	0.09	0.44	0.2	2	1322b
Milk, whole	1C	159	8.5	8.5	12.0	288	227	0.1	122	351	350	0.07	0.41	0.2	2	1320b
Vegetables																
Asparagus[b]	4															47b
Green beans, frozen, french style	½C	14	1.2	0.1	3.1	19	25	0.5	1	99	443	0.07	0.08	0.5	10	194c
Beans, lima (frozen)	½C	84	5.1	0.1	16.2	17	77	1.5	86	362	195	0.06	0.03	0.9	15	173c
Beets	½C	27	1.0	0.1	6.1	12	20	0.5	37	177	15	0.03	0.04	0.3	5	385b
Beet greens,[b] spinach, collards (cooked)	½C	22	2.5	0.4	3.5	111	34	1.4	33	260	6133	0.07	0.14	0.6	36	393a, 2170a, 807a, 492c
Brussels sprouts,[b] frozen	½C															
Cabbage, raw	1C	21	1.7	0.2	4.2	25	34	0.5	12	189	200	0.06	0.06	0.4	47	512c
Cauliflower	½C															831a
Corn on cob, 5" (boiled)	1	70	2.5	0.8	16.2	2	69	0.5	–	151	310	0.09	0.08	1.1	7	846a
Peas, green, frozen	½C	55	4.1	0.3	9.5	15	69	1.5	92	108	480	0.22	0.07	1.4	11	1530c
Potato, French fried (2" to 3½" diameter)	10	137	2.2	6.6	18.0	8	56	0.7	3	427	–	0.07	0.04	1.6	11	1789b
Potato, sweet, mashed	¼C	73	1.1	0.3	16.8	21	30	0.5	7	155	5038	0.06	0.04	0.4	11	2250c
Potato, white, baked (2" diameter)	½C	59	1.7	0.1	13.3	6	41	0.5	3	316	–	0.07	0.03	1.2	13	1787d
Pumpkin,[b] carrots, winter squash	½C	37	1.1	0.3	89	27	32	0.5	10	261	6757	0.04	0.08	0.6	7	1832d, 620a, 2201a

Rutabagas, mashed	½C	42	1.1	0.1	9.9	71	37	0.4	5	201	660	0.07	0.07	1.0	31	1920b
Summer squash[b]	½C															2192a
Celery, stalks	3															637c
Cucumbers, slices	16	9	0.7	0.1	2.1	19	17	0.6	18	133	290	0.03	0.04	0.3	6	942d
Lettuce, shredded	1C															1256c
Tomatoes,[b] canned and juice	½C	24	1.2	0.2	5.2	8	23	0.9	200	269	1028	0.06	0.04	0.9	20	2284d, 2288d
Tomatoes, fresh (2⅗" diameter)	1	20	1.0	0.2	4.3	12	25	0.5	3	222	820	0.05	0.04	0.6	21	2282c
Turnips, mashed	½C	26	0.9	0.3	5.7	41	28	0.5	39	216	–	0.05	0.06	0.4	26	2353b
Fruits																
Apple (2½" diameter)	1	61	0.2	0.6	15.3	7	11	0.3	1	116	100	0.03	0.02	0.1	4	13d
Applesauce, unsweetened	½C	50	0.3	0.3	13.2	5	6	0.6	3	95	50	0.03	0.01	0.1	1	28c
Banana, medium	½	51	0.7	0.1	13.2	5	16	0.4	1	220	115	0.03	0.04	0.4	6	141b
Berries[b] (blue, black, raspberries)	½C	46	0.8	0.4	10.9	19	15	0.8	1	113	118	0.02	0.04	0.4	10	424b, 418a, 1851a
Cantaloupe (¼ of 6" diameter)	1C	48	1.1	0.2	12.0	22	26	0.6	19	402	5440	0.06	0.05	1.0	53	1358c
Citrus fruit:																
Orange[b]/grapefruit juice	½C															1421c, 1053b
Orange, small	1	49	0.8	0.1	11.8	19	19	0.3	1	189	158	0.08	0.3	0.3	49	1437b, 1061a
Grapefruit	½															
Cherries, large	10	47	0.9	0.2	11.7	15	13	0.3	1	129	70	0.03	0.04	0.3	7	663b
Grapes	12	41	0.4	0.2	10.4	7	12	0.2	2	104	60	0.04	0.02	0.2	7	1085a
Pears, water pack	1	50	0.4	0.4	1.8	8	10	0.4	2	136	–	0.02	0.04	0.2	2	1504e
Raisins (1½ T)	½ oz.	40	0.4	–	10.8	9	14	0.5	4	107	–	0.02	0.01	0.1	–	1846c
Strawberries	1C	55	1.0	0.7	12.5	31	31	1.5	1	244	90	0.04	0.10	0.9	88	2217e
Watermelon, diced	1C	42	0.8	0.3	10.2	11	16	0.8	2	160	940	0.05	0.05	0.3	11	2424c
Bread and Crackers, Enriched																
Biscuit (2" diameter, 1¼" high)	1	103	2.1	4.8	12.8	34	49	0.4	175	33	–	0.06	0.06	0.5	–	410a
Cornbread, piece (2½" × 2½" × 1½")	1	178	3.8	5.8	27.5	133	209	0.8	263	61	130	0.10	0.10	0.8	–	1350d

TABLE 1 Calculation of Food Energy Intake, Nutritive Value of Common Foods[a] *(Continued)*

	AMOUNT	CAL	PRO-TEIN (g)	FAT (g)	CARBO-HYDRATE (g)	CAL-CIUM (mg)	PHOS-PHORUS (mg)	IRON (mg)	SOD-IUM (mg)	POTAS-SIUM (mg)	VITA-MIN A (iu)	THIA-MIN (mg)	RIBO-FLAVIN (mg)	NIA-CIN (mg)	AS-CORBIC ACID (mg)	USDA HAND-BOOK NO. 456/ REF. NO.
Frankfurter roll (6")	1	119	3.3	2.2	21.2	30	34	0.8	202	38	–	0.11	0.07	0.9	–	1902c
Graham crackers	2	55	1.1	1.3	10.4	6	21	0.2	95	55	–	0.01	0.03	0.2	–	914b
Hamburger bun (3½")	1	119	3.3	2.2	21.2	30	34	0.8	202	38	–	0.11	0.07	0.9	–	1902c
Muffin, plain (2" × 1½")	1	118	3.1	4.0	16.9	42	60	0.6	176	50	40	0.07	0.09	0.6	–	1343b
Saltines (2½" square)	4	48	1.0	1.3	8.0	2	10	0.1	123	13	–	–	–	0.1	–	916d
Soda crackers (2½" square)	5	65	1.3	1.8	10.0	3	13	0.2	156	16	–	–	–	0.1	–	918d
White or whole wheat bread	1	76	2.4	0.9	14.1	24	27	0.7	142	29	–	0.07	0.06	0.7	–	461b
Cereals, Enriched																
Bran flakes, 40%	½C	53	1.8	0.3	14.1	10	63	6.2	104	68	825	0.20	0.25	2.1	6	441
Corn flakes	¾C	73	1.5	0.1	15.9	–	7	0.4	188	22	885	0.22	0.26	2.2	7	866a
Farina, cooked	½C	51	1.6	0.1	10.6	5	15	–	176	11	–	0.05	0.03	0.5	–	992
Grits, corn	½C	62	1.4	0.1	13.5	1	13	0.4	251	14	75	0.05	0.04	0.5	–	863a
Oatmeal, cooked	½C	66	2.4	1.2	11.6	11	68	0.7	262	73	–	0.09	0.02	0.1	–	1391
Rice, cooked	½C	74	1.4	0.1	16.4	7	19	0.6	256	19	–	0.08	0.01	0.7	–	1872a
Wheat, puffed	1C	54	2.3	0.2	11.8	4	48	0.6	1	51	–	0.08	0.03	1.2	–	2458
Pasta, Enriched																
Noodles,[b] macaroni, spaghetti	½C	91	3.0	0.6	18.3	7	41	0.7	1	43	–	0.11	0.07	1.2	–	1378c, 1299c, 2159c
Meat, Poultry, Fish																
Beef,[b] Lamb, Veal	1 oz	79	7.4	5.2	–	3	32	0.8	16	74	2	0.03	0.07	1.6	–	353d, 1185e, 2370e
Beef liver	1 oz	65	7.5	3.0	1.5	3	135	2.5	52	108	15130	0.07	1.19	4.7	7.7	1267a
Bologna (1 slice, 4½" diameter)	1 oz	86	3.4	7.8	0.3	2	36	0.5	369	65	–	0.05	0.06	0.7	–	1982g
Chicken, light meat	1 oz	50	9.4	1.0	–	3	80	0.4	19	123	17	0.01	0.02	3.5	–	682d
Cod,[b] haddock, halibut (broiled)	1 oz	48	6.9	1.8	0.5	8	73	0.3	40	121	80	0.01	0.02	1.4	–	795d, 1118d, 1104d

Food	Amount															Ref.
Ham, cured	1 oz	92	6.3	7.1	—	3	52	0.8	227	71	—	—	0.06	1.1	—	1779f
Hot dog	1	139	5.6	12.4	0.8	3	60	0.9	495	99	—	0.15	0.09	1.2	—	1994c
Pork, fresh	1 oz	103	6.8	8.1	—	3	73	0.9	17	78	—	0.07	0.07	1.6	—	1716c
Shrimp	1 oz	37	7.7	0.4	0.2	37	84	1.0	—	39	20	0.26	0.01	0.6	—	2045c
Tuna, canned in oil	1 oz	82	6.9	5.8	—	2	83	0.3	227	85	26	0.01	0.02	2.9	—	2323h
Egg, large	1	82	6.5	5.8	0.5	27	103	1.2	61	65	590	0.05	0.15	—	—	968b
Cheese																
Cheddar, domestic	1 oz	113	7.1	9.1	0.6	213	136	0.3	198	23	370	0.01	0.13	—	—	646p
Cottage cheese, small curd, creamed	½C	112	14.3	4.4	3.1	98	160	0.3	241	90	180	0.03	0.26	0.1	—	647d
Peanut Butter	2T	188	8.0	16.2	6.0	18	122	0.6	194	200	—	0.04	0.04	4.8	—	1499f
Dried Beans and Peas																
Navy beans,[b] kidney beans, split peas	½C	114	7.5	0.4	20.6	32	123	2.2	8	342	15	0.12	0.07	0.8	—	115b, 161d, 1533a
Fats																
Bacon, crisp, slices	2	86	3.8	7.8	0.5	2	34	0.5	153	35	—	0.08	0.05	0.8	—	126d
Cream,[b] light, 20% or half & half	1T	26	0.5	2.5	0.7	16	13	—	7	19	100	—	0.02	—	—	929b, 928b
French or Italian dressing[b]	1T	75	0.1	7.6	1.9	2	2	0.1	267	8	—	—	—	—	—	1932b, 1936b
Margarine/butter[b]	1t	34	—	3.8	—	1	1	—	46	1	160	—	—	—	—	1317d, 505d
Mayonnaise,[b] salad dressing	1T	83	0.2	8.8	1.3	3	4	0.1	86	3	35	—	—	—	—	1928b, 1940b
Oils	1T	120	—	13.6	—	—	—	—	—	—	—	—	—	—	—	1401j
Nuts																
Unsalted peanuts, pecans, walnuts, almonds	2T	103	2.9	9.6	2.9	20	64	0.5	19	102	5	0.07	0.05	1.0	—	1496b, 1536j, 2421e, 81
Desserts																
Brownies, with nuts (1¾" × 1¾" × ⅞")	1	97	1.3	6.3	10.2	8	30	0.4	50	38	40	0.04	0.02	0.1	—	813
Cake, chocolate (3" × 3" × 2")	1 piece	322	4.2	15.1	45.8	65	121	0.8	259	123	130	0.02	0.09	0.2	—	525c
Cake, plain (3" × 3" × 2")	1 piece	313	3.9	12.0	48.1	55	88	0.3	258	68	150	0.02	0.08	0.2	—	534b

TABLE 1   Calculation of Food Energy Intake, Nutritive Value of Common Foods[a] *(Continued)*

	AMOUNT	CAL	PRO-TEIN (g)	FAT (g)	CARBO-HYDRATE (g)	CAL-CIUM (mg)	PHOS-PHORUS (mg)	IRON (mg)	SOD-IUM (mg)	POTAS-SIUM (mg)	VITA-MIN A (iu)	THIA-MIN (mg)	RIBO-FLAVIN (mg)	NIA-CIN (mg)	AS-CORBIC ACID (mg)	USDA HAND-BOOK NO. 456/ REF. NO.
Chocolate pudding	½C	193	4.1	6.1	33.4	125	128	0.7	73	223	195	0.03	0.18	0.2	–	1823
Cookies, chocolate chip	2	99	1.1	4.4	14.6	8	24	0.4	84	28	26	0.01	0.01	0.1	–	818b
Custard, baked	½C	153	7.2	7.3	14.7	149	155	0.6	105	194	465	0.06	0.25	0.2	–	948
Gelatin dessert	½C	71	1.8	–	16.9	–	–	–	61	–	–	–	–	–	–	1032b
Ice cream, vanilla	4 fl. oz.	129	3.0	7.0	13.9	97	77	0.1	42	121	295	0.03	0.14	0.1	–	1139d
Pie, apple (9" diameter)	⅙ pie	302	2.6	13.1	45.0	9	26	0.4	355	94	40	0.02	0.02	0.5	1	1566c
Sherbet, orange	4 fl oz	130	0.9	1.2	29.7	16	13	–	10	21	60	0.01	0.03	–	2	2041b
Vanilla wafers	5	93	1.1	3.2	14.9	8	13	0.1	51	15	25	0.01	0.02	0.1	–	833b
Sweets																
Milk chocolate	1 oz	147	2.2	9.2	16.1	65	65	0.3	27	109	80	0.02	0.10	0.1	–	587
Molasses,[b] jams, jelly, maple syrup	1T	52	0.1	–	13.4	16	3	0.8	2	17	–	–	0.01	–	–	2050b, 1149e, 2049d
Soft drinks	6 fl oz	72	–	–	18.5	–	–	–	–	–	–	–	–	–	–	404a
Sugar	1T	46	–	–	11.9	–	–	–	–	–	–	–	–	–	–	2230b

[a]Approximate values. All values have been rounded to the nearest decimal point.
[b]Average value for the group of foods listed.
[c]Dash indicates a true amount of nutrient that contributes to serving size.

From U.S. Department of Agriculture "Nutritive Value of American foods," in *Agriculture Handbook No. 456* (Washington, DC: U.S. Government Printing Office).

TABLE 2 Moderately High Fiber Diet

Breakfast
½ c. stewed prunes
1 c. shredded wheat cereal
½ c. milk
hot beverage

Lunch
2 oz. sliced turkey
2 sl. whole wheat bread, with lettuce, tomato, and mayonnaise
½ c. applesauce
beverage

Dinner
3 oz. chopped beef
½ c. mashed potatoes
½ c. peas
1 small banana
beverage

Snack
1 c. milk
fresh orange

TABLE 3 Foods Which Have a High Nutrient-to-Calorie Ratio

1. Skim milk
2. Cheese (from part-skim milk)
3. Cottage cheese
4. Lean meat, poultry, and low-fat fish
5. Fortified breakfast cereals
6. Whole wheat enriched bread
7. Orange juice and other citrus fruit juices
8. Fresh fruits, e.g., oranges, grapefruit, cantaloupe, banana
9. Green, leafy vegetables, e.g., spinach, broccoli
10. Dark yellow vegetables, e.g., carrots, squash

TABLE 4 Average Sodium and Potassium Content of Common Foods

The following tables are reprinted from the second edition of the U.S. Dietary Goals. The Goals recommend restricting salt intake to about 5g a day, which effectively means reducing sodium intake to about 2g (2000 mg). No recommendation is made for the daily consumption of potassium, but people taking diuretics, instructed by their physicians to eat foods high in potassium to replace losses, may be interested to see what foods contain large amounts of this mineral.

FOOD	WEIGHT (g)	SODIUM (mg)	POTASSIUM (mg)
Meat, fish, or poultry, cooked without added salt			
Average	30	33	125
Clams, soft	100	36	239
Clams, hard	100	205	311
Crab, canned	100	1000	110
Crab, steamed	100	456	271
Flounder	100	237	587
Frankfurters (2)	100	1100	220
Frozen fish (cod)	100	400	400
Haddock	100	177	348
Kidneys, beef	100	253	324
Lobster, canned	100	210	180
Lobster, fresh	100	325	258
Oysters, raw	100	73	121
Salmon, canned	100	522	349
Salmon, saft-free, canned	100	48	391
Scallops, fresh	100	265	476
Shrimp, raw	100	140	220
Shrimp, frozen or canned	100	140	200–312
Sweet breads	100	116	433
Tuna, canned	100	800	240
Tuna, salt-free, canned	100	46	382
Cheese			
American cheese	30	341	25
Cream cheese	30	75	22
Cottage cheese	30	76	28
Cottage cheese, unsalted	30	6	–
Low-sodium cheese (cheddar)	30	3	120
Egg			
Whole, fresh and frozen (1)	50	61	65
Whites, fresh and frozen	50	73	70
Yolks, fresh	50	26	49
Milk			
Buttermilk, cultured	120	135	192
Condensed sweetened milk	120	135	377
Evaporated milk, undiluted	120	142	364
Powdered milk, skim	30	160	544
Low-sodium milk, canned	120	6	288
Whole milk	240	120	346
Yogurt (skim milk)	100	51	143

TABLE 4   *(Continued)*

FOOD	WEIGHT (g)	SODIUM (mg)	POTASSIUM (mg)
Potato			
White, baked in skin	100	4	323
White, boiled	100	2	285
Instant, prepared with water, milk, fat	100	256	290
Sweet (canned solid pack)	100	48	200
Breads			
Bakery, white	25	127	26
Bakery, whole wheat	25	132	68
Bakery, rye	25	139	36
Low-sodium (local)	25	4	25
Plain muffin	40	132	38
English muffin	57	215	57
A-protein rusk (1)	11	4	5
Graham crackers (2)	14	93	53
Low-sodium crackers (2)	9	10	11
Vanilla wafers (5)	14	35	10
Yeast doughnut	30	70	24
Cake doughnut	35	160	32
Cereal, dry			
Kellogg's Corn Flakes	30	282	15
Puffed Rice	15	trace	7
Rice Krispies	30	267	15
Special K	30	244	17
Puffed Wheat	15	trace	21
Shredded Wheat	20	1	52
Kellogg's Sugar Frosted Flakes	30	200	19
Sugar Pops	30	67	22
Bran Flakes	30	118	151
Cereal, cooked without added salt			
Corn grits, enriched, regular	100	1	11
Farina, enriched, regular	100	2	9
Farina, instant cooking	100	7	13
Farina, quick cooking	100	190	10
Oatmeal or Rolled Oats	100	2	61
Pettijohn's Wheat	100	trace	84
Rice	100	5	28
Rice, instant	100	trace	trace
Wheat, rolled	100	trace	84
Wheatena	100	trace	84
Fat			
Bacon (1 strip)	7	73	17
Butter	5	49	3
Margarine	5	49	1
Mayonnaise	15	90	5
Mayonnaise, low-sodium	15	17	1
Low-sodium butter	15	1	3
Unsalted margarine (Fleishman's)	5	1	1
Vegetable oil	15	0	0

TABLE 4 Average Sodium and Potassium Content of Common Foods *(Continued)*

FOOD	WEIGHT (g)	SODIUM (mg)	POTASSIUM (mg)
Sugar substitutes			
Saccharine (¼-gr tablet)	1	1	0
Sucaryl	500‡	0	0
Sweet-10	500‡	0	0
Adolph's	500‡	0	0
Morton	500‡	0	0
Diamond Crystal	500‡	0	0
Beverages			
Beer	100	7	25
Chocolate syrup (2 tsp)	10	5	29
Coca-Cola	100	4	1
Coffee, instant (beverage)	–	1	50
Cranberry juice	100	1	10
Diet Seven-Up	100	10	0
Egg nog, reconstituted	240	250	630
Fresca	100	18	0
Frozen lemonade, reconstituted	100	trace	16
Gingerale	100	6	2
Hot chocolate (Carnation 1 pack—6 oz water)	100	104	190
Kool-Aid, reconstituted	240	trace	0
Meritene, reconstituted	240	250	740
Pepsi Cola	100	2	4
Royal Crown Cola	100	3	trace
Seven-Up	100	9	0
Sprite	100	16	0
Tab	100	5	0
Tea, instant (beverage)	–	trace	25

Fresh fruits and fruit juices are naturally very low in sodium and thus are not listed individually in this table.
*In teaspoons.
†Average serving.
‡In milligrams.

FOOD	SODIUM (mg)
*Group I Vegetables (0–20 mg/100 g, average 7.4 mg)***	
Asparagus	7
Broccoli	12
Brussels sprouts	14
Cabbage, common	14
Cauliflower	9
Chicory	7
Collards	16
Corn	2
Cow peas	1
Cucumbers	6
Eggplant	1
Endive	14
Escarole	14

TABLE 4 *(Continued)*

FOOD	WEIGHT (g)	SODIUM (mg)	POTASSIUM (mg)
Cream			
Coffee Mate	1*	4	27
Half-and-half	30	14	39
Heavy whipping cream (30 percent)	30	10	27
Poly-perx	30	–	–
Sour cream (Sealtest)	30	13	43
Table cream (18 percent)	30	13	37
Whipped topping	30	4	6
Gravy			
Low sodium	30	10	25
Regular	30	210	28
Peanut butter			
Cellu, Salt free	15	1	100
Regular, made with small amounts of added fat and salt	15	91	100
Desserts			
Baked custard (Delmark)	120	128	174
D'zerta	120	35	0
Gelatin	120	51	1
Ice cream (4-oz cup)	60	23	49
Sherbet	60	6	14
Water ice	60	trace	2
Cakes			
All varieties except gingerbread and fruit cakes (both mixes and recipes)	50†	123	50
With low-sodium shortening and baking powder	50†	10–20	75–150
Pies			
All varieties except raisin, mince (⅛ of 9-inch pie)	320†	375	180
Candy			
Hard candy (1 equals 5 g)	100	32	4
Gum drops (8 small equals 10 g)	100	35	5
Jelly beans	100	12	1
Salt			
1 g NaCl—packet salt	–	400	–
5 g NaCl—1 tsp	–	2000	–
Salt substitutes			
Diamond Crystal	500‡	1	220
Co-salt	500‡	0	185
Adolph's	500‡	0	241
McCormick's	500‡	0	234
Morton	500‡	0	250

FOOD	SODIUM (mg)
Green peppers	13
Kohlrabi	6
Leeks	5
Lentils	3
Lettuce	9
Lima beans, not frozen	1
Mushrooms, raw	15
Mustard green	10
Navy beans	7
Okra	2
Onions	7
Parsnips	8
Peas, dried, split, cooked	13
Peas, green	1
Potatoes, baked in skin	4
Potatoes, boiled, pared before cooking	3
Radishes	18
Rutabagas	4
Squash, summer or winter	1
String beans	2
Sweet potato	10
Tomatoes	4
Turnip greens	17
Wax beans	2
Yams	4
Group II Vegetables (23–60 mg/100 g, average 40 mg)	
Artichoke	30
Beets	43
Black-eyed peas, frozen only	39
Carrots	33
Chinese cabbage	23
Dandelion greens	44
Kale	43
Parsley	45
Red cabbage	26
Spinach	50
Turnips	34
Watercress	52
Group III Vegetables (75–126 mg/100 g, average 81 mg)	
Beet greens	76
Celery	88
Chard, Swiss	86

This table assumes the use of fresh vegetables without salt added in cooking. The amount of salt added to canned and frozen vegetables can vary. *Agricultural Handbook No. 8* from the USDA estimates that canned vegetables average 235 mg sodium per 100 g edible portion. Frozen vegetables range from almost no sodium to as high as 125 mg sodium per 100 g edible portion.
**A 100-g portion for most vegetables is about a ½-c to 1-c serving.
Select Committee on Nutrition and Human Needs, *Dietary Goals for the United States,* 2nd Ed. (Washington, DC: U.S. Government Printing Office, 1977), pp. 80–83. The Senate's tables are taken from information in U.S. Department of Agriculture, Agricultural Research Service, Composition of foods: Raw, processed, prepared, *Agricultural Handbook No. 8* (Washington, DC: U.S. Government Printing Office, 1963).

TABLE 5   Low Fat, Low Cholesterol Foods of Animal Origin

	SERVING SIZE	CHOLESTEROL (mg)	FAT (g)
Milk and Milk Products			
Milk, skim	1 c	7	–
Milk, 2 percent	1 c	15	4.9
Cottage cheese[1]		5	1.0
Yogurt[2]		6	0.9
Ice cream	½ c	5	2.5
Meat and Fish			
Beef, lean, cooked[3]	3 oz	100	6.7
Lamb, lean, cooked	3 oz	100	7.3
Cod, cooked	3 oz	100	3.0
Fish, cooked	3 oz	54	0.9

[1]uncreamed
[2]made from partially skimmed milk
[3]boiled, steamed, baked or broiled (no fat added)
Low fat diet = selection of foods listed above plus bread, cereals, breakfast rice, fruit and vegetables to give ≤ 50 g fat/day.
Low cholesterol diet = selection of foods listed above plus bread, cereals, breakfast rice, fruit and vegetables and *all* vegetable margarine to give ≤ 200 mg cholesterol/day.
Values, converted to domestic measures, are from A. A. Paul and D. A. T. Southgate, McCance and Widdowson's 4th Revised Edition of MRC Special Report No. 297, HMSO (London, 1978), and from E. M. N. Hamilton and E. N. Whitney, *Nutrition Concepts and Controversies* (St. Paul, New York, Los Angeles, San Francisco: West Publ. Co., 1979).

TABLE 6   High Fiber Foods

FOOD	DIETARY FIBER (g/100 g)
Cereals	
Wheat bran	44.0
All-bran	8.4
Shredded wheat	12.3
Special K	5.5
Whole wheat bread ("whole meal")	8.5
Crispbread rye	11.7
Fruits	
Apples, raw (flesh only)	2.0
Bananas	3.4
Prunes, stewed with sugar	7.7
Vegetables	
Broccoli, cooked	4.1
Carrots	3.1
Peas	5.2
Spinach	6.3

Values are from A. A. Paul and D. A. T. Southgate, McCance and Widdowson's 4th Revised Edition of MRC Special Report No. 297, HMSO (London, 1978).

Class Projects

1. Students visit an elderly individual in the community or in an institution to find out about this person's life and about the circumstances which have determined his or her present situation. The individual is questioned about food purchases, preparation, and diet. Following the informed consent of this individual, a conversation is taped between the individual and the student or between the individual, the caregiver, and the student which can be played back in class and used for instructional purposes. The elderly client or patient can be selected by the instructor or by the student with approval from the instructor.

   Practical experience has shown that these tapes have their greatest teaching value when the instructor plans discussions of:
   a. History taking
   b. Difficulties the elderly have in obtaining food
   c. Problems of dietary assessment in the elderly
   d. Determinants of independent living

   Students should give a short preamble before playing their tape to explain whom they were interviewing; their relationship, if any, to this individual; where and when interview took place; and the constraints on the interviewing process.

2. A senior citizen comes to the class and participates in a discussion group. Best use of this is when the senior is particularly interested in the subject to be discussed and wants information on a nutrition or diet-related problem.

3. Students take supervised field trips to:
    a. A skilled nursing home
    b. An intermediate care home
    c. A domiciliary care unit

    Visits are planned to include attendance at staff meetings where patient care plans are discussed (including dietary); observations of patients or residents at meal times; inspection of kitchen facilities, menus, and recipe manual; and meeting with staff members, including dietary staff, nurses, physical therapist, occupational therapist, social worker, and physician.

4. Students prepare and give an in-service instruction on a nutrition-related topic to:
    a. Home health aides (working with geriatric patients)
    b. Meals-on-Wheels driver/volunteer

5. Students conduct a discussion group at the Senior Citizens Center on a nutrition topic chosen by the audience.

6. Students give brief nutrition talks at a congregate meal center. Appropriate topics are:
    a. How to avoid high-sodium intake
    b. What foods are rich sources of potassium and why you need them
    c. Good buys at the supermarket
    d. How to understand food labels (with a magnifying glass)
    e. Why's and wherefore's of dietary fiber

7. Students prepare a diet instruction for an elderly patient who is:
    a. A diabetic
    b. Constipated
    c. A cardiac patient recently discharged from the hospital with congestive heart failure

8. Students deliver Meals-on-Wheels.

9. Students spend a day with the public health nurse visiting elderly patients.

10. Students visit the Office for the Aging to find out about local services, state and federal services for the elderly, and the characteristics of the population over 65 years of age in their community.

Essay Questions

Questions are based on an assigned text or case history. Students are expected to solve one or more than one essay-type problem(s) following classroom instruction based on specific chapters of the book. Problem-solving abilities that should be acquired through these exercises include:

1. Knowing how to assess the coping skills of elderly clients and patients
2. Being able to explain the difference between the aging process and diseases commonly occurring in the elderly
3. Showing why geriatric diseases can increase the susceptibility of the elderly to nutritional disorders
4. Understanding nutritional survey methods
5. Finding the means to assess the nutritional needs of geriatric patients
6. Deciding why the older patients change their eating habits
7. Knowing how to measure food intake in the elderly
8. Understanding how to select reliable methods for geriatric nutritional assessment
9. Knowing the signs of nutritional deficiencies
10. Being able to plan practical diets for the elderly, including those who need to lose weight, those who are constipated, and those who are likely to develop congestive heart failure
11. Having the competency to examine orders for medications and decide whether one or more of the drugs prescribed could be causing an eating disorder or a nutritional deficiency

12. Being able to offer advice to elderly patients on food distribution programs or other nutrition-support services in your area

QUESTIONS

1. A 68-year-old man complained of increasing fatigue and numbness of the extremities. Neurological examination showed absence of deep-tendon reflexes and diminished vibratory and proprioceptive sensation in all extremities. The hemoglobin level was 5.4 g/dl, leukocyte count was $2.2 \times 10^9 1$, and platelet count was $150 \times 10^9 1$. The blood smear showed hypersegmented granulocytes. Aspirated marrow demonstrated marked megaloblastosis. The MCV was 125 fl. The serum cobalamin level was 42 pg/ml and the serum folate level was 14.4 ng/ml. Schilling's test results were compatible with absence of intrinsic factor.

   What is the diagnosis? Discuss the relationship between this patient's nutritional deficiency and the aging process. Describe the Schilling test.

2. A 75-year-old woman who has had a stroke has been in an acute care hospital for four weeks. The medical resident thinks she is ready for discharge since, although she cannot get out of bed, her medical condition and weight are stable. She has edema of her lower back and a pressure sore over the sacrum. The medical resident asks the clinical nutritionist if his plan for this patient's discharge is justified. The nutritionist examines the patient and checks the lab reports, which indicate that the plasma albumin is 2.1 g/dl.

   Discuss the nutritional diagnosis, its possible causes, and the appropriate management of the case.

3. Discuss the major constraints on the provision of Recommended Dietary Allowances for men and women who are ≥ 75 years of age.

4. You are asked to make recommendations on where a 76-year-old man should go after his discharge from an acute care hospital where he has been treated for congestive heart failure. His physician has prescribed a strict low-sodium diet.

   Discuss the factors that would influence you in deciding whether he should be discharged to his own home or sent to a geriatric care facility.

5. Following the death of her husband, Mrs. Brown, who is 72, goes to live with her son and daughter-in-law. In the next three months she loses 25 pounds in weight. The daughter-in-law becomes concerned because of the weight loss and because she notices that Mrs. Brown is "not eating her meals" and seems to have "no appetite."

   How would you investigate the causes of weight loss and anorexia in this woman?

6. In a grant application, a physician states that he intends to study the caloric and nutrient intakes of a group of homebound elderly women using a 7-day dietary record. You are asked to comment on his proposed

methodology and to offer an alternate method for dietary assessment of this sample population.

Write a critique of his proposal, indicating why you have reservations about this method and why you are suggesting another way of obtaining the necessary dietary information.

7. In the intermediate care section of a nursing home where patients eat their meals together, 10 of the 50 patients are found to be anemic during the last three months. All of these patients are arthritic.

Find out the cause of these patients' anemia. Describe what investigations you would make, related to their diet, to their other health problems, and to the drugs they are taking.

8. Abnormal lab reports are often overlooked in nursing homes. Since physicians may not be able to visit geriatric facilities daily, a system has been proposed by which a physician's assistant would be trained to visit each area facility daily to check lab reports for grossly abnormal values which require prompt attention. The assistant would then notify the doctor of serious hypokalemia (Isiadinso, O. O. A., "Physician's assistant in geriatric medicine," *N.Y. State J. Med.*, 78 [1979], 1069–1071).

Discuss causes of these metabolic abnormalities commonly occurring in the nursing home population.

9. *The New York Times*, May 13, 1981:
"While there is no guarantee that changing your life for the sake of your health will keep you hale and hearty for the biblical three-score and ten or longer, you can certainly increase the odds of living a long and healthy life by reducing the lifestyle risks most strongly associated with premature death and disability. And the changes involved need not diminish the pleasures of living, though they sometimes mean exchanging one source of pleasure for another."

Give a concise account of the "lifestyle risks" related to nutrition and the diet which you believe are most strongly associated with premature death and disability.

10. Mr. Jones has been given a low-fat, low-cholesterol diet after his second myocardial infarct. He develops a severe athlete's foot 2 months later, for which griseofulvin is prescribed by a dermatologist. When Mr. Jones returns to the dermatologist for a follow-up, he complains that his athlete's foot has not improved. Assuming that Mr. Jones has been careful to take the griseofulvin after his breakfast and dinner, explain why you think his condition has not gotten any better.

11. You have been asked to give four 15-minute talks on nutrition at the nearby Title IIIC Congregate-Meal Center. Choose four topics which you would like to discuss with this audience and explain the goal and plan of each talk.

12. A number of different support services are available which allow home-bound elderly to live more or less independently. Discuss alternate means whereby food purchase and preparation may be provided for handicapped people.

Resource Materials*

Gerontology

MARKIDES, K. S., ED., *Aging and Health: Perspective on Gender, Race, Ethnicity and Class*. London: Sage Publications, 1989.

SLESINGER, D. P., M. McDIVITT, and F. M. O'DONNELL, "Food patterns in an urban population: age and sociodemographic correlates," *J. Gerontol.*, 35 (1980), 432–41.

WILLIAMS, J. B., H. MUNLEY, and L. EVANS, *Aging and Society*. Chicago: Holt, Rinehart & Winston, 1980.

Drugs

BROCKLEHURST, J. C., ED., *Geriatric Pharmacology and Therapeutics*. London: Blackwell Scientific Publications, 1984.

BROWN, C. H., *Handbook of Drug Monitoring*. Baltimore: Williams & Wilkins, 1990.

ROE, D. A., *Handbook on Drug and Nutrient Interactions: A Problem-Oriented Reference Guide for Dietitians*, 4th Ed. Chicago: The American Dietetic Association, 1989.

RAFFAEL, P. R., J. K. COOPER, and D. W. LOVE, "Drug misuse in older people," *The Gerontologist*, 21 (1981), 145–50.

Nursing Homes

KAHN, K. A., W. HINES, A. S. WOODSON, and G. B. ARMSTRONG, "A multidisciplinary approach to assessing the quality of care in long-term care facilities," *The Gerontologist*, 17 (1977), 61–66.

*Includes reference texts, manuals, and supplementary teaching aids.

KATZ, P. R., and E. CALKINS, *Principles and Practice of Nursing Home Care.* New York: Springer Publications, 1989.

Community Care

PETERSEN, M. D., and D. L. WHITE, EDS., *Health Care of the Elderly: An Information Source Book.* London: Sage Publication, 1989.

Health Status

AKHTAR, A. J., and G. A. BROE, "Disability and dependence in the elderly at home," *Age and Aging,* 2 (1973), 102.
HAMDY, R. C., *Geriatric Medicine.* Philadelphia: Bailliere Tindall, 1984.
LAWRENCE, P. S., "Patterns of health and illness in older people," *Bull. N. Y. Acad. Sci.,* 49 (1973), 1100.
SHANAS, E., "Health status of older people: cross-national implications," *Amer. J. Public Health,* 64 (1974), 261–64.

Functional Assessment

KANE, R. A., and R. L. KANE, *Assessing the Elderly.* Lexington, MA: Lexington Books, 1981.
LAWTON, M. P., "Functional assessment of elderly people," *J. Amer. Geriat. Soc.,* 19 (1971), 465–81.

Nutrition Guidelines

National Research Council, Diet and Health. Washington, DC: National Academy Press, 1989.

Nutrient Requirements

MUNRO, H. N., "Nutrition and aging," *Brit. Med. Bull.,* 37 (1981), 83–88.

Bibliography

METRESS, S. P., and C. S. KART, *Nutrition and Aging: A Bibliographic Survey.* Monticello, IL: Vance Bibliographers.

Programs

HARPER, J. M., G. R. JANSEN, C. T. SHIGETAMI, and A. L. FREY, "Menu planning in nutrition programs for the elderly," *J. Amer. Dietet. Assoc.,* 68 (1976), 529–34.
KOHRS, M. B., "Recommendations for nutrition programs for the elderly," *J. Amer. Dietet. Assoc.,* 75 (1979), 543–46.

Medical Ethics

BUTLER, R. N., "Protection of elderly research subjects," *Clin. Res.,* 28 (1980), 3–5.

Food and Special Diets

COALE, M., *Meal Planning and Exchange Lists.* 80 slides. Audiocassette, 22-minute script. Department of Family Practice, Medical University of South Carolina, 171 Asley Ave., Charleston, SC 29403.

DIABETES EDUCATION CENTER,   *Convenience Food Lists.* 1979. 4959 Excelsior Blvd.,
Minneapolis, MN 55416.
GENERAL MILLS,   *Meal Planning for the Golden Years.* Rev. 1979. Box 1113, Min-
neapolis, MN 55416.
NATIONAL ACADEMY OF SCIENCES,   *Sodium-Restricted Diets and the Use of Diuretics.*
1979. 2101 Constitution Ave., N.W., Washington, DC.
SIMKO, M. D., C. COWELL, and M. S. HREHA, EDS.,   *Practical Nutrition: A Quick
Reference Guide for the Health Care Practitioner.* Rockville, MD: Aspen Publica-
tions, Inc., 1989.

Glossary of Medical Terms

Alzheimer's disease Presenile dementia
ariboflavinosis Riboflavin deficiency
ataxia Loss of ability to walk straight
cachexia Wasting
candidiasis Yeast infection
cheilitis Inflammation of the lips
cheilosis Redness and fissuring of lips associated with B vitamin deficiency
cirrhosis Replacement of liver cells with fibrous tissue—commonly, alcohol-related liver disease
cor pulmonale Heart condition secondary to chronic disease of the lungs
decubitus ulcer Bed sore
dermatitis Inflammation of the skin
dermatosis Skin disease
diverticulitis Inflammation of one or more colonic diverticula
diverticulosis Condition of the colon associated with single or multiple pouches
dyspnea Breathlessness
emphysema Condition in which the air sacs in the lungs become distended or ruptured
glossitis Inflammation or loss of normal surface of the tongue
gluten-sensitive enteropathy (*syn.* celiac-sprue syndrome) Malabsorption syndrome caused by gluten intolerance
hemiplegia Paralysis of one side of the body
hemolysis Destruction of red blood cells
icterus Jaundice
intertrigo Superficial dermatitis of folds of skin
koilonychia Spoon-shaped nails associated with iron deficiency

metastasis   Deposit of cancer in a secondary location

myxedema   Condition associated with failure of thyroid function

neoplastic disease   Cancer

Parkinson's disease   Chronic disease of the central nervous system associated with tremor

paraplegia   Paralysis of lower portion of the body

pellagra   Niacin deficiency

pemphigoid   Blistering disease with epidermal cell cohesion intact

pemphigus   Blistering disease with loss of cohesion of epidermal cells

Plummer-Vinson syndrome   Chronic iron deficiency plus premalignant changes in the throat or esophagus

psychosis   Any mental disease with or without deterioration of intellectual functioning in which individual lacks insight into his or her own condition

purpura   Bleeding into the skin

scurvy   Vitamin C deficiency

seborrhoeic dermatitis   Scaly, red condition of the skin of the face, scalp, chest, or skinfolds

stomatitis   Inflammation or loss of normal lining of the mouth

systemic sclerosis (*syn.* **scleroderma**)   Generalized connective tissue disease

thyrotoxicosis   Overactive thyroid with increased metabolic rate

uremia   Toxic condition associated with failure of kidney to function

Wernicke-Korsakoff psychosis   Thiamin-dependent syndrome associated with acute and chronic psychosis, usually in alcoholics

Answer Key

Chapter One

1. a,b,c,d,e
2. c
3. a
4. b,c
5. a,b,d
6. b,c,d

Chapter Two

1. a,c,e
2. a,c,d
3. a,b,d
4. b,c,d
5. b,c,d
6. d,e

Chapter Three

1. b,c,d
2. d
3. b,c,e

4. Independently living—a,d
   Institutionalized or
   hospitalized—b,c,e
5. c

Chapter Four

1. e
2. b,e
3. e
4. b
5. a,b,c,d

Chapter Five

1. a,c
2. a,b,c
3. a,b,c,d—do
   e—do not
4. a—iv
   b—ii
   c—v
   d—i
   e—iii

5. b,c,e
6. c

Chapter Six

1. a—triceps skinfold thickness
    b—proxy for stature height
    c—assessment of hydration and
        anemia
    d—nutrient analysis of diet
    e—immunological assessment
2. Symptoms—a,b,e,g,i
    Signs—c,d,f,h,j
3. c,d
4. b,d,e
5. a
6. c

Chapter Seven

1. c,d,e
2. a
3. a—i or iii
    b—i or iii
    c—i, ii, iii
4. Acute—a,c,e,g,h
    Chronic—b,d,f,i,j
5. a-thiamin
    b—vitamin C
    c—vitamin D
    d—niacin
    e—vitamin B_{12}

Chapter Eight

1. a,b,d,e
2. a,c,d,e
3. a,c,d,e

4. a,c,d
5. c

Chapter Nine

1. b,c,d,e
2. c,d,e
3. a,c
4. a,b,c,d,e
5. c,d
6. a,b,c,e

Chapter Ten

1. b,e
2. a,b,c,e
3. b,c
4. a—iii
    b—i
    c—iv
    d—v
    e—ii
5. a,b,d,e
6. b,d,e

Chapter Eleven

1. Hypertension; diabetes; coronary
    artery disease
2. c,d,e
3. d,e
4. a. Diabetes care should be part
    of the community-based health care
    system.
    b. Insulin should be available
    to all diabetics requiring it.
    c. Intensive efforts should be
    made to reduce risk factors.
5. c

Index